Animal Behavior and Welfare

Animal Behavior and Welfare

Chris Dunn

Larsen & Keller
www.larsen-keller.com

Animal Behavior and Welfare
Chris Dunn
ISBN: 978-1-64172-504-0 (Hardback)

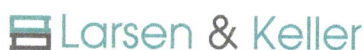

☲ Larsen & Keller

Published by Larsen and Keller Education,
5 Penn Plaza,
19th Floor,
New York, NY 10001, USA

Cataloging-in-Publication Data

Animal behavior and welfare / Chris Dunn.
          p. cm.
Includes bibliographical references and index.
ISBN 978-1-64172-504-0
1. Animal behavior. 2. Animal welfare. 3. Animal psychology.
4. Animals--Social aspects. I. Dunn, Chris.
QL751 .A55 2020
591.5--dc23

For more information regarding Larsen and Keller Education and its products, please visit the publisher's website www.larsen-keller.com

Table of Contents

Preface

Animal welfare is the scientific study of the welfare of animals. Some of the measures used by this discipline are immunosuppression, reproduction, disease, longevity, behavior and physiology. There are several issues which are related to animal welfare such as behavioral enrichment, animal testing, abandoned pets and blood sports. Animal welfare considers that the animals are sentient and their well-being should be considered. Animal rights is the extension of this belief, where it is believed that all non-human animals are entitled to the possession of their existence. This book provides comprehensive insights into the field of animal welfare. It also presents researches and studies performed by experts across the globe. Coherent flow of topics, student-friendly language and extensive use of examples make this textbook an invaluable source of knowledge.

A foreword of all Chapters of the book is provided below:

Chapter 1 - Animal welfare includes measures of longevity, immunosuppression, behavior, physiology and reproduction for the well being of non-human animals. The topics elaborated in this chapter will help in gaining a better perspective about the strategies and assessment of animal welfare; **Chapter 2** - There are many issues and problems faced by animals living in the environment. It includes farming practices, ivory trade, poaching, animal testing, habitat loss, climate change, blood sport, etc. This chapter has been carefully written to provide an easy understanding of these problems faced by animals; **Chapter 3** - Animal behavior deals with the study of interaction between animals and their environment. Animal ethics examine the human-animal relationships. Animal rights and ethics are the essential components of animal welfare. This chapter discusses about animal behavior, rights and ethics to provide an in-depth understanding of the subject; **Chapter 4** - The welfare of farming animals is important for animals to live a longer, healthier and active life. Welfare of goats, pigs, hens, cows, horse, etc. have been studied under it. This chapter closely examines the aspects associated with the welfare of farming animals to provide an extensive understanding of the subject; **Chapter 5** - Animal health focuses primarily on ensuring that the animals are healthy, disease-free and well looked after. Diseases like anthrax, black-leg, blue tongue, rinderpest, footrot, calf scour, etc. are common in animals and their treatment practices fall under the domain of disease management. This chapter delves into the concept of animal health and disease management to provide an in-depth understanding of the subject.

I would like to thank the entire editorial team who made sincere efforts for this book and my family who supported me in my efforts of working on this book. I take this opportunity to thank all those who have been a guiding force throughout my life.

Chris Dunn

Animal Welfare: An Introduction

Animal welfare includes measures of longevity, immunosuppression, behavior, physiology and reproduction for the well being of non-human animals. The topics elaborated in this chapter will help in gaining a better perspective about the strategies and assessment of animal welfare.

Animal welfare refers to the relationships people have with animals and the duty they have to assure that the animals under their care are treated humanely and responsibly.

The term "animal welfare" is being used increasingly by corporations, consumers, veterinarians, politicians and others. However, the term can mean different things to different people. Understandably, in the past, veterinarians and farmers have seen animal welfare chiefly in terms of the body and the physical environment (shelter, feed, etc.). If an animal is healthy and producing well, it is faring well. Animal welfare has also focused on the body, using physiological measures, such as endorphins, plasma cortisol and heart rate, to examine how the animal is coping with its environment. However, there are limitations to seeing animal welfare only in terms of the body. One limitation is that genetics and the environment can produce desirable physical outcomes, even though the animal's mental state is compromised. For example, a canine breed champion may have perfect conformation and be in perfect health, but it may be very anxious in its home environment. Another limitation is that some physical parameters (heart rate, plasma cortisol) are difficult to interpret, because they can be increased by both positive and negative experiences, such as the presence of a mate and the presence of a predator.

The above would suggest that animal welfare includes not only the state of the animal's body, but also its feelings. Most would agree that animals have feelings (fear, frustration) and it has been proposed that animal welfare consists entirely in feelings and that these have evolved to protect the animal's primary needs. Thus, if an animal feels well, it is faring well. A feelings-based approach to animal welfare typically measures behavioral outcomes, such as willingness to "work" (pushing open a weighted door) and behavioral signs of fear or frustration.

A third view of welfare, linked to the feelings-based approach, is that animals fare best if they can live according to their nature and perform their full range of behaviors. Physical suffering, such as feeling cold and mental suffering, such as the fear induced by being preyed upon, may be acceptable. Sectors of the general public favor the "natural living" approach, however, as with physical and mental aspects of welfare; animal welfare scientists have largely discounted this as the sole basis for ensuring optimal welfare. Instead, they propose that the physical, mental and "natural-living" aspects of welfare are interrelated and are all of ethical concern. Thus, the most widely accepted definition of animal welfare is that it comprises the state of the animal's body and mind and the extent to which its nature (genetic traits manifest in breed and temperament) is satisfied. However, the three aspects of welfare sometimes conflict and this presents practical and ethical challenges.

The situation of laying hens illustrates how the physical, mental and natural aspects of welfare can conflict and the difficulty in agreeing on how best to compromise among them. Disagreement occurs because the form of compromise that is acceptable to different animal-oriented groups depends on their values and is complicated by the need to consider legitimate human interests (those of the farmer in earning a living).

In the case of laying hens, noncage systems have been advocated, so that the birds might live more according to their nature and thus avoid the frustration of close confinement in barren cages. However, cannibalism is common in noncage systems, perhaps because hens are not adapted to living in the large groups involved in noncage systems. These systems can also carry a greater risk of disease and are more labor intensive than are conventional cages. These difficulties can be managed somewhat (cannibalism can be controlled by beak-trimming, which is itself questionable, because it causes neuromas and chronic pain, but conventional cages have been considered more desirable in both financial and humane terms. Veterinarians have accepted this compromise, which is consistent with their focus on animals' physical welfare and with their role in helping farmers to provide affordable food. However, conventional cages do not permit hens to express their nature (roost at night, dust-bathe and lay eggs in seclusion). This limitation has contributed to the view that conventional cages are unacceptable and that hens bear too many of the costs of egg production without sufficient benefit. The European Union (EU) has ruled that barren cages be phased out of all member countries by 2012 and that more space be provided for birds in the interim. This ruling represents a new compromise among the physical, mental and natural aspects of hen welfare. The ruling also involves human compromise in that the potential increase in the production costs under alternative systems is estimated at 5% to 50%, depending on the system used which will increase the cost to consumers. The premise of the ruling is that animal welfare is a public good that society must pay to protect. However, some animal welfare scientists argue that there is insufficient scientific evidence to justify the ruling and that welfare may be worse because of it. Other scientists support the ruling, arguing that it is inadequate husbandry and the current market conditions that can reduce welfare under the housing systems required by the EU ruling. Both sides represent a compromise, the acceptability of which depends not only on scientific evidence, but also on values.

Strategies to Improve Animal Lives

There are many way to improve the lives of animals and animal welfare, some of them are discussed below:

- Volunteer at your local city/county animal shelter or rescue group in your community.

- Foster a cat or cog until they get adopted. Contact your animal shelter or local rescue group. They all need fosters and you will save an animal's life each time you foster.

- Microchip your pet: Microchips are inexpensive and will dramatically increase the chance that your pet will be found if they are lost or there is a disaster. Increase the chance you will be reunited with them.

- Adopt don't shop: Adopt a rescue cat or dog from your local animal shelter or rescue group— and you will be saving two lives—the life of the dog or cat you adopt and the space that opens up for another dog or cat in the shelter or rescue group. Breeders add more pets into a system where 8 million individual cats and dogs are euthanized every year in U.S. shelters.

- Get kids involved with animals: Visit animal sanctuaries, animal rescue groups on adoption days and join activities that support the wellbeing of animals in your community.

- Sponsor KIND News: You can sponsor giving KIND News to elementary schools across the nation that teaches young children humane education.

- Prepare a disaster kit for your pets. Emergencies can come suddenly and you want to be prepared. Keep emergency pet supplies, pet food (wet and dry), pet first-aid kit, extra medications, photocopies of medical records, photos of your pets, bottled water and an emergency kit in your home and in case of evacuation.

- Arrange a safe haven: Make arrangements in the event of an evacuation by identifying evacuation locations for your pets. Have a list of vets ready that offer boarding kennels, identify hotels outside your area that accept pets and ask friends and family outside your immediate area if they would be willing to take in your pets.

- Set up a pet trust: Have a plan in place for if and when you become incapacitated or die. A living trust, pet trust or pet protection agreement (PPA) can protect your pet. Set one up today and designate a caregiver to take your pet from your home if you suddenly become incapacitated. Many pets die in owner's homes or are given to animal shelters and are euthanized.

- Spay & neuter your pets: Domestic dogs and cats are routinely euthanized in animal shelters across the U.S. at a rate of over 8 million individual animals per year. It's a tragedy, unnecessary and a complete waste of an animal's life. Spaying, neutering and rescuing from shelters—not buying from breeders, will solve the euthanasia rates in our shelters.

- Help feral cats in your community: Help the plight of homeless, abandoned and feral cats. Learn to trap-neuter-return (TNR) and volunteer for cat rescue groups who are active in spaying and neutering and feeding these cats. Volunteer to feed feral colonies needed food and water every day that depend on our humane support.

- Give monthly: Donate monthly or when you can to animal protection charities that support their welfare and fight cruelty.

- Watch animal documentaries: There are many enlightening, informative and powerful animal documentaries available today that provide insight into animals and ways humans are impacting them and their world.

- Go fur free: Buy faux fur. Be sure to check the labels that it is faux and not raccoon dog fur from China.

- Avoid buying leather, reptile skin, & duck/goose down. These are all the result of the cruel treatment of animals. Try to buy replacements like artificial leather or pleather and polyester-filled comforters and jackets.

- Go bird watching: Get a pair of binoculars and visit a park or go on a hike to see the diversity of nature and the beautiful birds around you.

- Visit animal sanctuaries: Take a tour of a local farm animal sanctuary or animal sanctuary near you. It's a fun way to learn more and pet the animals.

- Volunteer at an animal sanctuary: Take a weekend—or a week and volunteer to help at an animal sanctuary. It will change your life.

- Get politically active: Learn about the many animal welfare issues at the state and federal level and how you can help. This is one of the most effective ways to help animals.

- Vote: Vote for legislators that support improving animal welfare, the humane care and treatment of animals and fight against animal cruelty.

- Write your legislators: Speak up about animal welfare issues that concern you. Write, email and call your state and federal representatives and senators. Be brief but express your concern. It counts and will make a big difference.

- Support wildlife in your yard: Create a wildlife sanctuary in your back and front yard, by choosing native and animal-friendly plants that attract hummingbirds, birds, bees, small wildlife and insects. Support wildlife and help them coexist with us.

- Hang bird feeders: Help bird populations hurt by development, climate change, drought and habitat destruction, by hanging bird feeders in your backyard. Birds need clean fresh water too. You can add attractive water fountains and bird baths. Keep feeders and baths clean regularly to avoid spreading infections amongst the birds.

- Be a friend to wildlife: Don't think of wildlife in your back or front yard as "trespassers or intruders," but instead as our wild co-inhabitants. They belong there and were living there well before we came.

- Be tolerant and generous: Use only non-lethal means if/when dealing with wildlife that has moved into your house. There are many non-lethal means to encourage them to leave and go back outside. These are kinder and better for them and you.

- Avoid using insecticides, herbicides or weed killers. These can be harmful and deadly to birds, wildlife and domestic animals. Use natural products without any toxins that are equally as effective and much better for the environment.

- Recognize that urban and suburban wildlife deserves their own home. Learn to live WITH the wildlife around you—be their friend not their foe. They need to be accommodated and are challenged and impacted by humans too.

- Put out water bowls in your backyard for wildlife. Protect them from dehydration, drought and severe and prolonged dry weather. They need our help.

- Support buying humane products & brands: Be a humane consumer and support a humane economy in shopping and buying decisions. Be a conscientious consumer about the products you buy and the brands you support.

- Purchase cruelty-free cosmetics & household products: Buy cosmetics and household products that DO NOT test on animals. Many cosmetic and household product brands cruelly test on animals that are intentionally poisoned, blinded and forced to suffer immeasurably. But many products are available today that are not tested on animals.

- Call the police: If you see an animal being abused in any way, call your local police and animal control officer immediately. Don't wait. Take photos if you can for evidence.

- Help neglected animals: You can help them by notifying your County or City Animal Control or Shelter and the police when you see an animal being seriously neglected – chained in a backyard without food and water; in a hot car; in extreme weather without protection; or know people who abandoned their pet and left them behind. Notify authorities and get help.

- Don't patronize entertainment that uses (and abuses) animals. Don't support businesses that use animals for entertainment. They are often confined in unnaturally small spaces, trained using abusive practices, forced to do what they don't want to do, transported long distances and have been forcibly removed from their natural environment.

- Sign: Commit to compassionate living and sign the evangelical statement on responsible care for animals. Join the new campaign by Christian leaders for Christians to take more responsibility to speak out against animal injustice, cruelty and abuse.

- Reduce or eliminate meat: Try to reduce your meat consumption. It's one of the biggest things you can do to help animals. Over 99% of the animals raised for meat are raised in inhumane factory farms that impose extremely cruel conditions on the animals that causes them deep suffering and misery.

- Reduce or eliminate dairy: Try to reduce your consumption of dairy. Dairy cows suffer some of the worst cruelty of all—from forcible over-production of milk, constant pregnancies, having every baby calf taken away from them at birth, they acquire painful diseases and conditions due to the production of too much milk that is entirely unnatural for their bodies and their calves are slaughtered at birth or forced into inhumane veal production. Choose plant-based milks and cheeses.

- Reduce or eliminate eggs: Egg-laying hens experience some of the worst, most cruel conditions of all as well, from force molting by starvation to produce more eggs, to being given hormones and drugs to increase egg laying 5 times what is normal for their bodies, weakening their bodies and the chronic and painful diseases that result.

- Become conscious of ways animals are used and abused today. Become more aware and active against any business or institution that forces animals to behave in ways that are unnatural, where they are made to suffer or are abused – such as rodeos, dolphinariums, roadside zoos, circuses, some amusement parks like Six Flags, etc. Avoid patronizing these and let them know that you are opposed to their treatment of animals for profit or entertainment.

- Sign up for email alerts: Sign up for email alerts and learn about animal issues from leading animal welfare groups or media such as PETA, HSUS, Mercy for Animals, World Animal Protection, The DoDo, PCRM, Animal Welfare Institute, CARE2, Humane Society International or any of the many other organizations that positively support animals.

- Sign the petitions: Sign and add your name to the animal protection petitions that circulate.

- Celebrate thanksgiving without a Turkey: That's right. Celebrate the day with all the other trappings. You can honor the purpose and meaning of the day by giving thanks, without killing a turkey for it.

- Distribute animal welfare literature: Join animal welfare groups and help them educate the public about animal cruelty by distributing flyers and brochures at events, stores and shopping centers.

- Donate your used Carto an animal welfare organization.

- Donate through a trust, living trust or will to an animal welfare organization.

- Take classes: You can learn through a wide variety of online workshops, webinars, certificate programs and credentialed programs given by the Humane Society Academy, part of the Humane Society of the U.S.

- Help in disasters: Get trained by your local county CART (County Animal Response Team) or national DART training programs to help animals in disasters.

- Teach kids in schools to learn about how to care for animals and the importance of recognizing abuse, neglect or cruelty. Help teach kids humane education.

- Give gifts that support organizations trying to help animal protection and welfare, such as the ASPCA, Humane Society of the U.S. and World Animal Protection.

- Don't do harm to animals. Yes, that seems obvious. Be part of the solution not the problem—by making a positive impact to individual and collective animals' lives—whether it's wildlife or domestic animals, by not harming or hurting them in any way.

- Spread the word: Ask friends and family to join you in your efforts to protect animals. Share and repost on social media – and spread the word to help animals.

Wildlife Habitat Assessment

Wildlife habitat assessment is the evaluation of the relative habitat conditions available to a focal group of wildlife. Assessments of wildlife habitat are predicated on the basic assumption that at some level wildlife is controlled by its habitat, because an organism's ability to survive depends in large part on the resources (e.g., food, water and cover) available to it. These resources are provided by the habitat in which organisms live. Thus, habitat conditions are often used as a surrogate to make inferences about the presence, abundance, fitness or productivity of wildlife populations, species or communities.

Each species is adapted to a fairly unique set of habitat conditions. For example, Swainson's warblers (Limnothlypis swainsonii) most often are associated with moist lowland forests that have a dense shrub layer, whereas brown-headed nuthatches (Sitta pusilla) prefer mature upland pine forests. These associations between wildlife species and their preferred habitats are often referred to as wildlife habitat relationships. The range of habitat conditions that are acceptable varies considerably among species. Swainson's warblers and brown-headed nuthatches tend to be restricted to the types, whereas many other bird species may be found virtually across the landscape. Species that occur only in a narrow range of conditions are habitat specialists, whereas those that tolerate a broader range are habitat generalists. It tends to be easier to assess or predict the habitat relations of specialists than of generalists.

The assumption that the presence or abundance of a species reflects the quality of a given location as habitat is not always valid. An important aspect of habitat quality is the contribution of the habitat to the reproductive fitness of the population and hence its ability to persist through time. In this regard, habitat quality may not be very well correlated with density. For example, in birds, territoriality may limit the number of breeding individuals that can occur in a particular forest stand, even one of optimal quality and relegate non-breeding individuals to areas of lesser quality. Density may actually be higher in the low quality stand where no reproduction occurs. Likewise, areas of potentially optimal quality may be completely unoccupied by species that are rare, simply because of a lack of individuals to fill available habitat. These considerations notwithstanding, as long as managers are alert to this possibility, the assessment of habitat conditions based on density still can be a useful tool in evaluating and understanding the impacts of habitat alteration.

Wildlife habitat assessment is conducted for a variety of purposes. A manager may simply want to assess the capability or likelihood that a given tract can support certain wildlife species. When declines in the abundance of a focal species are noted, wildlife managers may assess habitat conditions to determine if some degradation in quality may be responsible. Often, it is desirable to be able to predict in advance the impact of proposed land management activities, such as timber harvest or prescribed burning, on the quality of wildlife habitat. Following is an overview of some considerations and common approaches to wildlife habitat assessment:

- Habitat Feature: Before undertaking any assessment of habitat, it is essential to understand the habitat relationships and preferences of the species of interest. Habitat characteristics can be considered as either macro or micro variables, roughly corresponding to the scale or perspective of measurement. Assessment of the quantity and quality of such variables, either formally or informally, can provide insights into the relative quality of habitat for wildlife.

- Macro Features: Characteristics of habitats that are described across relatively large areas or within a landscape context usually can (and sometimes must) be assessed remotely via the use of tools such as geographic information systems (GIS), satellite imagery or aerial photography. Examples of such variables include stand or patch size, shape and age, amount of edge, vegetation cover type and distance to other important features such as water, roads, cliffs, caves or neighboring nesting/roosting sites.

- Micro Features: Some habitat features that describe more site-specific conditions must be directly assessed on-site. Forest inventory databases are available in some situations (e.g., the U.S. Forest Inventory and Analysis database), but the data recorded in such inventories may be of limited use if collected for other purposes or if very specific features are needed. Micro habitat features most often include measures of vegetation structure and composition, though soil and topographic conditions are also critical to some species. In forested habitats, vegetative conditions are usually the most important habitat components for wildlife. Vegetation structure includes both vertical and horizontal aspects of density (e.g., stem density, foliage volume) and particular preferred plant species may need to be considered. Other specific features like snag size and density (for cavity nesting birds and small mammals), burrows (for small mammals, reptiles, amphibians and invertebrates) or the availability and quality of preferred browse plants (for deer) may be measured.

Wildlife Habitat Models

A tremendous body of literature exists on wildlife habitat modeling. The purposes of such models range from enhancing our understanding of species' ecology and the habitat factors that affect their distribution and abundance to predicting future distribution and abundance under different scenarios affecting the habitat. Many approaches to modeling and many types of models have been developed. General model types include (but are not limited to) statistical empirical models, habitat relationship models, simulation models, GIS-based models and expert (or knowledge-based) models.

Wildlife Habitat Relationship (WHR) Matrix Models

WHR matrix models are simply tables that relate each of any number of wildlife species to habitat types. The quality of each habitat type for each species may be indicated simply as suitable or unsuitable or it is often given as a qualitative categorical rank, such as marginal, suitable or optimal. These ranks may be derived from field studies, professional judgment or a combination of both. While WHR matrix models lack detail and tend to predict more species as present than actually are, they can be useful in quickly assessing potential habitat capabilities across many species.

Forest stand growth and yield models designed for silvicultural purposes and models of ecological succession are often used to assess wildlife habitat. Predictions of future vegetation conditions from such models can be cross-walked to the general habitat types of WHR matrix models to produce an assessment of future habitat potential.

Habitat Suitability Index (HSI) Models

HSI models have been used by the U.S. Fish and Wildlife Service and other agencies to assess the quality of habitat for individual species of importance. The output is a suitability index that ranges from 0 to 1. This value represents the geometric mean of a set of environmental variables that are perceived to have the greatest impact on the species' presence, abundance or productivity. Thus, the basic structure of an HSI model is $HSI = (V_1 \cdot V_1 \cdot ... V_n)^{1/n}$, where the V's represent the environmental variables. Although HSI models have many shortcomings and have been heavily criticized, they constitute a repeatable assessment procedure and values can be compared among management alternatives.

HSI models frequently are used in habitat evaluation procedures (HEP), wherein an HSI score is determined for a habitat and multiplied by the area of the habitat to produce a "habitat unit." Habitat units for the species can then be compared among locations or management alternatives.

Spatially Explicit Models

GIS models that use geographically referenced information on habitat conditions in conjunction with models of species response can be used to simulate the impacts of habitat alteration, disturbance and changes in landscape structure. Such models have gained popularity, as they can be combined in the GIS environment with different model types, both theoretical and quantitative, to produced much more specific output on species response than more general model types like WHR matrix or HSI models.

Model Accuracy and Applications

Perhaps the greatest shortcoming of most wildlife habitat models is the uncertainty of their accuracy. Validation of wildlife habitat models involves testing model predictions against actual field data. This process can be difficult or impossible when model structure and output is subjective or otherwise non-quantifiable in real-world terms such as density or survival or reproductive rates. However, there is growing recognition in the wildlife literature of the necessity of validating predictive models. Without an assessment of accuracy, model predictions remain only hypotheses to be tested.

Nevertheless, assessments of wildlife habitat are crucial in order to understand wildlife and habitat relationships and to adjust our forest management practices to favor desirable species, deter undesirable species and minimize adverse impacts of habitat modification on wildlife and biodiversity.

Human-wildlife Conflict

Human–wildlife conflict (HWC) occurs when the needs of wildlife encroach on those of human populations or the needs of human populations encroach upon those of wildlife. More broadly, interactions between wildlife and humans can cause damage or costs to both and lead to conflicts between different groups of people (human–human conflicts) over wildlife and how it should be managed.

Conflicts between humans and wildlife and between humans over wildlife, have occurred since the dawn of humanity. However, in many regions these conflicts have intensified over recent decades as a result of human population growth and the related expansion of agricultural and industrial activities. Conflicts have also arisen due to the growth of some wildlife populations and the presence of certain species (e.g. red fox, wild boar) in urban environments, as well as a recurrent inability of institutions to manage such conflicts effectively. Climate change is exacerbating these conflicts through, for example, increased competition for water and habitats. Changing human values and attitudes are also shaping wildlife management approaches, where ecocentric, protectionist views of wildlife may not recognize or accommodate the needs of those living with wildlife.

HWC cannot be detached from the context of conflicts between groups of people about how to manage wildlife, which have marked the history of conservation. For example, centuries of urbanization have led to radical agrarian dissent and resistance to dominant urban cultures and values in many places. The implementation of protectionist conservation policies has often aggravated feelings of disenfranchisement and injustice among rural communities, as well as frustration toward wildlife authorities. Problems are particularly severe when the wildlife species concerned are of major conservation importance and the conservation objectives are at odds with those of local communities.

Impacts of HWC can range from injury and death, loss of crops and livestock, damaged infrastructure, disease transmission (to humans and also to wildlife) and school absenteeism of children to guard crops at home or too scared to walk to school, to reduced farm productivity for farmers who are spending more time guarding their crops and other intangible social costs such as stress. As a result of these negative impacts, wildlife species may be killed in retaliation, with a risk of population declines. In certain cases, indiscriminate killing of non-problematic wildlife or habitat destruction may also take place as an expression of resentment or hostility toward conservation and wildlife management authorities.

Local solutions should therefore take into account the histories of past interventions and their outcomes, including monitoring to enable appropriate modifications because perceptions, as well as the populations and activities of both humans and wildlife, change over time.

Safety and Security

Large carnivores and large herbivores are responsible for most attacks on humans, often leading to injury or death. Deaths may occur when people are in or near waterways, for example when travelling, fishing or fetching water; while protecting crops and water against wild animals (usually at night); or when people encounter injured animals whose normal sense of caution is impaired. The fear of conflict restricts people's freedom of movement and access to resources and can induce high levels of stress and feelings of insecurity.

Road accidents caused by wildlife and bird–aircraft collisions occur worldwide and can also result in human death and injury.

Food Security and Livelihoods

Across the world, crops are subject to damage caused by wildlife, from deer to kangaroos, geese or elephants. While crop damage can have a negative impact on economies and livelihoods, food security is typically most vulnerable in developing countries, where it can depend on the result of a single cropping season. The fear of loss of crops to wildlife can also be a severe limitation for growing specific crops (for example, where birds feed on sunflower seeds just before cultivation), with consequences for land-use practices and commercialization of food products at local, regional and national level. Consequences are particularly serious where government responses (such as compensation) are non-existent, inadequate or ineffective.

A high density of large ungulates (hoofed mammals) in forests can endanger the sustainability of forest management by eating tree bark as well as small trees, which can affect forest succession and lead to a polarization between forest and wildlife management.

The loss of livestock can also damage livelihoods. For rural populations, domestic animals may be an important resource or the only source of income. Predation on livestock often forces rural communities to adopt new mechanisms to protect stock, such as building enclosures or introducing guard dogs.

Large herbivores often compete for food or water, particularly in arid regions. This is the case for guanacos in South America, deer in North America and wildebeest in Africa. Actions taken to decrease native herbivore populations can significantly change population sizes and predators and affect the people who also rely on the resources, such as local pastoralists.

Transmission of Diseases to Livestock and Humans

Many wild species can play a major role in disease transmission to/from domestic animals due to their abundance, wide distribution and close proximity to these animals with which they frequently share pasture and watering points. Common livestock diseases such as brucellosis and bovine tuberculosis can adversely affect wildlife populations and in some cases lead to infections that are much more difficult to control than in livestock. Diseases in wildlife can cause severe problems for domestic animals but diseases in domestic animals can also devastate wildlife populations and threaten biological diversity.

Of the growing list of human pathogens, 61 percent are zoonotic. Of emerging infectious diseases, 75 percent are zoonotic originating principally from wildlife. Over the past four decades, agents responsible for pandemics such as Human Immunodeficiency Virus (HIV) and other diseases that cause high case-fatality rates (e.g. Ebola virus (EBOV), Severe Acute Respiratory Syndrome (SARS), Middle East Respiratory Syndrome Coronavirus (MERS-CoV), other coronaviruses and brucellosis) have been reported to have emerged from wildlife reservoirs through consumption of wild meat.

As the populations of many wildlife species decline, their conservation importance increases. In such cases, needs of local communities may clash with conservation objectives. For example, some species of large carnivores such as lions, hyenas and wolves have been eliminated from extensive parts of their former ranges due to HWC. Today, illegal killing, including poisoning, shooting and trapping, remains a major threat to these species. It can not only affect population viability, but may also have broader environmental impacts.

Experience and Knowledge

Causes of Human–wildlife Conflict

In dealing with HWC, it is crucial to address both the relationship between wildlife and humans and the underlying conflicts over wildlife among people with different values, objectives and experiences. Reducing impacts may not reduce conflict if the underlying causes are not addressed.

An important source of conflict lies in the competition between growing human populations and wildlife for the same declining resources. The transformation of forests, savannah, wetlands and other ecosystems into agricultural or urban areas as a consequence of increasing demand for land, food production, energy, water and raw materials, has led to a dramatic loss of wildlife habitats. War, civil unrest and climate change can force people to seek shelter in or procure resources from, protected areas, in which they may exert a strong pressure on natural resources and enter into competition with wildlife. Illegal hunting for food and the death of herbivores as a result of drought can reduce prey populations, forcing predators to turn to livestock. The growing interest in eco-tourism and increasing presence of humans in protected areas may exacerbate conflicts between humans and wildlife.

In some areas, by contrast, conflicts between wildlife and local communities have been sparked by success in species recovery such as for crocodiles and by efforts to reintroduce large carnivores and raptors, as well as a recurrent inability of institutions to mitigate such conflicts effectively.

The conflicts between people over wildlife often reflect real or perceived injustices around who bears the cost of living with wildlife and who benefits from its conservation. Where local communities who experience HWC do not have a say in management decisions, concerning hunting or fencing for example, they may resent wildlife management and conservation authorities and organizations and retaliate by killing wildlife. This may be exacerbated by being excluded from the tangible benefits of conservation, for instance where communities adjacent to protected areas are excluded from using natural resources in these areas and see benefits flowing to others, while they bear the risks and livelihood impacts of wildlife.

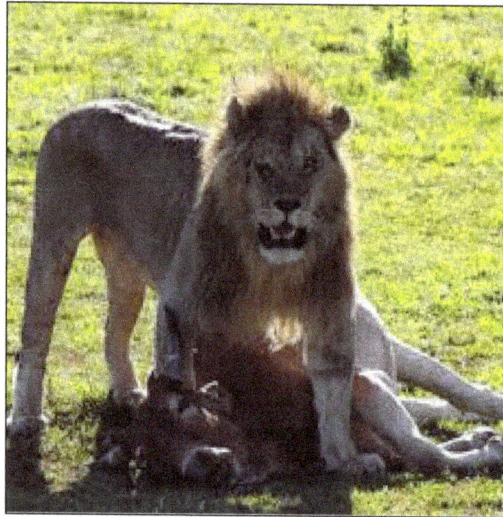

The intrinsic or learned characteristics of wildlife, such as food preferences, migration patterns, wariness or predation behaviour can also influence conflicts. Generally, lower tolerance is ascribed to wildlife with larger body sizes, that occur in large groups or herd sizes, forage or hunt nocturnally, chronically raid, that are habituated to human environments and cause extensive damage per incident (e.g. raiding on mature crops, predation on adult livestock, surplus killing). Moreover, the risk of wildlife damage is higher when (i) crops/livestock are unconfined and unprotected, (ii) natural prey is scarce or well-defended, (iii) landscapes provide adequate cover for predatory wildlife (e.g. are forested) and (iv) when wildlife and crops/livestock are in close proximity.

Addressing Human–wildlife Conflict

There are various approaches that may be taken to address conflicts over wildlife and the costs imposed by wildlife on humans. Approaches to addressing the human dimensions of the problem are addressed here first, followed by a summary of technical approaches to reducing impacts of wildlife. In most cases, however, the process of developing a response jointly with local communities affected by wildlife will be crucial. Important aspects of the process include identifying and meaningfully engaging key stakeholders (including conservationists and veterinarians) throughout the process, mapping out the conflict and ensuring it is well understood, testing and adapting strategies, ensuring effective communication, building trust and coproducing knowledge and working closely with the affected local communities.

Shared governance, education and awareness-raising is crucial. Communities are likely to be less resentful and more tolerant of wildlife populations and the damage they cause where they are involved in the related planning and management and where the costs of living with wildlife are offset by benefits from their sustainable use and conservation. For instance, communities may be granted co-management rights over protected areas. They may be consulted in or given responsibilities for the development of wildlife management plans. They may be legally recognized as stewards of wildlife on their own land and enabled to retain the benefits from tourism (including hunting tourism). They may be granted rights to hunt wildlife themselves or to harvest fuel wood, timber, mushrooms or fodder in wildlife areas. They may be entitled to receive a proportion of revenue from tourism in neighbouring protected areas or be supported in selling handicrafts or other goods and services to tourists, among other strategies. Such approaches may foster more positive attitudes to wildlife and toward wildlife management and conservation agencies and organizations, cooperation in conservation actions and willingness to tolerate impacts of wildlife.

Education about wildlife and particularly the benefits of wildlife populations may also lead to changed attitudes with an increased appreciation of wildlife and tolerance of wildlife damage. However, education alone is unlikely to change attitudes where wildlife populations impose significant net costs.

Recognizing the often extensive knowledge of wildlife held by local communities can improve the management of wildlife and inform conservation efforts. Empowering rural communities with a shared understanding of animal behaviour and information about past conflicts, patterns in seasonality, breeding seasons and habitat preferences, as well as practical skills and tools, may help them to deal with dangerous wild animal species and acquire new approaches for defending their crops, water and livestock. Over time, more effective engagement of the local populations may result in a change of behaviour and contribute to reduced risks, improvements in local livelihoods and a reduction in their vulnerability.

The payment of compensation in the event of loss is usually confined to a specific category of loss, such as human death, livestock loss or area and type of crop loss. These schemes may be funded by governments or conservation organizations. All are designed to increase damage tolerance levels among the affected communities and prevent them from taking direct action themselves. Such schemes, however, do not always function effectively in practice, due to factors such as lack of resources, low compensation, inbuilt incentives to abuse the system, excessive transaction costs, delays in acknowledging damage or processing claims or failure to address the root causes of the conflict.

Insurance schemes are an innovative compensation approach where farmers pay a premium for cover against a defined risk, such as livestock depredation. Those who suffer damage are then compensated from the accumulated pool of resources. Voluntary relocation of local communities, where appropriate land alternatives and incentives are available, to areas offering better access to natural resources and improved socioeconomic opportunities, may offer a solution to managing conflict. This approach is virtually never used in developed regions. Great care must be taken to ensure that justice and human rights are fully respected and that communities give free prior informed consent to relocation and that their socioeconomic needs are met in the new area in the long term.

Good land-use planning will be critical in the long term in managing human–wildlife impacts. Land-use planning techniques for managing human–wildlife interactions may include relocating agricultural activity out of wildlife range, grouping crop fields and moving them from the forest edge closer to dwellings and reducing the encroachment of human settlements into wildlife range by repositioning the boundaries of protected areas or creating buffer zones.

Land-use interventions can alter environmental resources for wildlife in ways that decrease impacts on human activities. For instance, the natural prey base of carnivores can be improved by protection or alternative water sources for wildlife species can be established. Where herdsmen are present to guard livestock, the rate of depredation is generally lower than in unsupervised free-ranging herds. Likewise crops can be protected against wildlife incursions. In both cases, however, people acting as guards may themselves become vulnerable to attack. Guard animals provide an alternative to a herder monitoring a flock.

Barriers, including fences (electric, normal wires, stone walls, steel bars), hedges and moats, if well designed, constructed and maintained, can be almost completely effective in preventing wildlife impacts. However, this approach is not always feasible and may prevent wildlife migrations or access to water resources.

Growing alternative crops that are less palatable to wildlife is an option in some contexts. Changes to livestock husbandry practices may reduce impacts, such as herding during the day, avoiding predators' home ranges, keeping livestock in predator-proof enclosures at night and (for example where crocodiles are present) watering them in secure enclosures.

Deterrents can be used to repel animals from the targeted resource. They can target several senses – hearing, sight, smell, taste and touch – and include smearing chili on wires, beating pots and letting off firecrackers. However, intelligent animals such as elephants may become quickly accustomed to such deterrents, which then cease to be effective.

Wildlife translocation, involving moving animals from a problematic zone to a new site, has been used with animals such as elephants, crocodiles and big cats. While sometimes effective, it is expensive, may simply export the problem elsewhere and, for animals with strong homing instincts, may lead to animals returning to the same area. In some cases where animals are territorial, another animal will often simply take its place.

Lethal control, through the killing of problem-causing animals can be carried out by three main groups of actors: public services, local communities and trophy hunters. Killing of individual animals, however, is often ineffective in reducing ongoing conflicts over and with, wildlife populations.

Challenges and Opportunities

Considering the current human population growth rate, the increasing demand for natural resources and the growing pressure for access to land, conflicts over human–wildlife interactions pose ongoing challenges that are likely to escalate.

Expectations of management should not be raised to the level of eliminating conflict. Rather, we need to learn how to effectively reduce or offset such conflicts to bring them to a level where communities are willing to tolerate long-term coexistence with wildlife.

No single approach is adequate to address HWC. Clear policies to prevent and deal with HWC may help establish options that can be implemented either by administrations (national or local), wildlife authorities, farmers and communities and the private sector. Policies should be designed through a joint approach involving all stakeholders and particularly local communities. Inclusive approaches, while often resource-intensive in terms of time and effort, are likely to be the best in designing transparent and workable strategies to prevent, reduce and manage HWC.

Conflict management should be an adaptive process. From a practical point of view, in order to carry out informed and cost-effective management decisions, the following aspects should be addressed in cooperation with affected local communities:

- Collection and analysis of information on HWC and on possible underlying causes, including scientific and local knowledge.

- Joint communication of findings to locals, managers and other stakeholders.

- Collective setting of objectives (and expectations) for management actions.

- Choice and implementation of conflict management approaches.

- Informed monitoring and evaluation of management decisions and processes, leading to adjustments where needed.

2

Problems and Issues Faced by Animals

There are many issues and problems faced by animals living in the environment. It includes farming practices, ivory trade, poaching, animal testing, habitat loss, climate change, blood sport, etc. This chapter has been carefully written to provide an easy understanding of these problems faced by animals.

Habitat Loss Effect

Habitat loss (degradation and destruction) and fragmentation (turning large areas of habitat into smaller disconnected patches) may result from direct land clearing, contamination and negative environmental affects due to human activities including agriculture, plantation harvesting, mining, building construction and other landscape changes.

Habitat loss poses major welfare risks including preventing safe animal movement across the landscape, restricting expression of normal behaviors and denying animals' access to basic needs such as food, water and shelter. Other impacts include stress, injury, illness, pain, psychological distress and death. It is estimated that over 50 million mammals, birds and reptiles are killed every year due to land clearing in Queensland and NSW alone. Furthermore, loss of animals from land clearing can cause negative ecological effects such as disruption of natural food chains. This can lead to further negative impacts on animals which may not have been directly affected by the initial land clearing.

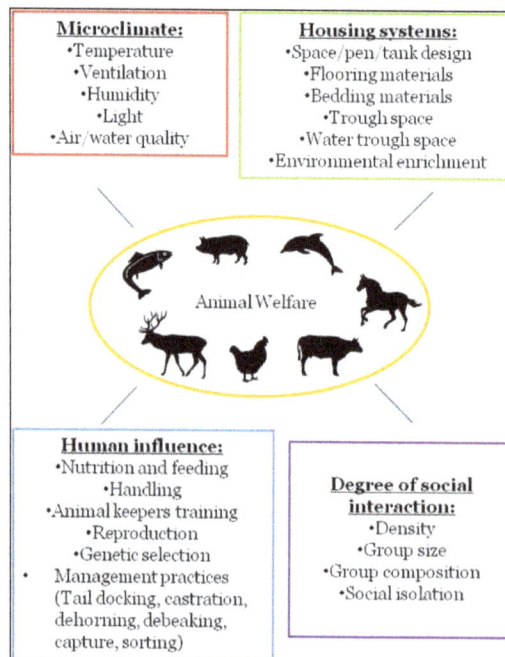

Farm Animals

Cattle and Small Ruminants

Ruminants belong to the order Cetartiodactyla, which encompasses numerous species and only a minority has been domesticated including cattle, sheep and goats. Although these are suited to different habitats, in intensive farming systems, domestication has led to exposure to different stressors potentially responsible of pathologies.

For centuries, cattle have been grown in a traditional manner, within small farms, mainly grazing. Since the second half of the nineteenth century, the continuous demand of protein products and the availability of grains and protein sources to low costs led to an intensive, highly specialized production system, where animals are "adapted" to meet the constraints caused by their housing conditions and the management practices, thus restricting their natural behaviors. Furthermore, individual selection for enhanced production traits has placed an even greater metabolic demand on these animals.

The microenvironment experienced by cattle in houses, on open feedlots or at pasture is determined by the microclimate. Beef cattle can tolerate and adapt to a wide range of air temperatures and metabolic heat production increases with increasing feed intake. Microclimate changes (e.g., inadequate ventilation, extreme temperatures, high relative humidity, ammonia concentration, etc.), affect the animal's immune response resulting in respiratory and enteric diseases, the major welfare problems in beef cattle.

The housing system could play an important role in cattle welfare. Loose housing systems allow more freedom of movement than tether systems, also offering the animals the possibility of experiencing more natural social behaviors. The resting area is one of the most important areas, especially in a cow facility. Lying down is a basic requirement and repeated deprivation is aversive to cows. Lying times are lower and standing times are higher when dairy cattle are forced to use hard surfaces. Particularly, in dairy cow, the poor hygiene and the materials of the bedding leads to udder problems, as manure may compromise cow comfort and increase the risk of intramammary infections. The type of flooring on which animals walk has been found to affect their welfare by impairing locomotion and increasing the occurrence of hoof disorders and lameness, which represent a major concern for the dairy industry because it negatively affects milk production. Beef cattle kept on slatted floors show a higher incidence of abnormal standing and lying movements and also a higher incidence of injuries than animals kept on concrete floor with fully or partially straw-bedded areas. A long duration of grazing periods, associated with frequent manure removal during the housing period, is probably a key factor for limiting the occurrence of podal lesions.

As far as social interactions are concerned, mixing and regrouping of cattle increase the incidence of agonistic behaviors and have also disadvantages from a health perspective. Older and more aggressive animals may cause trauma and continuous and severe stress to lower ranking calves (bullers). Small and young animals are more prone to diseases if kept with larger and older animals. For these reasons, groups should be made up with animals of similar age, weight and sex. Moreover, overcrowding and the reduced space at the manger are one of the most critical factors negatively affecting cattle welfare by increasing competition among pen-mates, causing the buller steer syndrome, decreasing the feed intake, reducing the time spent resting, eating and ruminating and increasing lesions, such as trauma on bones and joints, osteoarthropathies, prepuce injury and tail-tip necrosis. In most intensive farming systems, the separation of the dairy calves from their mother in the period immediately after birth may have negative consequences for the health and welfare of cows and calves. Particularly, the socialization of calves may profit from staying with the dam, preferentially in a group.

Husbandry practices can have a tremendous effect on cattle provoking an increase in the prevalence of stress responses and physical injuries. In fact, a positive attitude of the stockperson in handling and taking care of the animals seems to improve cattle welfare. The age of the farmers is also responsible for the less efficient management and consequently poor welfare of the animals. Not well-trained milkers may produce teats injuries that predispose to mastitis.

Furthermore, the welfare of any animal clearly depends on the provision of sufficient food to supply principally energy (Net Energy [NE]), proteins, amino acids, fatty acids, minerals and vitamins, which are essential for the functions of life (maintenance, growth, activity and reproduction). Failure to provide sufficient NE and optimal amounts of specific nutrients can lead to severe loss of body condition, infertility and severe metabolic disorders. Growing beef cattle, housed, yarded or on feedlots and presented with high energy and low fiber rations ad libitum are at risk of digestive disorders. The most common of these ones is subacute ruminal acidosis, which occurs when the fermentation rate and hence the volatile fatty acid production exceed the buffering capacity of the rumen, but it is possible to observe also fatty liver, ketosis, displaced abomasum, liver abscesses and laminitis. Unnatural foraging regimes, possibly exacerbated by restrictive environments, are thought to elicit stereotypic oral behavior in cattle, such as tongue-rolling, object-licking, chain-chewing or bar-biting.

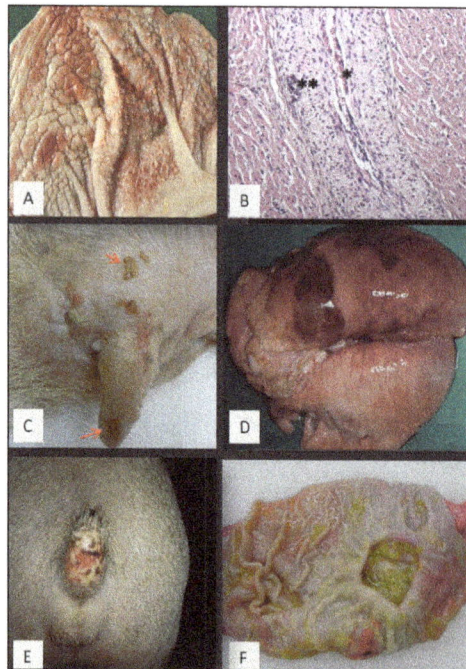

(A) Beef cattle—abomasitis due to improper nutrition. (B) Beef cattle—heart. Arteriosclerotic alterations: Diffuse intimal hyperplasia (*), medial smooth muscle cells reoriented and with disseminated vacuolar degeneration of the cytoplasm, moderate medial hypertrophy/hyperplasia (**). Histological section stained with H & E. Original magnification 20×. (C) Goat—udder. Traumatic teat injuries caused by milking. (D) Pig—lung. Pulmonary sequestration due to Actinobacillus pleuropneumoniae infection. (E) Pig—tail-biting lesions. (F) Pig—gastric ulcer due to improper nutrition.

Basically, the major farming systems of small ruminants are those based on pasture (extensive-grazing), the indoor ones (intensive-industrial) and the semi-intensive. The negative impact of intensification of breeding systems can be observed at several levels. However, limited studies on the small ruminant welfare have been carried out, since they are considered very rustic animals able to cope with prohibitive environmental conditions and inadequate management practices, without harming their welfare and productive performances. This aspect has been overrated for many years considering that also in sheep and goats, stress can impair growth rate, wool growth and feed conversion efficiency, also leading to the development of multi-factorial diseases such as mastitis, laminitis and metabolic disorders and increasing the frequency of abnormal behaviors (aggressive behavior), stereotypies and vocalizations.

The microclimate is fundamental in preventing respiratory diseases. Indeed, animals allocated in hot and dusty environments are more prone to develop bacterial or viral pneumonia. Additional stressors could be found in the extensive systems, such as climatic extremes, that may evoke a decrease in feed intake efficiency and utilization, disturbances in water, protein, energy and mineral balances, enzymatic reactions, hormonal secretions and blood metabolites.

The housing system is fundamental for small ruminant welfare too, only few animals are reared in extensive production systems in which animals are free to move and perform their physiological and behavioral functions; most of them are housed only during the night and in the periods when grazing is not feasible. In any case, it is fundamental to understand that maintenance of good hygiene conditions, correct dimensioning of structural parameters and adoption of proper management practices are important in either type of system.

With regard to social interactions, separation of goats/sheep from the group and re-introduction (e.g., for shearing or milking) and introduction of goats/sheep into established groups are stressful. One measure to reduce the effects of separation and re-introduction is to enable the (separated) goat/sheep to still hear and smell the other goats.

Human-animal interaction is a key factor also in the welfare of small ruminants too and it is not unusual to find shepherds who have no specific skills or are not aware of the welfare standards of the animals. An inadequate milking may produce teat injuries which is why specific training of farm crews should therefore be encouraged. Finally, an inadequate pasture in terms of quality and quantity can lead to nutritional unbalance with liver disease, enzootic ataxia, pregnancy toxemia, hypocalcaemia, diarrhea and enterotoxaemia.

Pigs

Genetic selection in domestic pigs has been widely exploited in order to achieve specific phenotypic characteristics. Many pigs are raised in intensive conditions and thus strongly conditioned by the environment where they live. Moreover, even free-ranging domestic pigs and wild boars may be strongly influenced by human activities. Several signs of suffering in swine have been described and they can be quantified using animal-based measures (ABMs). Furthermore, researches on pig welfare and ABMs led to the identification of "iceberg indicators" such as body injuries and ear and tail lesions. These indicators can be a proxy of "disturbed habitat" which is strongly influenced by microclimate and management. Microclimate heavily affects the stress conditions for pigs, particularly in intensive farming where different age groups require different microclimate standards (air, temperature and humidity). If ventilation and air quality are not optimal, respiratory disorders, such as pneumonia and pleuritis from opportunistic pathogens, may occur, thus increasing the mortality. Variations in temperature and humidity (outside the thermal comfort) result in abnormal behaviors. For example, distressed pigs show increased huddling due to excessive cold weather and panting due to excessive hot weather.

Proper management is the key to maintain suitable habitat conditions for both intensive and extensive pig farming. Housing systems affect both animal behavior and physical conditions. In the intensive farming, floor types (e.g., slatted or solid), space allowance and availability of bedding material influence incidence of bursitis, erosions, lameness and shoulder ulcers. Moreover, the type of flooring directly affects the hygiene of the pig's body and the risk of developing enteric disorders. In the extensive farming, pigs must always have access to proper shelters; otherwise, outbreaks of severe enteric and respiratory disorders will occur increasing also the mortality rating. Appropriate structures and adequate space allowance for activities such as resting, feeding and drinking are directly related to social behavior and interactions. Indeed, the environment in which pigs are confined influences the degree of social interactions. When a new group of pigs is formed, a stable social hierarchy is usually established in 1 or 2 days. During this initial phase, negative interactions arise and their outcomes may be observed mainly as wounds on the body. Once the hierarchy is established, negative interactions drastically subside while positive interactions (e.g., grooming, sniffing, nosing and liking) and exploratory behaviors become prevalent. Nevertheless, rearing conditions typical of intensive housing systems can exacerbate inappropriate behaviors such as stereotypies (e.g., sham chewing) and negative interactions (e.g., ear and tail biting). Human influence on genetic selection and daily management is one of the most important variables which can exacerbate consequences of "disturbed habitat." Indeed, daily management errors, such as improper nutrition or feeding, may lead to severe conditions like gastric ulcers or toxic states (e.g., salt poisoning) which can cause high mortality. Clear differences in the body condition scores of pigs of the same age are also a direct consequence of inadequate feeding. Genetic selection has led to great production results improving parameters such as reproductive performances, meat production, daily weight gain and feed conversion ratio. However, this intense selection has made pigs less able to adapt to certain environmental situations (e.g., thickness of the subcutaneous fat layer), with organs at the limit of physiological potentiality (e.g., heart), leading to an increased risk of pathologies such as hernias and mulberry heart disease. Pigs are also selected to be more prolific but, without adequate assistance, there is a drastic increase of newborn piglet mortality. Finally, human influence on pig management has repercussions on infectious diseases, which negatively affect pig health, such as colibacillosis, polyserositis, enzootic pneumonia, post weaning multisystemic wasting syndrome and porcine reproductive and respiratory syndrome.

Equines for Meat Production

Equine meat consumption depends on cultural and traditional customs. Since it is a niche product, scientific community has made little efforts to define the main factors responsible for a "disturbed habitat". Equine breeds specifically selected for meat production do not exist and genetic selection focused more upon preserving and improving traits related to horses' morphology and performance. Therefore, although equines' domestication dates back to 5000 years ago, these species still retain the ancestral characteristics of their progenitors and feral equine populations can provide information about many aspects of equine behavior (e.g., social and foraging behavior). Considering the most important microclimate factors that negatively affect the equine habitat, insufficient ventilation and inadequate air quality may cause an increased exposure to gaseous ammonia and airborne dust that contain high levels of organic particulates including mite debris, microbes and vegetative material with varying content of endotoxins. The inhalant exposure to those irritant factors is implicated in the pathogenesis of chronic inflammatory pulmonary disorders such as inflammatory airway diseases (IAD) and recurrent airway obstruction (RAO).

Equines reared for meat production are housed in conditions that markedly differ from those in which they evolved. As a consequence, those animals attempt to adapt to the conditions in which they are kept performing functionless and repetitive activity known as stereotypic behaviors that include crib-biting, wind sucking, box walking and weaving. Therefore, using equine stereotypies as welfare indicators should lead to perform management changes to enhance equine's welfare.

Bedding is an essential component in the housing of the equine stabled. Bedding should be dry, clean and not dusty, providing comfort, allowing animals to express their natural behavior of lying and resting and also avoiding the risk of hoofs and skin lesions.

Regarding the equines' opportunity to perform normal behaviors, it is important to guarantee an adequate space allowance to prevent aggressive reactions that might lead to stress competition for resources and for hierarchy establishment with consequent physical injuries. Indeed, wild horses live in relatively stable harem bands, so the overcrowding and the high rates of regrouping of intensively farmed horse may cause an increase in aggressiveness and injuries. On the contrary, in nature, donkeys adapt easily and their social organization depends on the availability of food and water resources. Therefore, the competition in the stabled donkeys, probably, could be increased if the available resources are not accessible to all.

Equines are grazing herbivores adapted to eating a forage-based diet. In nature, horses and donkeys spend about 16 hours per day foraging over wide distances and this is essential for the health of their gastrointestinal tract and for their behavioral needs. On the contrary, equines in the breeding farms are fed high-energy, low-fiber concentrates and this lack of foraging opportunity along with the high amount of concentrate feedstuff has been directly linked to the onset of gastrointestinal disorders such as gastric ulcerations and colic. Equine gastric ulcer syndrome (EGUS) is reported in domesticated horses mainly involved in athletic endeavors. EGUS prevalence and severity have been correlated with the type of training and management practice. Common known risk factors have been identified in intense exercise, high grain-low roughage diet, water deprivation, fasting, hospitalization and overdose of NSAIDs. In particular, excessive ingestion of carbohydrates causes a rapid proliferation of the hindgut gram-positive bacteria Streptococcus bovis and Streptococcus lutetiensis that lead to very acidic conditions with pH lower than 4. Low pH in the large intestine causes the death and lysis of a large number of bacteria and the release of the toxic components which are absorbed from the gut into the bloodstream and may cause the development of laminitis.

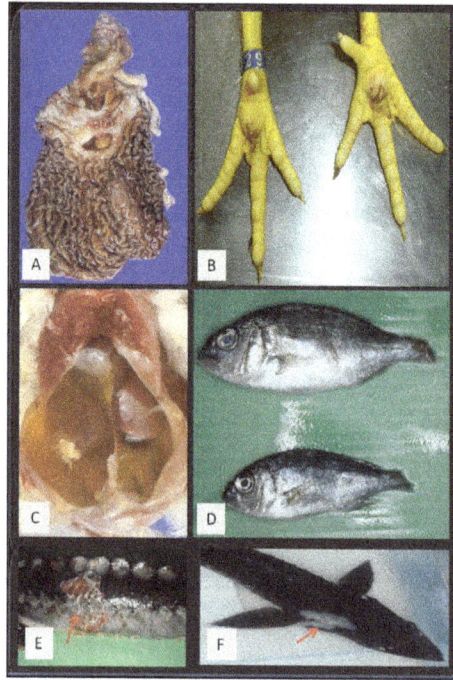

(A) Horse—gastric ulcer due to improper nutrition. (B) Chicken—footpad dermatitis. (C) Chicken—ascites. (D) Sea bream (Sparus aurata)—peduncle mutilation caused by bite in overcrowding breeding conditions. (E) Sturgeon (Acipenser spp.)—skin erosion caused by an inappropriate and traumatic manipulation. (F) Sturgeon (Acipenser spp.)—dark color and a skin whitish patch due to Flavobacterium spp. infection. Evidence of stress and opportunistic infections.

Poultry

The concept of "disturbed habitat" in poultry farming can be almost entirely related to the continuously increasing production levels of the breeding programs, which are focused on increasing the growth rates and decreasing the feed conversion ratios of the animals. These management procedures lead to remarkable imbalances between the high potential productivity of birds (as a result of the targeted genetic selection) and their ability to physiologically adapt. These imbalances are frequently associated with homeostatic dysregulation and pathological changes of organs that supply the energy for production and maintenance (liver and cardiovascular system) or muscle tissue severely forced to obtain a fast weight increase. The other "disturbed habitat" conditions may strictly depend on microclimate alterations or management defects related to housing system and degree of social interactions.

With regard to the microclimate alterations, heat stress is the most common physical environmental stressor that can lead to alterations in the intestinal epithelium integrity and microbiota composition (with development of necrotic enteritis), hyperthermia, heat exhaustion and death. Multiple behavioral, physiological and health issues, such as reduced feed consumption, neuroendocrine disorders, electrolyte imbalance and systemic immune dysregulation, which in turn will negatively affect nutrient uptake and utilization, growth and survival rate, are also frequently observed. Modern broiler hybrids seem to be particularly susceptible to heat stress, since the high body heat resulting from their great metabolic activity may exacerbate this phenomenon. Metabolic disorders resulting from other microclimate alterations (such as cold, hypoxia and light/dark hour changes) are less frequent and quite nonspecific.

Management defects related to housing conditions and social interactions among animals are strictly related to each other. One of the most frequent welfare problems in broiler chickens is contact dermatitis (i.e., hock burns, breast burns and foot pad dermatitis), which is caused by continuing contact and pressure of the skin of the breast, hocks and feet against humid and soiled bedding. In particular, footpad dermatitis (FPD) has the greatest relevance. It is also known as pododermatitis and represents a condition that is characterized by inflammation and necrotic lesions, ranging from superficial too deep on the plantar surface of the footpads and toes. Deep ulcers may also lead to abscesses and thickening of underlying tissues and structures. Several environmental factors such as litter material, moisture depth and amendments, drinker design and management and stocking density may influence FPD development. Indeed, a straw, wet, thin and acidifier-added litter and small drinker cups and higher stocking densities have been reported to be associated with a greater incidence of FPD. Feather-pecking, which is defined as a nonaggressive behavior whereby birds peck at and pull out the feathers of conspecifics, represents one of the most significant welfare concerns in laying hens resulting in feather damage, feather loss, wounds, pain, cannibalistic pecking and death. Development of feather-pecking has been associated with different causative factors, one of the most important being the inhibition of foraging behaviors (such as ground-pecking or lack of environmental stimuli) and lack of early life access to litter.

The selection procedures focused on a high growth rate may cause specific diseases of the energy-supplying organs (in particular the intestine and the liver), as a result of the developing imbalances between oxygen supply and oxygen requirement. In particular, fatty liver-hemorrhage syndrome (FLHS) is frequently observed in laying hens, while broiler chicken gut may show malabsorption syndrome. High growth rates, as well as high body weights and low levels of activity, are also frequently associated with the development of lameness of various degrees of severity. It is most prominent in rapidly growing males, with leg deformities such as angular bone deformity (valgus-varus), dyschondroplasia and spondylolisthesis (kinky back) accounting for 65–80% of the noninfectious causes of lameness in broiler chickens. Modern fast-growing strains may also present an increase in skeletal muscle myopathies, such as white striping and wooden breast. In turkeys, focal avascular or ischaemic necrosis (osteochondrosis) of articular cartilage, avulsion fractures and ligament damage at the intertarsal joint or femorotibial joints and spontaneous fracture of the femur may also occur. Finally, pulmonary arterial hypertension (PAH, also known as ascites syndrome and pulmonary hypertension syndrome) is one of the most common diseases observed worldwide in fast growing broilers. This disease can be attributed to the fast growth-related imbalances between cardiac output and the anatomical capacity of the pulmonary vasculature to accommodate ever-increasing rates of blood flow, as well as to an inappropriate degree of constriction maintained by the pulmonary arterioles. Other common cardiovascular diseases associated with rapid growth are the sudden death syndrome (SDS) in broilers and hypertrophic cardiomyopathy (HCM), spontaneous turkey cardiomyopathy (STC) and aortic dissecting aneurysm in turkeys.

Fish

Fish class is the biggest and the most differentiated among vertebrates. Fishes are adapted to different extreme situations as their evolutional success depends on their ability to thrive in a variable medium: water. One of the most remarkable examples of the strict connection between fishes and water is the fishes' inability to regulate their internal temperature (ectothermic animals). Nowadays aquaculture is one of the more sustainable and economically favorable sources of animal protein. Studies on the effect and pathological results of the fishes' "disturbed habitat" are well known due to common compromised (naive) situations. Considering wild habitats, we must sentence that they are strongly impacted by human activity (pollution, overfishing and introduction of non-indigenous organisms) and this makes it difficult to define what is to be considered normal, not normal or sub-normal for fishes in a specific situation. In farmed animals, the effect of "disturbed habitat" can sometimes become more evident and dramatic than into the wild. Moreover, the severity of a given disease is dependent on the intricate interaction of numerous variables of the host, the pathogen and the environment, among which the environment is the less-known factor. In addition, early signs of suffering in fishes are difficult to relate to a specific disease by inexperienced staff. Commonly, acute stressed fishes show color changes because the melanin pigmentation in skin is under neuroendocrine control in fish and it is thus affected by hormones such as epinephrine involved in the first step of stress reaction. If a stress factor persists for a longer time, other hormones, such as cortisol, become dominant (chronic stress). The chronic stress induces immunodeficiency that causes a higher incidence of opportunistic disease outbreaks.

Among abiotic ambient factors, there are all the physical and chemical water parameters such as temperature, conductivity, salinity, turbidity, hardness, dissolved oxygen and other gasses, pH, ammonia and other nitrogen compounds, metals, pesticides, etc. Fishes can handle an open range of variations for each parameter without showing recognizable signs of disease or suffering, thus accumulating chronic stress. Out of these ranges, water quality parameters can influence acute stress along with high mortality showing or not respiratory symptoms. More frequently, considering the synergistic effect of water-quality parameters, only subclinical evidences like a reduction of productivity and reproduction, dissimilarity of age classes (for wild stocks) or a higher impact of some infectious agents or tumors (if a carcinogenic pollutant is suspected) can be noted. Focusing on the farm self-pollution, due to organic wastewater and nitrogen compound discharge (e.g., ammonia), a direct damage at the fish gills (acute gill disease) is evident due to decreased dissolved oxygen. This acute gill disease is easily detected in fishes with an acute respiratory distress shown by a higher frequency of gill opercula movements. On the contrary, in case of prolonged mild problems, fishes develop a "chronic gill disease" characterized by a fusion of secondary lamellae and a typical fish silhouette called "snake head shape" due to the contrast between a large and triangular head, deformed for the enlarged opercula and a thin body. In fact, the low level of oxygen blood saturation causes a growth failure for the inability to optimally metabolize food nutrients.

The housing system in aquaculture management must take into consideration the different biology, ecology and natural behaviors of individual fish species. The space, design, composition material for tanks, pools, basins and nets, water source, flow and change, lighting and photoperiod, etc. must be taken into account. An inappropriate housing system determines lower growth performances and a higher incidence of opportunistic diseases due to chronic stress. The degree of social interaction among fishes, with the main critical point of the animal density, is different in extensive farming when compared to the intensive one: the first is closer to a wild condition while the second is richer of health-limiting conditions. In nature, high animal density happens only for short times (i.e., migration for the reproduction or for feed) but in farmed fishes is a constant need. Over-density causes traumatic lesions by bite (skin erosion, ulcers and body mutilation) and fast deterioration of water-quality parameters. Similar consequences can be observed as a result of husbandry practices, such as selection, artificial reproduction, handling, transport and net confinement, especially if carried out without suitable tools or by unskilled workers. Infections caused by opportunistic bacteria or fungi (Oomycetes) such as Flavobacterium spp., Columnaris disease (fin or skin rot) or Saprolegnia spp. (water mold infection) can develop into skin or gill injuries. Sometimes, if fish density is high and the water quality and exchange low, parasites such as barnacles or motile ciliates can also provoke a massive outbreak with evident skin hemorrhages and erosions. At the same time, also common aquatic bacteria such as motile Aeromonas spp., Pseudomonas spp. or Vibrio spp. can cause septicaemia characterized by skin, gills and internal organ hemorrhages, pop eyes and skin ulcerations. Regarding feeding, as fish are ectothermic, periods of food deprivation may be less detrimental than in endotherms. For this reason, temporary starvation prior to transport, treatment of disease or any other kind of handling procedures is highly recommended to reduce physiological stress. However, an inappropriate food composition or feeding procedure can generate gut problems like enteritis and size inhomogeneity in the fish stock.

Zoo and Wild Animals

The literature merges concepts and definitions of modern zoos and aquaria as "centers for education and conservation." In this sense, their animals are considered as "ambassador guests" or even stakeholders of the zoological institutions. Husbandry procedures impact directly on the welfare of every managed animal species and should be carried out with "human care" regardless of the context, artificial, semi-natural or wild; this highlights the importance of precise estimation of the resources provided to the animals, by humans.

But, is this always the case? Advocacy groups often claim that animals would only live a good life "worth living," if they were left into the wild. In reply to this controversy stands the extremely relevant anthropic detrimental influence on the environment and a precise definition of "ex situ" as: "conditions, under which individuals are spatially restricted with respect to their natural spatial patterns or those of their progeny, are removed from many of their natural ecological processes and are managed on some level by humans".

This concept has created a lot of confusion in the years, on whether the artificial environment could really provide excellent welfare conditions, to be evaluated directly on each individual. Welfare indicators in fact, vary among and within species and depend directly on human interests and uses of them. This is particularly true for nondomestic species where individual case relevance is rare, fragmented and often requiring comparison with their wild counterpart.

For this reason, modern zoological institutions tend to mimic the irreplaceable wildlife observations and provide the animals with environmental resources extrapolated from previous ex situ experiences and consolidated in best practice guidelines. Careful attention is paid to animal management processes, starting from animal acquisition and transport, quarantine and acclimation and introduction into social group. Exhibits with multiple species must take into consideration social compatibility, both intra and interspecific. The density and distribution of most species should be compatible with the space provided, allowing the expression of natural behaviors and guaranteeing individual safety, thus avoiding undesired dominance and aggression.

Zoo and aquarium "artificial habitat" construction takes into consideration the preparation of controlled microclimate systems. For example, indoor air temperature, ventilation and filtered aeration prevent transmission of respiratory pathogens (Aspergillus spp., Mycobacterium spp., etc.) in most air breathing species. Appropriate lighting and photoperiod allow a natural circadian rhythm to regulate hormonal cycles, reproduction and molt in most species. For aquatic and semi-aquatic species, the installation and management of "Life Support System" provides computerized systems to control filtration, disinfection and chemical/physical water parameters suitable for the species maintained. Mechanical filtration removes particulate solid matters and the complex system of biological filtration avoids direct contact with all the toxic compounds originating from nitrogen life cycle. Water temperature control is mandatory since it could literally limit survival of species originating from different climates. Inappropriate levels of pH, salinity and hardness might lead to chronic stress or even death. Water disinfection and oxidation must be under strict control to avoid damages or losses from accidental increased redox potential, lethal for fish and invertebrates and seriously damaging skin and eyes of aquatic reptiles and mammals.

Health affects the animal's welfare and the quality of its life. Veterinary programs address general and specific issues such as nutrition, reproduction and management of geriatric individuals. Unbalanced diets can lead, for example, to abnormal growth, gout or hypovitaminosis, to even impossibility to thrive. Poor fitness affects breeding and lifespan, but also physical appearance and behavior of the individuals, influencing the human perception of their role for conservation or "ambassadors of the species." Zoos and aquaria maintain animals in good physical, social and mental health, to fulfill their mission and promote ex situ conservation.

Wildlife is also strongly influenced by human impact on the environment, only from a different perspective. The correlation between "disturbed habitat" and pathology is in fact not always clear, nor evident for wild animals; disease and death are in fact processes of the normal circle of life and can be considered as unnatural problems only when caused by human interference. As stated by the World Association of Zoo and Aquaria in Caring for wildlife: "We affect animals by destroying their habitats, polluting their environment, introducing invasive species into their ecological systems, building structures in flight-paths, tilling the land, cutting trees, driving cars, burning fuel".

An increased food demand, an intensification and mechanization in agriculture, including use of chemical products, led to a widespread decline in farmland biodiversity and remarkable change of landscapes and habitats. The use of pesticides facilitates farmers' work, thus menaces the environment and its living creatures. In the European rice fields, the butterfly Lycaena dispar, an important environmental indicator, is in decline due to the massive use of herbicides; and similar events occurred in Japan as well. "The European Red List of Saproxylic Beetles" highlights the importance of these beetles in the forest ecosystems and their dependence on dead and decaying wood. They are involved in numerous processes but often ruined by the wrong perception that deadwood is a sign of neglected forest management.

The effects of climate warming are recognized by everyone and lead to desertification in many countries, provoke unprecedented disastrous events and affect ecosystems and species survival around the world, including our own. Glaciers melting at an increasing speed directly affect polar bears (Ursus maritimus) and Arctic environment, leading to disappearance of their habitat and food resources.

Invasive species became a very relevant problem: The gray squirrel (Sciurus carolinensis), introduced in the last century in Europe, is a threat to the native red squirrel (S. vulgaris). Gray squirrels compete for resources and, in Britain, are a reservoir for a virus highly pathogenic for red squirrel, inducing a disease-mediated competition between the species. Other countries could face the same problem in future: In Japan, S. vulgaris is a common pet with high risk of uncontrolled release and impact on the native S. lis. The introduction of the popular American pet red-eared slider caused similar threats imposing major conservation activities to preserve the native European pond turtle.

Artificial lights can affect plant's photosynthesis, circadian rhythm, visual perception and spatial orientation and can disorient many nocturnal species. Preys around lamps attract bats that also become more detectable by birds of prey. New road constructions are welcomed with enthusiasm, but they fragment habitats and represent insuperable dangerous barriers for crossing animals.

Coexistence between domestic and wild species can spread transmissible diseases. Infectious keratoconjunctivitis originates from infected livestock and passes to alpine chamois (Rupicapra rupicapra) and alpine ibex (Capra ibex) that graze close to each other. Another type of challenge is represented by the return of wolves in the Alps, since farmers do not tolerate their predation on livestock. The authorities promote preventive measures and compensation for the damage, but the conflict is strongly due.

Overexploitation of natural resources is a worldwide-recognized problem and animal collectors have a huge impact on biodiversity. Oriental medicine utilizes parts of wild animals (tigers, rhinos, sharks, seahorses, etc.). The indiscriminate fishing of the totoaba, a very popular fish, whose swim bladder represents an unremarkable black market value, has brought the small cetacean vaquita on the verge of extinction.

Animal Welfare and Environmental Issues

Animals in the wild face many challenges. Predators, food shortage, social competition and intricacies, weather, illness – all these threaten their health and survival and hamper their reproductive efforts. For any species and any individual, the natural environment is complex and in an ever-fluid state as a result of fluctuating physical conditions and the actions of cohabiting living beings. Animals are adept at turning challenges into opportunities, sometimes through mastery in a specific task, sometimes through flexibility of response, yet such capabilities are often not enough to stay fit, survive and reproduce. Challenges are intrinsic and natural yet, if they are too severe or too many, animals fail to cope with them and their individual welfare deteriorates, frequently to the point of premature death.

By contrast, animals in captivity often live in simple, monotonous and predictable environments, where they are challenged infrequently or not at all. One might expect this to be an improvement: the animal can relax and get on with its life. But could it go too far the other way – might animals also suffer from a lack of environmental challenge? How much of a welfare problem is the fact that captive animals live in barren environments that give them very little opportunity to engage actively with meeting the needs of their own life?

Before turning to this question, it is necessary to look at how wild-living animals deal with challenges. Some challenges come with little novelty but still demand a lot of attention, time or energy because they pose an important threat or opportunity. For instance, coping with seasonal temperature stress or defending a position in a stable dominance hierarchy is serious challenges, but the aspect of novelty may not play an important role in them. Animals can overcome these challenges by being masters in specific behavioural or physiological tasks and responses. Other challenges are highly unpredictable, such as predator attacks, sudden turm oils in social situations or random changes in food accessibility. Such challenges are much more likely to present animals with novel problems, for which they must be able to find new solutions.

We use the term competence to denote the whole array of cognitive and behavioural experience, tools and strategies that an animal possesses at any given moment to deal with novel challenges. How do animals acquire and enhance such competence? As for any biological trait, animals inherit genetic predispositions that feed into and support the different aspects of competence. These predispositions unfold through developmental maturation and sensory experience and by learning through interaction with the hard-and-real everyday striving for food, security, partners, social ties etc. However, if competence could be stepped up only as a result of reaction to external events, the process would be haphazard and risky. It may be too late to start looking for a solution when the challenge is already arriving. Therefore, it is also worth it for the animal to invest in the future, i.e. to expend time and energy in exposing itself to a degree of risk in order to have better chances at dealing with unexpected events later on. Many animals hoard food or build body reserves for lean times – but they also gather information and train their own abilities for later times and moments of need.

Here, we label as agency the propensity of an animal to engage actively with the environment with the main purpose of gathering knowledge and enhancing its skills for future use. In other words, agency is the intrinsic tendency of animals to behave actively beyond the degree dictated by momentary needs and to widen their range of competencies. In goal-oriented behavioural sequences such as foraging, mate seeking and predator avoidance, the animal will mostly use existing skills, whereas through agency-based patterns such as exploration and play, it is building novel competencies. In reality, however, these two aspects of a day's ongoing problem-solving activities are often intertwined, because features of the environment are rarely sharply divided into 'old' and 'new' challenges and the animal's response will often be a mixture of reactive and proactive decision making. One could say that agency and competence reflect, respectively, the procedural (more proactive) and functional (more reactive) aspects of the animal's ability to prepare for, discern and resolve challenges that are meaningful to it in the context of its ecological niche.

Facets of Agency/Competence

First, the environment is rich and complex. Most animal species live in complex ecosystems that offer a plethora of stimuli and their inter-contingencies. Only few of the apparent associations between environmental features reflect true causal links and even fewer can be harnessed, but the utility of those few can be pivotal. For instance, food can often be discerned only through very subtle or highly complex cues. Therefore, animals need a highly developed ability of associative learning.

Secondly, elements of the natural environment, especially other organisms, often resist attempts to harness them. For example, plants and animals defend themselves from being eaten through structural and behavioural defences, such as hard shells or poisonous skins or stings. Thus, animals need to learn how to overcome such hindrances effectively and to develop good operant or instrumental learning capability.

Thirdly, the environment continually presents the animal with new objects, situations and events. It is important to learn more about the nature of these as soon as possible and it is safer to do this when other challenges are not looming; therefore animals tend to react to novel objects with inspective exploration.

Fourthly, most wild animals live in an open world. That is, they live in an environment where there is a possibility to expand their horizon of knowledge and activity – a valuable resource could be hidden just behind the next bush or stone. Therefore, in addition to inspective exploration, inquisitive exploration is a fundamental element of the animal's competence.

Fifthly, from the animal's perspective, the environment is highly probabilistic. That is, because of the intrinsic variability of so many features of the environment, the same action by the animal works on some occasions but not on others. This probability may change in time and it may also contain a hidden regularity or combination of contingencies that the animal might be able to detect through more intense engagement. In order to allocate its time, energy and attention efficiently, the animal should be motivated to track the environment's stochasticity, i.e. it would have to be able to assess uncertainty and update this information regularly

Sixthly, many sources of environmental variability, especially those generated by other animals, interfere with the animal's activities and this often leads to lack or loss of control over its own movements and actions. Therefore, animals possess not only species and situation-specific skills but also a general behavioural, cognitive and emotional flexibility. One prominent way to train for the unexpected is through play.

Lastly, but not least, others living in the natural environment are also knowledgeable. Conspecifics and other organisms also gather and appraise information about the environment and it is often faster, more precise and more efficient to use, share and combine this available knowledge than to rely solely on one's own experience and assessment. Therefore, animals are adept at observational and social learning and at communicating with others around them in general.

The list of challenge types here does not aspire to be comprehensive but it shows that in order to live and reproduce in the natural world, animals need a large array of behavioural and cognitive activities, such as associative, operational/instrumental and social learning, information gathering and updating, flexibility in the face of atypical events and loss of control and, generally, a sophisticated capacity for communication. These facets continuously interact with and enhance each other; for instance, regular patrolling in order to update information can reveal novel features in the environment that stimulate exploration, which, in turn, may produce incentives to employ operational learning, e.g. on a potential food source. The concepts of agency and competence can thus best be regarded as denoting the animal's ability to integrate these various facets into effective, intelligent conduct that will optimize its survival and wellbeing. Such a view sits well with the growing tendency among scientists no longer to regard 'intelligence' as the prerogative of a select few so called 'higher' animal species, but rather as a systemic characteristic of adaptively behaving organisms.

The Expression of Agency/Competence in Problem Solving, Exploration and Play

Here, we focus on problem solving, exploration and play as examples of prominent facets of agency/competence. These three facets illustrate well how agency and compentence are intertwined, although functional competence-oriented aspects are more pronounced in problem solving, while procedural agency-based aspects prevail in play.

Problem Solving

Problem solving comes into action when previously applied behavioural solutions no longer work to attain a goal such as obtaining food. The animal then switches back to appetitive behaviours and modifies them, but also engages 'off-line' higher levels of cognitive control where representations of the world beyond the current sensory input as well as memories of the animal's own past actions, successes and failures are stored. So problem solving is initially driven by an external situation, but it triggers cognitive processes that have many degrees of freedom and that may well continue beyond the instant when the animal solves the actual problem.

Harlow was one of the first to demonstrate that problem solving itself is intrinsically rewarding to animals when he showed that rhesus monkeys will manipulate and learn to open a complex six-step mechanical puzzle even when no explicit reward is given for either manipulating or solving the puzzle. Recent evidence for an intrinsic motivation for problem solving came from Langbein, who taught dwarf goats to discriminate between sets of visual shapes with water as a reward. When the goats were later presented both with freely available water and water attained through the cognitive task, the goats still oriented about one-third of their drinking activity towards the cognitive task. Such data illustrate that problem solving encompasses an element of active cognitive engagement that goes beyond the immediate problem at hand and that animals continue to exercise even when the problem no longer exists.

This propensity appears to have longer term beneficial consequences for the animal's ability to cope with its environment. For instance, Bell rearranged the spatial configuration of the living environment for laboratory rats frequently for several weeks and made it more complex every 10 days. Rats living in this dynamic, enriched and cognitively demanding space were subsequently shown to be faster learners in spatial memory and danger avoidance tasks than control rats. Another example is a study by Ernst, who provided individual pigs with an automated feeding system that summoned them to the feeding station by individually distinct acoustic stimuli. Pigs cognitively challenged in this way showed fewer aberrant behaviours in the home pen and less fear in a novel environment than conventionally fed pigs, indicating an improvement of their coping abilities.

Exploration

Exploration is a form of behaviour that appears to be directly aimed at gathering information. If, for example, we observe a laboratory rat placed into an unfamiliar arena or cattle entering a new pasture, what we are likely to see is the animals moving around inspecting all kinds of stimuli in their new surroundings. However, animals not only explore in response to new situations, but also go out and actively seek novel stimuli, which are often referred to as 'inquisitive exploration'. For instance, piglets prefer to visit places where they can expect novel objects to places where they will encounter familiar objects. Thus, exploration has its own motivation that is expressed, for instance, in the strong rebound of explorative activity that can be observed when animals housed in impoverished conditions are presented with a novel object or situation.

The motivation for exploration probably evolved because animals need to reduce the environmental uncertainties that they are constantly faced with in the wild. Cohen argue that the trade-off between the exploitation of known resources and the exploration of new alternatives is governed by a complex interplay of brain systems in which the forebrain cholinergic and adrenergic systems monitor the expected and unexpected forms of environmental uncertainty, medial frontal brain structures report about rewards and costs and the locus coeruleus noradrenergic system integrates these inputs and shifts the behaviour either towards exploitation or exploration. Intensive research is also being pursued on many other aspects of exploration such as evolutionary modelling or the social dimension of information gathering. Seppanen for example, review evidence that animals explore the environment not only directly but also indirectly, through paying specific attention to cues and signals from both conspecific and heterospecific animals. The common theme of all such research is that active gathering of information brings animal's crucial advantages for the future and they are therefore well equipped and strongly motivated to engage in it.

Play

One of the defining features of play behaviour is that it is a spontaneous, intrinsically motivated, self-rewarding activity that is being performed for its own sake rather than to achieve a consummatory goal such as to obtain food, escape a predator or gather information. It has, therefore, always been assumed that play has deferred, long-lasting positive effects on the development of young animals. More recently, it has been documented that play can also have immediate functions. For instance, domestic dogs seem to confirm their dominance relationships during play and post-pubescent laboratory rats use social play initiation to maintain friendly relationships with the dominant male. Nevertheless, the delayed, lasting functions of play are still considered very important. It seems that what animals mainly learn and train for in play are not so much physical fitness/endurance (which fades away quickly) or specific skills such as prey catching in cats or fighting proficiency in meerkats, as these seem to mature to full function even if play is prevented or reduced, but rather various kinds of general physical and psychological flexibility. This is underscored by the facts that the neurobiology of play is distinct from that of 'serious' adult types of behaviour such as social, sexual or aggressive behaviour and that play repertoires include many elements totally dissimilar to 'serious' behaviours.

Play has several features that channel it towards creating novelty: Play elements are incomplete, exaggerated or awkward compared with elements used in 'serious' contexts; play elements follow each other in variable sequences; and many play elements have a self-handicapping character, that is, they put the playing animal into unnecessary disadvantageous positions and situations where the animal loses control over its movements. For instance, vigorous and variable head rotations, torso twists and body pirouettes are among the most widely occurring elements of play analysed the kinematics of play head rotations in Hanuman langurs (Presbytis entellus) and found that they include different, sometimes extreme positions of the head that follow each other in variable sequences; vision is most probably blurred during such rotations owing to the high angular velocities. Spinka specifically suggested that one major and widely present function of play is to train for unexpected situations and mishaps, i.e. to practice in a 'relaxed field' how to handle, behaviourally and emotionally, situations where external forces kick the animal out of control and routine. Deprivation of play fighting during rat ontogeny does not take away specific social or cognitive skills but, rather, impairs the ability of the animals to calibrate their emotional response; hence, play-deprived animals are unable to apply their motor, social or cognitive skills effectively in challenging situations.

These examples from different fields of behavioural research indicate and support that animals possess a general skill to initiate and persist in, interaction with their environment in a way that appears directly beneficial to a range of specific skills and their ability to cope with adverse, restrictive conditions.

Agency Responds to Appropriate Challenge

The examples of agency/competence in the preceding sections illustrate that an animal may be intrinsically motivated to engage with the environment, but still requires certain conditions to be met before it will do so. Not all types and levels of challenge elicit exploration or play equally it seems that a moderate degree of challenge is most likely to evoke a positive interactive response. To capture this, Hebb proposed a model in which he linked the occurrence of explorative behaviour to optimal levels of arousal, postulating that too little novelty would fail to arouse the animal's attention, whereas too much would startle or frighten it into a fear or stress response. This idea was further developed by Inglis, who, suggested that an animal prefers the greatest degree of discrepant input to occur when it is best able to assimilate that input. Watters takes this notion further in a zoo context, arguing that apparently paradoxically, zoo animals are most motivated to interact with types of enrichment that produce a pay-off that is uncertain, i.e. that is neither guaranteed nor highly improbable. For example, play behaviour tends to be stimulated by environments that are slippery or otherwise tricky to such a degree that full control over the animal's own movements becomes difficult, yet the risk of injury or serious mishap is small, such as is the case for shallow water, fresh snow, sloped terrains, thin flexible branches or swinging suspensions.

Not only is agency best stimulated by intermediate levels of challenge, it also affects the animal's competence most positively at such levels. This notion is akin to the idea of 'eustress': the idea that moderately challenging environments can evoke a stress response in the animal which in the longer term has a positive effect on its survival and welfare. Summarizing such information, Meehan and Mench propose the notion of 'appropriate challenge', defined as 'problems that may elicit frustration, but are potentially solvable or escapable through the application of cognitive and behavioural skills'. Figure illustrates this notion. If challenges are too strong for the skills of the animal, fear will freeze agency; if challenges are not up to the skills, boredom will result. An appropriate level of challenge stimulates agency and this engagement, in turn, enhances competence. The type and relative level of challenge may also influence the type of agency in which the animal will engage. For instance, relatively high levels of uncertainty or novelty may incite exploration, but as the confidence of the animal with the situation grows, exploration may give way to play.

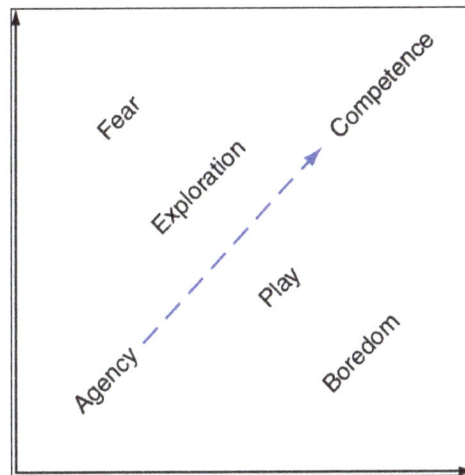

Schematic depiction of the relationship between the strength of a challenge and the strength of an animal's skill.

Importance of Agency/Competence for Welfare

Agency and competence are clearly important for the survival and reproductive success of wild animals. But do these abilities also play an important role for the welfare of captive animals whose survival and concomitant needs are mostly met by the captive environment? In the following paragraphs, we argue that there might be a threefold positive relevance of agency/competence for animal welfare. In figure we illustrate our argument with the simplifying assumption that feelings (i.e. sentient experiences) are at the core of animal welfare, although more complex approaches that also include health, naturalness and indeed the wholeness of the animal may be more appropriate.

First, there is growing evidence that expressions of agency are rewarding for animals independently of any functional outcome that they may have. We know, as argued above, that animals will engage in solving problems without any apparent form of external reward and this suggests they may enjoy the process of learning itself. For example, pigs, cattle, chickens and other species engage in what is known as 'contra free loading'; that is, they will make an effort to work for a reward even if the reward is also available freely. Combining a cognitive task with a food reward in an otherwise barren environment can lead to overeating in rats and goats; this also supports the rewarding value of such tasks over and above obtaining food. Physiological evidence in support of such value comes from a study by Kalbe and Puppe, who found that long-term cognitive enrichment for pigs in the form of an operant feeding system significantly affects gene expression of reward-sensitive cerebral receptors in the amygdalae of the animals concerned.

In addition, a number of studies indicate more directly that the process of problem solving affects an animal's mood. Hagen and Broom set five heifers (the experimental animals) the task of learning how to open a gate to gain access to a food reward and matched these animals with five control heifers for which the gate opened automatically the moment that the experimental animals had succeeded in opening the gate. Detailed comparison of fluctuations in the heart-rate and behavioural vigour of the two animal groups led the authors to suggest that progression of the problem-solving process in experimental animals was associated with raised arousal and agitation and that this may in turn reflect an awareness by the animal of its progress in learning – in other words, an understanding of and excitement about, 'getting there'. Whether this was mainly a positive or negative excitement (i.e. frustration or enjoyment) cannot be told from these quantitative data. A qualitative assessment approach addressing an animal's 'body language', such as developed by Wemelsfelder, may shed further light on the actual experience of such experimental animals. Langbein in a study of instrumental learning in dwarf goats, also looked in detail at correlations between the learning process, learning success and physiological indicators such as heart rate and heart rate variability. Like Hagen and Broom, they suggest that the observed response patterns reflect a process of understanding of and gaining control over, the task – a process they interpret in terms of 'positive stress'. Yet this term still reflects an abstract scientific understanding; what precisely this means for the actual experience of the animals requires more direct qualitative investigation of their behavioural expression.

Expressions of agency other than problem solving appear to be similarly self-rewarding. Play routinely tends to be considered as self-rewarding because it does not result in any obvious goal and often emanates a sense of relaxed and intensive in the-moment enjoyment. Common ravens, for example, will fly upside down, slide down snowy slopes on their backs, play tug of war or play 'pass the stick' in mid-air; Siberian ibex kids may jump into the air from overhangs and perform two or three neck twists and heel kicks before landing; and domestic piglets can stimulate each other into a playing frenzy in which the whole litter sprints around barking excitedly. Such behavioural examples are complemented by evidence that the performance of play instigates an increase in brain opioid levels.

Exploration, too, is positively valued by animals, even when the acquired information has no immediate use for feeding, sexual behaviour or other actions leading to consummatory rewards. Wood-Gush and Vestergaard demonstrated that piglets select an arena containing a novel object rather than one containing a familiar object, even though neither object was of any utility. Moreover, the piglets displayed an increase of locomotor play near the novel objects, indicating their positive experience from the exploration. Newberry showed that domestic chickens value the possibility of exploring novel objects of zero utility as much as the exploitation of non-essential resources such as peat moss or straw bale.

The second way in which agency may benefit welfare stems from the self-building nature of agency/competence. The idea is that because animals benefit from being as competent as possible and because exercising agency engenders competence, animals will get 'drawn into' agency-based activity through positive competence–reinforcement loops. Inglis and Inglis and Langton showed that mathematical modelling of behaviour based on such starting points could indeed simulate empirically observed behaviour in, for example, studies of contra freeloading and latent learning. Csikszentmihalyi is an author well known for his studies of the interaction between competence and happiness in humans, which resulted in what he calls a 'theory of flow'. This theory posits that a person's experienced happiness is a function of the interaction between perceived challenge and skill levels. If the level of challenge is perceived to be higher than the level of skill, a person will try to learn new skills, while if perceived skills are greater than the challenge, he/she will seek more challenge. Thus, perceived challenge and skill chase each other, which, Csikszentmihalyi argues, leads to 'reorganization and growth in the order and complexity of consciousness' a process subjectively experienced as 'flow'. The greatest experience of 'flow' and the greatest associated happiness, arise when both perceived challenges and skills are high and the person is intensely engaged with what he or she is doing through focused attention and sustained concentration and activity. So for animals as well, opportunities to initiate and maintain meaningful cycles of behavioural and cognitive effort are likely to produce a similar feeling of 'flow' and thereby contribute significantly to their longer term welfare.

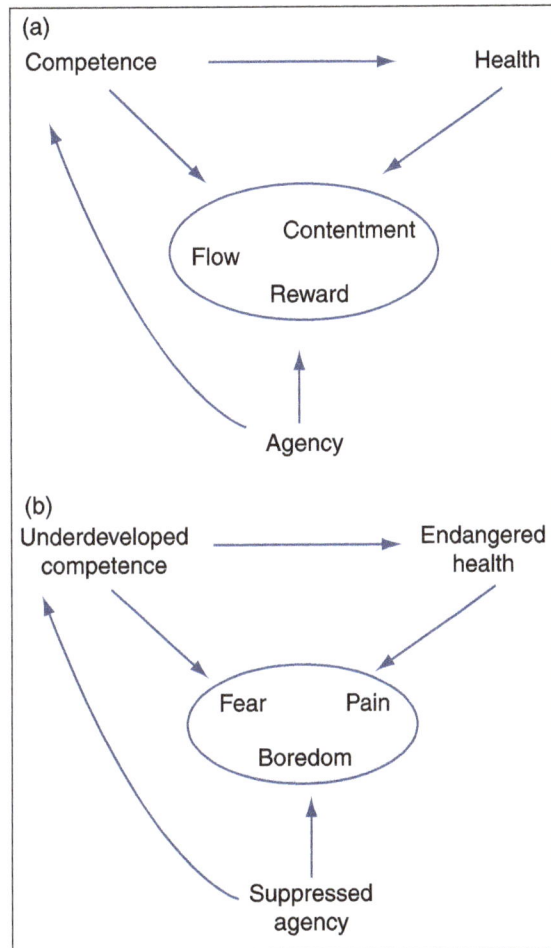

Welfare effects of agency (a) expressed and (b) suppressed.

The third welfare effect of agency arises from the influence that increased competence potentially has on an animal's physical health and fitness and thereby on positive feelings such as contentment. In the first place, increased levels of interaction and mobility may have direct physical benefits, such as stronger bones, stronger muscles, a stronger heart and higher physical endurance, while improved sensorimotor coordination has been shown to lead to greater neural complexity and plasticity which, in turn, may enhance physical fitness and rehabilitation. More generally though, through the skills and information that they acquire, active animals are likely to be more confident and perform better in fulfilling their daily needs – ending up better fed, better protected and socially better positioned than animals that are highly restrained. Evidence is growing that such general improvement of an animal's ability to cope can affect its health and fitness even in captive environments; for example, rats exposed to spatially demanding tasks are subject to lower mortality rates while pigs taught to discriminate between sounds to obtain food showed faster wound healing and better overall immunity than pigs not exposed to these challenges. So allowing an animal to exercise agency not only affects its immediate welfare, but is also likely to improve its longer term physical health and fitness.

The Consequences of Suppressed Agency/Competence in Restrictive Environments

What happens when animals adapted to deal with the vagaries of natural environments are born and raised in simple, restrictive captive environments? Does this affect their expression of agency/competence and concomitantly, the richness of their behaviour and experience? Also, most importantly in the context of this book: what are the consequences of such behavioural and cognitive changes for their welfare?

Agency is intrinsic to the way animals behave and animals will therefore engage with their environment even if it is unchallenging, restrictive and unresponsive. However, such environments will limit the frequency and diversity with which agency is expressed. For instance, enclosures are often much too small to allow animals to go out and look for novelty and prevent the expression of inquisitive exploration; at best, an opportunity for inspective exploration may occasionally arrive. Equally, if social partners are few, of the wrong category or absent altogether, an animal will not be able to engage in social play with the animal's agency suppressed this way, its development of competence will soon hit a limit too and the animal's scope for interaction will remain limited and stagnant.

There is considerable evidence indicating that animals housed in restrictive environments show reduced behavioural diversity both in their home pens and in response to novel objects and use a large proportion of their time lying down, sleeping or dozing. They may also spend extended periods of time in motionless sitting or standing, often with drooping heads and ears, half-closed eyes, abnormally bent limbs or pressed against a wall or stall division. Such passive postures have been characterized qualitatively as apathetic, helpless or depressed. In addition, certain behaviour patterns appear to become less versatile and more fixed and compulsive in their execution; stereotyped pacing in captive polar bears, for example, has been linked to the frustration of their freedom to patrol, while food-related stereotypies in intensively farmed animals are linked to, among other factors, the prevention of foraging. Stereotyped animals may also show an overly aggressive and fearful reaction to novel or unexpected events.

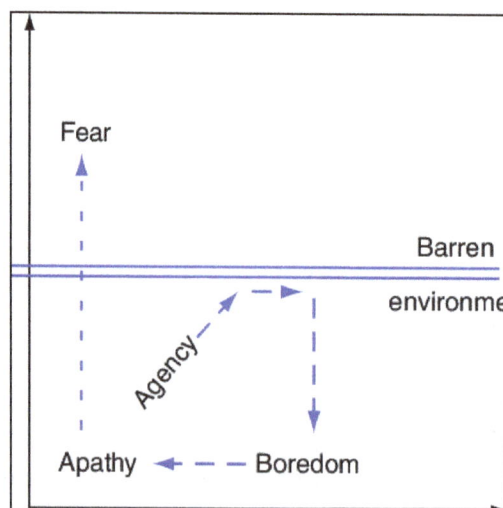

Effects of suppressed agency on animals living in barren environments.

Thus, captive animals may be physically mobile and respond to perceived stimuli, but the question is whether such activity is reflective of normal agency. Do the animals interact resourcefully and playfully with their environment, are they busy and absorbed in organizing their lives? The passive, unvaried and sometimes rigid nature of behavior patterns that are, as discussed in the paragraph above, observed in captive animals, suggests this may not be the case. Wemelsfelder proposes that such characteristics, in their multifaceted complexity, reflect a chronic disruption of 'flow' in the organization of an animal's behaviour and with that a potential suppression or even dismantling, of its agency. Animals are prevented from sustaining activities that they are motivated to perform and so their engagement with the environment deteriorates and the versatility and flow of their behaviour dries up.

What are the welfare consequences of such deterioration? First, the suppression of agency will directly affect an animal's emotional state in various ways. For a start, inability to express agency will deprive animals of experiencing the positive feelings that accompany agency. In recent years, there has been increasing emphasis on the importance of the positive aspects of welfare for an animal's well-being, related for example to social interaction or exploration and play.

Welfare is no longer viewed solely in terms of functional health and the absence of suffering, but also in terms of positive experiences or, generally, good 'quality of life'. Here, the expression of agency was described as being associated with the positive interest and excitement of exploration and problem solving, the relaxation and enjoyment of play and the contentment and happiness of experiencing sustained competence and 'flow'. Depriving animals of opportunities for agency would therefore deny them a source of naturally sustained positive experience. Clearly, more research is needed to investigate whether and under what circumstances, animals experience states of pleasure, enjoyment or contentment.

In addition, various authors have suggested that the suppression of agency is also associated with an experience of boredom and, in the longer run, perhaps also with states of depression and helplessness. Glanzer argued that suboptimal levels of information processing induce boredom, but adds that animals growing up in impoverished environments may adjust to such conditions and not acutely suffer. Inglis postulates as well that animals may get used to discrepancies between expected and actual levels of novelty and although initially bored, may eventually settle down. So one could argue that passivity in captive animals could be seen as an adaptive strategy or life history avenue designed for highly predictable environments. However, the question is to what extent such assertions correspond with actual observed behavioural processes in captive animals. Wemelsfelder, argues that a multifaceted range of behavioural symptoms in captive animals reflects chronic disruption of behavioural 'flow' and that, as such, this should not be regarded as a form of functional adaptation. Rather, in analogy with human behavioural organization, such symptoms may be considered indicative of chronic boredom and depression or general psychological atrophy. Early discussion of this condition in animals was provided by McFarland, who characterized states of chronic behavioural deprivation and indecision as 'limbo'. In the more recent experimental literature, the term boredom is frequently used to interpret the observed effects of impoverished environments on animal welfare. Therefore, if we can accept that through active engagement with their environment animals experience meaning and enjoyment in what they do, then there seems to be no reason why chronic disruption of such engagement should not be experienced as debilitating, boring or even depressingly dull.

A second way in which declining agency may affect welfare is through the consequences of underdeveloped competence, such as heightened fear and anxiety and compromised social coping. Not exercising competence may lead animals to regress in their ability to develop appropriate expectancies and act upon these; they become less well able to classify and evaluate perceived environmental stimuli and will be less ready to deal with challenges once they arise. As a consequence, unexpected or novel events will startle and arouse animals more and they will fail to exploit the novel information available. Laboratory animals, for example, may adjust poorly to experimental procedures which involve transport and handling while for farm animals, arrival at a slaughterhouse, with its crowded, noisy, unfamiliar conditions, may be particularly stressful. Rats and pigs deprived of natural amounts of play during early periods of ontogeny have compromised ability to solve social conflicts and therefore experience more prolonged and more intense fights. Thus, rather than living in quiescent adjustment to their barren surroundings, animals from impoverished backgrounds may be overwhelmed by events when they arise, fail to cope and experience intense fear or anxiety.

A third potential implication of declining agency for welfare lies in health-related effects. Animals living permanently in impoverished surroundings may heal from injuries less well and are therefore likely to experience more pain. Farm animals living in more restrictive systems generally suffer from a higher incidence of painful production-related diseases, such as mastitis and lameness in dairy cows or leg problems in pigs. To what extent these deleterious health effects are indeed a result of the effects of impoverished agency remains to be established.

Is the Expression of Agency/Competence the Same in all Animals?

The ability of animals to act competently in a challenging environment does not imply that animals always tackle challenges in innovative or complicated ways. In everyday tasks, animals use well-proven strategies, long-adopted behavioural routines, simple rules of thumb and direct cues from the environment whenever possible. For instance, after dwelling in a locality for some time, the process of motor learning trains the animal to move quickly and efficiently through the environment, with little further cognitive processing. Also, animal species, populations and individuals often specialize on a limited diet, even though other types of food in the environment are available and potentially equally rewarding. So many everyday tasks are performed in a skilled, routine way and yet the mastery of routine is complemented by the astuteness and flexibility of competence (when challenges arise) and by the self-driven dynamism of agency.

Notwithstanding the fundamental value of agency, its expression can differ to considerable extent between species, age groups, gender categories and individuals. In other words, the quantitative balance between application of routines and the utilization of competence- and agency-related behaviours varies across species, animals and situations. For instance, among non-human primate species, the proportion of time devoted to social play ranges between 1 and 22%, a variation that correlates closely with differences in relative volume of the amygdala and hypothalamus, two brain regions involved in the organization of social and emotional responsiveness. In polygynous and promiscuous mammal species, males engage more frequently in social play than females, whereas in monogamous species there is no difference between the sexes. Even in closely related species, the amount and complexity of play can differ considerably, such as between the Norway rat and domestic mice or between kaka and kea parrots. Such variations can be due to the different demands of species niches. For instance, migratory garden warblers explore more over a wide area, perhaps because they need to find food quickly during short stays on stopover sites, while the related resident Sardinian warblers are much less keen to explore widely.

However the amount of everyday expressions of agency is not in any obvious way related to the apparent intelligence of a species. For instance, wild-living orangutans are renowned for their tendency to spend several days on one tree with abundant fruits just sitting, eating and sleeping, while some reptiles, such as monitor lizards, may be agile learners when it comes to novel ways for acquiring food. Ontogenetic variation in agency can also be prominent. During the later phases of ontogeny, expressions of agency should theoretically decrease because the shortening remainder of lifespan diminishes the value of future competence in relation to the current costs of agency. Indeed, declining levels of exploratory behaviour after the prepubertal peak have been documented in rats and mice. Some facets of agency are mostly expressed during a well-defined period of ontogeny. For instance, play has a typical inverted U-shaped ontogenetic occurrence with the highest levels during the juvenile period in mice, rats, cats and pigs.

Furthermore, the expression of agency varies considerably within age and gender categories of the same species. It has long been recognized that individual animals respond to challenges in different ways and this fact has been the focus of intensive study over the past two decades, often under headings such as 'individual difference', 'coping style' or 'temperament', although where such studies include the tendency of animals to explore, play and be sociable, researchers are more likely to speak of 'personality dimensions'. From such differences, it follows that restrictive environments and their inhibiting effect on agency may affect some individuals more than others and will certainly affect different individuals in different ways. Research with captive orangutans for example, has indicated that animals scoring highly on 'extraversion' and 'agreeableness' personality factors and low on 'neuroticism' factors also score highly on a subjective well-being questionnaire.

Finally, even within one individual animal, the propensity to explore, play or patrol may vary with different locations, seasons, times of day or even moods. Theoretically, an animal should engage in such behaviours if and when this is likely to provide benefits that are greater than the costs, relative to the other things that it could be doing. In times of nutritional hardship, many mammalian species will dramatically reduce their engagement in play, focusing instead on essential foraging and maintenance behaviours. It has been suggested that, in this light, play may be considered a 'luxury behaviour'. While there may be clear prioritization of life-sustaining and reproductive behaviours over play and possibly over other types of agency in many instances, agency-type behaviours are often reinstated at an early occasion, indicating that they do have long-term fitness benefits.

Moreover, agency-type behaviours, including play, may actually increase during tense times, such as pre-feeding periods or crowded indoor housing, because they enhance competence through, for instance, relieving tension or signalling friendly intentions. The term 'luxury behaviour' is also misleading from a welfare point of view because it disregards how systematically important agency type behaviours are for the positive side of animal welfare.

As we argue throughout this chapter, the continuous opportunity to engage in agency and thus to enhance competence is fundamental for the welfare of any animal. However, the variability in quantity and quality of agency expression that we have just discussed indicates that how specifically welfare will be compromised as a result of the suppression of agency in captive environments depends very much on the species and category of animals.

The Integrated Nature of Agency and Competence

We have discussed different expressions, functions and benefits of agency and competence. However, it is important to note that in the end agency is an integrative capacity that works across specific modules of organization. The neuroscience literature also agrees that there are common neuromotivational pathways connecting specific modules and integrating emerging information into anticipatory, flexible, reward-sensitive patterns of behaviour. Yet, in the neuroscience literature that discusses such integrative systems, one seldom finds references to agency and competence. 'Integration' is not necessarily conceived as something actively done by the animal, but rather as something that happens in the animal, a systemic feature of behavioural organization which can at best be regarded as possibly a 'higher-order' neural state. This may perhaps seem a small semantic disparity, but philosophically it lies at the heart of what it means to talk about agency. Philosophical discussions of agency tend to centre around the question to what extent, if at all, humans and animals can be considered 'do-ers', that is, 'authors' of their own conduct.

Traditionally, in this context, agency is seen as yet another signifier of the human–animal divide: humans behave intentionally, with insight and foresight and hence can be held responsible for their conduct, whereas animals behave instinctively, blindly and cannot. In recent times, however, this ground has begun to shift. Animal intentionality, the question of whether or not animals act 'knowingly', is the subject of a rapidly growing field of research covering an ever-widening range of species. In this field, a wide range of evidence supporting the cognitive mediation of animal behaviour has emerged, such as, for example, evidence for foresight in pigs; yet scientific opinion on the extent to which such mediation reflects 'true understanding' remains deeply divided. There is much talk about 'lower-order' and 'higher-order' levels of intentionality, with recent studies proposing that it is not basic cognition, but 'metacognition', an ability apparently shown by few animal species that reflects true intentionality. At present, it remains extremely difficult to find criteria of any kind that unambiguously distinguish 'true' from 'apparently' intentional behaviour and discussions of what such a distinction might imply continue with unabated vigour.

But there is also a second way in which traditional views of agency are shifting. In this, the notion of agency is used to emphasize the integrity of the whole animal and to discuss critically mechanistic/informational models that typically separate ('lower') bodily behaviour and ('higher') mental processing of information into different conceptual realms. Cognitive approaches have, for example, been criticized for over intellectualizing agency, making application to animals less likely. A more holistic approach would regard animals generally as integrated sentient beings and, in this context, the notion of agency would not primarily refer to the direction of action by thought, but to the centrality of the whole animal in directing action. Such a notion does not encounter the need to distinguish between 'blind' and 'knowing' behaviour, because it regards all behaviour as sentient and all animal sentience as embodied and thus views sentience and intelligence as fundamental and gradually evolving properties of behavioural organization. Whether or not this is a reasonable, scientifically acceptable proposition is a question that goes to the heart of what it means to do science; clearly, there is not the space here to discuss that question at any length. One advantage of this approach for animal welfare, however, is that an animal's experience is conceived as an integrative aspect of its behavioural expression and hence becomes more directly observable and more amenable to description and interpretation, than it would have been if it were purely regarded as an 'internal mental state'.

The material discussed here is not meant to support any of these approaches in particular – we have drawn equally on physiological, health-related, behavioural and cognitive studies. That theme was to discuss and provide scientific support for the propensity and ability of animals to engage proactively with their environment and to learn to deal skilfully and flexibly with novel and existing challenges. We think this ability is real and that in addition to more specific abilities, plays a vital role in ensuring an animal's health and quality of life. Taking agency seriously as a topic for ethology and for animal welfare science and practice is bound to lead to more incisive observation of how animals behave and therefore to inform the philosophical debate in scientifically relevant ways.

Stress and its Impact on Farm Animals

The term stress has been derived from the Latin word stringere, meaning to draw tight. In the 1920s and 1930s, the term was occasionally used for harmful environmental agent that could cause illness. Walter Cannon used it in 1934 to refer to external factors that disrupted homeostasis. The novel usage arose out of Selye's 1930s experiments wherein he referred stress as a condition and stressor to the stimulus causing it. Stress is a reflex reaction revealed by the inability of an animal to cope with its environment, which may lead to many unfavorable consequences, ranging from discomfort to death. It covers the behavioral and biological responses to a wide range of abiotic stressors such as social interactions or rough handling, common farm practices (castration, dehorning, teeth clipping, shoeing, weaning crowding etc) improper feeding, exposure to adverse climatic conditions, exercise, work and transport etc. Stressors can originate from within an individual (endogenous) or from the environment (exogenous). Stress-triggering stimuli are not necessarily painful but psychological states, such as fear or anxiety also activate physiological responses. Once animal perceives a threat, it develops behavioral, autonomic, endocrine or immune response to maintain homeostasis. In case animal is unable to withstand stress, the consequences will be abnormal biological functions and development of pathologies. Stress responses are related not only to the nature and the intensity of the triggering stimulus, but also to individual response tendencies or temperament.

The body systems which are mainly involved in the process of adaptation to the environment are endocrine system for long-term responses and nervous system for sensory inputs and short term responses. When an environmental pressure exceeds to that which animal's adaptive mechanisms can accommodate, stress related disease occurs. Many theories have been postulated to explain the organism's physiological response to stress. Hans Seyle proposed the general adaptation syndrome which provided the first comprehensive biological theory of stress. He proposed three stages which constituted alarm, resistance and exhaustion. When the threat or stressor is identified or realized, the body's stress response is a state of alarm. In this stage that animals react by fighting or fleeing. If the stressor persists, the body tries to adapt to the strains or demands of the environment. Exhaustion is the third and final stage when all of the body's resources are eventually depleted and the body is unable to maintain normal function. If stage three is extended, the immune system is exhausted resulting to development of psychosomatic disease, immunosupression, reduced efficiency of production and reproduction. It affects ability to perform and make animals susceptible to physio-pathological disorders.

Impact of Stress

Impact of stress on growth, production, reproduction and disease outcome in farm animals has been studied by various workers.

Growth and Production

Growth and production performances of animals are adversely affected by different kinds of stressors. Increased levels of glucocorticoids in response to stress stimulate hypothalamic secretion of somatostatin, which inhibits growth hormone (GH) secretion from the anterior pituitary. It is obvious that growth of animal is affected by these stress hormones. Transportation stress in animals has been established to cause reduction in their body weight. During transportation the physiological alterations such as electrolyte imbalance, increased respiration rate and heart rate, dehydration, energy deficit and related catabolism have been reported. Besides transportation, heat stress has also been scientifically established to produce negative impact on the growth performance of animals. Different species, breeds and individuals depending upon their physiological states have comfort zones of temperature tolerance. Beyond these limits, the animals require extra energy for thermoregulation.

Therefore, less energy is available for growth and production performances. Heat associated with high humidity or drought remains the most stressful condition for animals. In heat-stressed animals, there is reduced feed intake, which has negative impact on growth and milk production. Heat stress in lactating cow leads to decline in milk production and protein content. The fall in milk yield in a hot environment is higher for older and more productive animals especially at the peak of lactation. The animals experiencing cold stress also have reduced milk yield but the decline is less when compared to heat stressed animals. High ambient air temperature and solar radiation have been shown to have negative impact on dry matter intake, average daily gain, carcass weight and fat thickness in beef cattle. Decline in feed intake ranging from 40 to 60% in 15-month-old buffaloes by variation of temperature and humidity has been reported.

Milk production traits in small ruminants have also been reported to have negative correlation with temperature or relative humidity. Different breeds of sheep have been reported to have variable tolerance for temperature and humidity. Solar radiations have a lesser effect on milk yield, but a greater effect on yield of casein, fat and clot firmness in the milk of Comisana ewes. High air temperature also affects the milk yield and milk components in goats. Lactating goats deprived of water during heat stress activate an efficient mechanism for reducing water loss in urine, milk and by evaporation, to maintain milk production for a longer time.

In heat stressed pigs due to reduced feed intake the milk yield of the sow decreases, hence growth, viability and survival of piglets also decline. In high ambient air temperature the heavier pigs reduce more appetite and growth. Because protein deposits require more energy than fat deposits, the carcasses are leaner at slaughter. In a study, decreased growth, carcass lipid quality and bacon quality in pigs housed at temperatures above the thermoneutral zone has been observed. Overcrowding further aggravates the condition whereas increasing the space alloca-tion for housing may ameliorate the negative effects of heat stress. Multiple concurrent stressors like high temperature, high stocking density and regrouping affect growth performance of pigs additively.

Environmental temperatures above 30 °C cause reduction in feed intake, body weight, carcass weight, carcass protein and muscle calorie content and high mortality in broiler chickens. In hens there is reduction of body weight and feed consumption due to heat stress. Egg production, egg weight, shell weight and shell thickness are considerably compromised by heat exposure.

Animal Reproduction

Stress has been reported to influence the animal reproduction adversely. The impact of stress on reproduction depends on the type of stress, genetic predisposition of the animals, timing and duration of the stress. Stress conditions such as infection, strenuous exercise and malnutrition have been reported to predispose to various reproductive pathologies like infertility or subfertil-ity, defective oocytes and consequent reduction in conception rates. Reproductive processes like expression of sexual behavior, ovulation and embryo implantation are controlled by neuroendo-crine system. The alterations in neuroendocrine responses as a result of stress are likely to influ-ence these processes.

Stress stimulates the hypothalamus, pituitary gland and gonads directly to affect gonadotropin-re-leasing hormone (GnRH) secretion into the hypophyseal portal blood. The hypothalamo-pitu-itary-adrenal axis is stimulated and produces corticotrophin-releasing factor (CRF) and arginine vasopressin. Corticotropin-releasing factor (CRF) interacts with GnRH-producing neurons, prob-ably through an opioidergic pathway, suppressing gonadotropin secretion. Leptin and adiponectin also provide feedback to hypothalamus for GnRH release. The corticotrophs produce neuropep-tides a adrenocorticotrophic hormone (ACTH), beta-endorphin and alpha-melanocyte-stimulat-ing hormone due to stress impact. ACTH acts on the cortex of the adrenal glands to stimulate the synthesis and secretion of glucocorticoids. Glucocorticoid feedback action on the brain also suppresses overactivity of the hypothalamopituitary-adrenal (HPA) axis. In addition, glucocorti-coid secretion is also believed to contribute to the stress-induced gonadal suppression by central actions on the pituitary or hypothalamus. The sympathoadrenal system consists of the sympathet-ic nervous system and the adrenal medulla. It is activated in response to stress and produces cat-echolamines (adrenalin, nonadrenaline and dopamine). Hormones that comprise components of the HPA axis, such as CRH, arginine vasopressin, ACTH and glucocorticoids have all been shown to inhibit GnRH/gonadotropin secretion at the hypothalamic and pituitary levels. CRH inhibits GnRH release in hypophyseal portal blood or GnRH pulse generator activity. Arginine vasopressin and ACTH are also reported to inhibit LH secretion by decreasing responsiveness of the pituitary to GnRH as well as decreasing GnRH release.

The effects of heat stress on the reproduction of dairy cattle have been studied extensively. Heat stress in the summer months lowers the conception rate of lactating dairy cows from 40-60% to 10-20%. It has negative impact on the anterior pituitary, preovulatory follicle, corpus luteum, embryo developments and endometrium resulting in low fertility and loss of fetus. Eestrus behavior in cattle and buffaloes is affected by heat stress in summers resulting in silent estrus or reduced estrus inten-sity and decreased duration. Heat stress damages ovarian follicles and causes a decrease in estradiol synthesis. This decrease in estradiol synthesis could influence expression of estrus, ovulation and the corpus luteum. It has been demonstrated that dairy cows in the summer had approximately one-half the number of mounts per estrus compared to dairy cows in the winter. Stress results in disturbance of spermatogenesis, decreased sperm fertility parameters and disturbed folliculogenesis. Catecholamines interfere with transport of gametes and decreases blood flow. Early embryonic loss in livestock is common due to stress. Prenatal maternal stress results in increased incidence of spontaneous abortion, preterm delivery and low birth weight. Maternal prenatal stress may induce overactivity and dysregulation of the HPA-system in the offspring. Cattle, sheep in heat stress exhibit reduced uterine and umbilical blood flows, resulting reduced fetal oxygen. Heat stress has also shown to have deleterious effect on estrus incidences, estrus intensity and embryo production in ewes.

The service period is increased because of stress arising due to milk fever or lameness in dairy cows. Stress due to transportation in dairy cattle reduces LH secretion in response to exogenous GnRH. In sheep, restraint and confinement enhances plasma cortisol concentrations and simultaneously decrease the pituitary's response to GnRH administration. Conditions, in which nutritional status is suboptimal, such as eating disorders, exercise-induced amenorrhea and functional hypothalamic amenorrhea, are associated with low serum leptin levels. GnRH pulse is highly affected by weight loss, decreased energy availability, altered body fat ratio. Although short-term fasting of adult cows in healthy body condition does not affect LH pulse frequency. Short-term fasting of peripubertal heifers leads to significant reductions in leptin gene expression and circulating leptin, along with decrease in LH pulse frequency.

Disease Susceptibility

It has been reported by many workers that various stressors increase the susceptibility to infection. Under stress conditions, pathogens like viruses or mycoplasma predispose the animals to secondarily bacterial infections, allowing opportunistic bacteria to become pathogenic. Increased risk of fatal bacterial respiratory infections following a primary viral infection has been observed in a wide variety of species. Viral–bacterial synergy has been established following human influenza epidemics and secondary bacterial respiratory infections leading to increased mortality. Stressors such as transportation have been associated with susceptibility to bovine respiratory diseases (BRD). The most intensively explored relationship of this kind has been that of exposure of calves to weaning and transportation and their subsequent susceptibility to shipping fever. BRD can be caused by a primary infection with a virus, commonly bovine herpesvirus-1 (BHV-1), followed by a secondary bacterial infection with Mannheimia haemolytica. The relationship between stress and mastitis in cattle is well documented. Infection by Mycobacteria, causative agent of tuberculosis is known to be increased by stress.

Glucocorticoids have been shown to increase the susceptibility of experimental mice to infectious agents L. monocytogenes, S. aureus, P. aeruginosa, Candida albicans etc. Nutritional imbalances, deficiencies can create various types of metabolic diseases like acetonemia, preganancy toxemia of cattle and sheep on deficient diets, hypocalcaemia of sheep, hypomagnesemia of cattle The sensitivity of animals to the environmental stress is greatest at times when they are already affected by metabolic stresses, late pregnancy, lactation etc. Three closely related stress syndromes occur in pigs. The porcine stress syndrome is common in commercial breeds of pigs used to raise low fat pork. It is characterized by acute death induced by stressors such as transport, high ambient temperature, exercise and fighting which lead to hyperthermia, dyspnoea, disseminate vasoconstriction and rapid onset of rigor mortis. These pigs are particularly susceptible to stress and if frightened may collapse or even spontaneously die. Malignant hyperthermia is drug induced stress syndrome characterized by muscle rigidity and hyperthermia occurring in the susceptible pigs following the use of halothane. Black muscle necrosis of pigs is another manifestation of porcine stress syndrome. Stress from metabolic problems may decrease the animal's resistance and compromise immune system function.

Indicators of Stress

Biological responses to a stressor have been used most frequently as indicators of stress. It is usually more informative to combine multiple indicators of stress to assess animal welfare. Behavioral and the immunological responses also serve as indicators of stress and welfare of animals.

Behavioral Changes

Changes in vocalization, motor activity or the expression of stereotypic behavior may be an early indication of a stressful situation. The effect of acute stress on the behavior of dogs was evaluated. Among the 58 examined dogs, 50 displayed at least one type of activity or posture indicative of stress. Among the activities or postures that indicate stress, vocalizations were the most common, followed by flattened ears, low tail, lowered body posture, paw lifting, digging oral manipulation of the cage, hiding, yawning, unresponsiveness and licking and grooming. Most dogs displayed multiple activities or postures. Males spent significantly more time vocalizing than females, while females adopted stress-related postures more often than males. Females displayed behavioral and physiological indicators of stress more often and for longer periods of time than males.

Ewes and lambs temporarily separated from each other express their distress by an increase in bleating and locomotor activity. Foals have been reported to increase general motor activity and vocalizations. Young piglets separated from their mother give distinctive and frequent squeals and sometimes try to jump out of their pen. These behavioral modifications help the animals to cope with the stress-inducing situation and communicate with each other. Dairy cows showed an increased percentage of the whites of their eyes, when their 4-day old calves were temporarily removed from them. Weaning creates a state of frustration, among young ones. It is a complex stressor as it includes dietary change, environmental change, social change and it prevents the animal from performing suckling.

Pigs, calves and cows try to avoid humans after they have experience of stockmen who hit, kick, prod, shock or threaten them. Pigs can be severely stressed by anxiety and fear caused by human handling. They can collapse and even die as a result. Hungry cows that were prevented from eating grass that they could see and smell showed their frustration by rolling their tongues, shaking their heads and opening their eyes abnormally wide. Vocalization, frequency of urination and defecation are increased in cattle due to acute stress. Incidence of stepping increases in isolation chamber or while being milked in unfamiliar surroundings. Increased movement is considered as sign of agitation in cattle. Hens have a particular 'frustration' call (the gakel call) when they are thwarted in getting to food, water, a dustbath or a nestbox. The birds show boredom and frustration by hyperactivity, aggression, stereotyped pacing and pecking. When stress becomes long-term, animals kept in confinement have been reported to carry out repetitive, apparently purposeless actions. These include the 'weaving' of horses kept in stalls, the bar-biting, tongue-rolling and head-waving of sows confined in narrow 'sow stalls' (gestation crates), the selflicking and tongue-rolling of calves confined in narrow 'veal crates', the repetitive pacing of zoo animals from one end of the cage to another. The cats show defensive vocalizations, inappropriate urination/defecation, pilo-erection, pupil dilation and hiding. Signs of stress in birds include depression, irritability, feather picking, increased pecking, abnormal vocalization and ruffled feathers

Hormonal Indicators

During stress, various endocrinal responses are involved to overcome stressful situations. The immediate endocrinal responses are symphatho-adrenomedullary system releasing catecholamines. The main biological stress responses are related to the HPA axis releasing corticosteroid i.e. cortisol, corticosterone, aldosterone in to blood. Corticotropic-releasing hormone (CRH), which acts on the anterior pituitary to synthesize and release ACTH, which in turn is released into the peripheral circulation to cause the release of glucocorticoids from the adrenal cortex. Plasma ACTH provides the direct determination of stress whereas cortisol provides the indirect criterion of stress.

Besides plasma, salivary and urinary cortisol levels are good indicators of stress. The disadvantage is that plasma cortisol levels naturally increase in the morning and decreases around midnight. Another disadvantage is that all types of stressors do not induce an increase in cortisol levels. Changes in cortisol levels do not occur in response to weaning stress. The complexity of diurnal activity, natural increase in cortisol, individual variability suggests the use of other markers as well to evaluate the stress response.

Fecal glucocorticoid analyses have been used in a wide range of studies as this is non-invasive measure of these stress hormones. Salivary alpha amylase has also been used as marker of stress.

Oxidative Stress Biomarkers

Oxidative stress is a condition associated with an increased rate of cellular damage induced by oxygen and oxygen derived oxidants commonly known as reactive oxygen species (ROS). Uncontrolled production of ROS that exceeds the antioxidant capacity of cells leads to oxidative stress. These ROS result in damage to nucleic acids, proteins and lipids leading to tissue damage cell death. Stressors, such as heat, toxins, ultraviolet rays, inflammation, infections, etc. can lead to the oxidative stress, with important consequences over the function, life and death of the affected cells.

Quantification of Oxidants and Antioxidants

Oxidative stress describes an imbalance between oxidants and antioxidants. It occurs in the presence of ROS in excess of available antioxidant buffering capacity. A free radical has unpaired electrons in the outer orbital and thus makes the specie unstable with affinity to react with other molecules for stability. Oxidant and antioxidant action can be observed directly by electron spin resonance and indirectly by quantification of dichlorofluorescein, a fluorescent product formed by reaction of non-fluorescent diacetate dye with oxidants. It can be measured by using a fluorescence plate reader, by microscopy or by flow cytometry. Electron spin resonance is not routinely used.

Estimation of the Antioxidant Enzymes and Redox Molecules

Changes in oxidative stress biomarkers, including superoxide dismutase, catalase, glutathione reductase, glutathione peroxidase, glutathione levels, vitamins, lipid peroxidation, nitrite concentration, nonenzymatic glycosylated proteins can be estimated. The two most important antioxidant biomarkers are GSH and ascorbate which are capable of regenerating other antioxidants to their active state. Decreased redox ratios of GSH–GSSH or ascorbate–dehydroascorbic acid indicates increased oxidative stress and decreased antioxidant status. The changes in lipophilic antioxidants vitamin E and coenzyme Q may also be measured along with GSH and ascorbate which are also biomarkers of oxidative stress. These compounds can be measured directly by high-performance liquid chromatography (HPLC) and spectrophotometry. Assays are also available to determine the activity of some antioxidant enzymes, such as catalase and superoxide dismutase. The overall antioxidant capacity can be determined by performing various tests like total antioxidant status, total radical-trapping antioxidant parameter, Trolox equivalent antioxidant capacity, ferric reducing-antioxidant power colorimetric assays and cyclic voltammetry.

Measurement of Oxidative Damage

Measures of oxidative damage have typically focused on the three major macromolecules: DNA, proteins and lipids. Oxidative modifications to DNA include base misincorporations, mutations, DNA strand breaks and cell death. Quantification of oxidised DNA damage is done by COMET assay. It assesses the number of DNA strand breaks in single cells semiquantitatively using gel electrophoresis. Oxidised nucleotides and nucleosides can be quantified by HPLC or mass spectrometry.

Protein oxidation leads to malfunctioning of enzymes incapable of performing their cellular tasks. Protein oxidation is estimated in terms of measurement of "protein carbonyls", which are produced by free radicalmediated oxidation of amino acids. A crude homogenate or a microsomal fraction is reacted with dinitrophenylhydrazine, which gives strong absorbance upon reaction with carbonyl groups. Increased absorbance at 370 nm is interpreted as an indication of increased protein oxidation.

Lipids are important constituents of the lipid bilayer of the cellular membrane and unsaturated fatty acids in particular are easily oxidised and may initiate chain reactions resulting in further oxidative damage. Polyunsaturated Lipids are more sensitive to oxidation. Lipid oxidation can be assessed by either the malondialdehyde (MDA) or isoprostane assays. Malondialdehyde is a breakdown product of lipids which can be quantified as a measure of lipid hydroperoxides. This is a crude assay known as thiobarbituric acid reactive substances (TBARS) assay which involves derivatisation with thiobarbituric acid, which is measured by spectrophotometer. More refined versions of the TBARS assay measure only the MDATBA2 derivative, by HPLC or determine MDA directly without derivatisation.

This assay predicts oxidative damage efficiently and has been shown to have very good correlation with other markers such as isoprostanes, which are the most reliable markers of lipid oxidation. Earlier, requirement of mass spectrometry being an expensive equipment limits the isoprostanes determination as a screening marker but nowadays, an ELISA based isoprostane assay has become commercially available. Changes in oxidative stress biomarkers, including superoxide dismutase, catalase, glutathione reductase, glutathione peroxidase, glutathione levels, vitamins, lipid peroxidation, nitrite concentration, nonenzymatic glycosylated proteins and hyperglycemia in diabetes is also reported.

Immunological Markers

The immune system is extremely sensitive to stress and therefore, immune variables can be used as indicators of stress. Several aspects of immune function are affected by various stressors, such as exercise, transport, tissue injury, infection etc. The effects of stress on immune function have been widely studied. Hormones induced in response to stress have effect on immune system of animals either by inhibition or proliferation of immune cells. Hormonal changes in response to stress, including rises in the plasma concentration adrenaline, cortisol, growth hormone and pro-lactin are known to have immunomodulatory effects. Cortisol levels are known to increase after a stressful event due to the activation of the HPA. It has been observed that cortisol can inhibit the functions of macrophages, mast cells, neutrophils, basophils and eosinophils. Glucocorticoids and ACTH have been shown to affect the proliferation of B and T cells, cytokine production and antibody production, chemotaxis of monocytes and neutrophils and NK cell cytotoxicity. Potential immunological markers in response to stress include lecukocyte responses to antigens, salivary IgA, neutrophil/lymphocyte ratio, CD4/CD8 ratio and plasma cytokines.

Strenuous exercise, like exhaustive endurance races in horses may cause detrimental effects on the immune system, by changing the cellular composition of peripheral blood. Exercise induced stress leads to substantial increase in the number of circulating leukocytes (mainly lympho-cytes and neutrophils), the magnitude of which is related to both the intensity and duration of exercise. There are also increases in the plasma concentrations of various substances that are known to influence leukocyte functions such as inflammatory cytokine, C-reactive proteins and activated complement fragments. Following recovery from exercise the blood neutrophil count continues to increase and the blood lymphocyte count decreases, it has been suggested that the neutrophil/lymphocyte (N/L) ratio can provide a good measure of exercise stress. T-lym-phocyte CD4+/CD8+ (helper/suppressor) ratio, secretory immunoglobulins such as salivary IgA and in vitro mitogen-stimulated lymphocyte proliferation are decreased in overtraining syndrome.

Neutrophilia and lymphopenia was also reported in cattle which have been transported. They also reported a decrease in antibody responses three days after transport and a decrease in lymphocyte blastogenesis in calves after transport. In a study, a 9 h transportation of young bulls induces a gene expression signature in blood neutrophils that increases their circulating numbers and may enhance their pro-inflammatory and antibacterial potential.

Macrophages and lymphocytes in bronchoalveolar fluid from young calves were changed in num-ber and function after short-term transport. Neutrophils are also targets of the stress response and are important in lung defense. Neutrophilia along with altered the neutrophil:lymphocyte ratio has also been observed during the weaning stress increasing the proportion of neutrophils. Chang-es in the neutrophil:lymphocyte ratio is thought to be a potential biological indicator of stress and disease susceptibility. It has been reported that corticosteroids decrease the accumulation of neu-trophils at a local inflammatory site such as neutrophil accumulation is important in clearance or resistance to bacterial infection. Increased susceptibility to infection as well as severity of disease due to altered immune function in stress response has been demonstrated in many species includ-ing humans, cattle and mice. T-helper 1 (Th1) cells are involved in cell-mediated immunity where-as Th2 cells are involved in antibody production. Inhibition of IL-12 synthesis and an increase in IL-10 production has been reported when peripheral blood leukocytes (PBLs) were treated with catecholamines in vitro. This shift in cytokine production causes a shift in T-helper (Th) cells from Th1 cells to Th2 cells. A shift away from a Th1 cell mediated response can result in increased sus-ceptibility to viral infections.

Genomic and Proteomic Markers

The involvement of genetic factors in neuroendocrine stress responses has been shown by selection studies. Divergent lines for HPA axis functioning have been obtained by genetic selection in poultry, pigs and turkeys. Considerable differences between breeds of pigs have been observed in cortisol levels both in basal conditions and under stress. To understand multiple responses studies are underway to map genomic areas, identify candidate genes, mutations and underlying genetic pathways responsible for such responses. Genomic regions responsible for phenotypic variation in stress conditions have been detected by using Quantitative trait loci (QTL) approach. The gene encoding corticosteroid-binding globulin (CBG), carrier of cortisol in plasma, had been mapped at chromosome 7 in Meishan and Large White crosses. Mutations in this gene have been found to influence cortisol levels, carcass composition and meat quality in pigs.

Phenotypic variation is not only associated with mutations but significant differences are also attributed to alterations in expression levels of clusters of genes. Nowadays, microarrays, serial analysis of gene expression allow the measurement of expression of thousands of genes at the same time in different tissues and provide unique possibilities to expedite large-scale analyses of gene expression. Changes at the transcription level do not always correlate with changes in expression of proteins but study of proteome can provide better understanding of the functioning inside body. Proteomics methodologies have sufficient resolution and sensitivity to identify candidate biomarkers. Proteomics techniques make it easier to identify changes or differences between a stressed and a healthy animal. High-throughput proteomic methods based on matrix-assisted laser desorption/ionization with time-offlight mass spectrometry (MALDI-TOFMS) analysis of tryptic 2D electrophoresis (2-DE) spot digest and peptide matching with available database have been used to study the protein biomarkers. This technique has been used to find the differential stress responses at protein levels in mandibular lymph nodes and oropharyngeal tonsils of European wild boars (Sus scrofa), naturally infected with Mycobacterium bovis .

The intergrated approach of combined OMICS has also been used to obtain proteomic, metabonomic and elemental profiles of bovine serum samples from stressed and control animals before and after a primary viral infection. Differential trends of protein, metabolite and element profiles were observed following a stress response by multivariate analysis. Proteomics profile analysis in rat liver has also been used to unravel the molecular mechanisms involved in the cellular responses to ionizing radiation. Comparison of the serum proteome yielded a new stress biomarker in pigs housed at higher density.

Animal Testing

An animal test is any scientific experiment or test in which a live animal is forced to undergo something that is likely to cause them pain, suffering, distress or lasting harm.

Animal experiments are not the same as taking your companion animal to the vet. Animals used in laboratories are deliberately harmed, not for their own good and are usually killed at the end of the experiment.

Animal Experiments

Animal experiments include:

- Injecting or force feeding animals with potentially harmful substances.

- Exposing animals to radiation.

- Surgically removing animals' organs or tissues to deliberately cause damage.

- Forcing animals to inhale toxic gases.

- Subjecting animals to frightening situations to create anxiety and depression.

Animals Used

Only vertebrate animals (mammals, birds, fish and amphibians) and some invertebrates such as octopuses are defined as 'animals' by European legislation governing animal experiments. Shockingly, in the USA rats, mice, fish, amphibians and birds are not defined as animals under animal experiments regulations. That means no legal permission to experiment on them is needed and they are not included in any statistics.

Animals used in experiments are usually bred for this purpose by the laboratory or in breeding facilities. It's a cruel, multi-million dollar industry. Cruelty Free International believes that all animals are equally important. A dog bred for research is still a dog who could otherwise live a happy life in a loving home.

Some monkeys are still trapped in the wild in Africa, Asia and South America to be used in experiments or imprisoned in breeding facilities. Their children are exported to laboratories around the world. The use of wild-caught monkeys in experiments is generally banned in Europe but is allowed elsewhere.

Horses and other animals such as cows, sheep and pigs are often supplied by dealers and may originate from racing stables or farms for use in animal experiments. The rules preventing the use of stray companion animals like dogs and cats vary from country to country.

Animal Suffering

A large proportion of animal experiments in the EU are reported to cause 'moderate' or 'severe suffering' to the animals - according to the researchers who carry them out. In the UK in 2018, 31% of animal experiments involved moderate or severe suffering.

Some experiments require the animal to die as part of the test. For example, regulatory tests for botox, vaccines and some tests for chemical safety are essentially variations of the cruel Lethal Dose 50 test in which 50% of the animals die or are killed very close to death.

Laboratories

Laboratories are no place for any animal. They are typically sterile, indoor environments in which the animals are forced to live in cages – denied complete freedom of movement and control over their lives. Some animals in laboratories are confined on their own, without the companionship of others.

Blood Sport

There is a growing issue about blood sports which includes animals. This is seen by many as cruel and inhumane activity and that of should be banned everywhere.

It is true that these cruel sports should be banned because every animal has their own rights to be treated well. Animals do not have the emotions to express their feelings like humans. The proponent of blood sports may see this as an entertaining pastime and lucrative business, but they should also consider the feelings, safety and wellness of those animals that they forced to fight. For instance, cockfighting, which is one of the most known blood sports particularly in the Southeast Asian countries, is popular because of the significant amount of price that it offers to the participants and organizers. As a result of this, the bigger the money they received, the more animals could get hurt or even killed.

This inhumane activity, furthermore, could also affect the relationship between people and animals. Dogs, for instance, are considered to be man's best friend but because of that dogfight is also a part of the modern bloodsport, this belief could be affected. If people will be exposed to this barbaric sport of dog fighting, they would treat their pets differently and their relationship will be affected. Instead of playing with their dogs and teaching them usual tricks, they would rather train their adorable animals how to fight and kill another of their kind. Therefore, the usual handling and caring of dogs will completely be changed in a negative way.

Cruelty to Animals

Animal cruelty can take many different forms. It includes overt and intentional acts of violence towards animals, but it also includes animal neglect or the failure to provide for the welfare of an animal under one's control. In addition to this, it is important to remember animal cruelty is not restricted to cases involving physical harm. Causing animals psychological harm in the form of distress, torment or terror may also constitute animal cruelty.

As a result of there being so many possible forms of animal cruelty, state and territory animal welfare legislation does not attempt to define it in an exclusive way; rather, animal cruelty is described generally as any act or ommission that causes unnecessary or unreasonable harm to an animal. Most animal welfare Acts will provide particular examples of cruelty. These may include:

- Torturing or beating an animal.
- Confining or transporting an animal in a way that is inappropriate for its welfare.
- Killing an animal in an inhumane manner.
- Failing to provide appropriate or adequate food or water for an animal.
- Failing to provide appropriate treatment for disease or injury.
- Failing to provide appropriate living conditions.

State and territory animal welfare legislation prohibits all forms of animal cruelty and imposes obligations on all animal owners to provide for the welfare needs of their animals. Breaching animal welfare legislation is a crime. Serious cases can result in large fines and imprisonment.

Hunting

Hunting may have played an important role, next to plant gathering and scavenging, for human survival in prehistoric times, but the vast majority of modern hunters in developed countries stalk and kill animals for recreation. Hunting is a violent and cowardly form of outdoor entertainment that kills hundreds of millions of animals every year, many of whom are wounded and die a slow and painful death.

Hunters cause injuries, pain and suffering to animals who are not adapted to defend themselves from bullets, traps and other cruel killing devices. Hunting destroys animal families and habitats and leaves terrified and dependent baby animals behind to starve to death.

Because state wildlife agencies use hunting, trapping and fishing licenses as a source of income, today's wildlife management actively promotes the killing of wild animals and joined by a powerful hunting lobby even sells wildlife trophy hunts to those who enjoy killing them. For instance, the California Department of Fish and Wildlife received $45,000 from the sale of a killing tag for California Desert Bighorn Sheep, sold at the 41st Safari Club International Convention in Reno, Nevada. Getting the trophy carcass is an unwritten guarantee.

Hunting Causes Pain and Suffering

A mere four percent of the human U.S. population hunts, compared to 22 percent - over 70 million people - who enjoy watching wildlife alive. Wild animal watchers spend over $20 billion more than hunters on their activities that respect, rather than harm animals.

Despite increasing public opposition, hunting is permitted on 60 percent of U.S. public lands, including in over 50% of wildlife refuges, many national forests and state parks; on federal land alone (more than half a billion acres), more than 200 million animals are killed every year (McCarthy).

Quick kills are rare and many animals suffer prolonged, painful deaths when hunters severely injure but fail to kill them. Bow hunting exacerbates the problem, evidenced by dozens of scientific studies that have shown that bow hunting yields more than a 50 percent wounding and crippling rate. Some hunting groups promote shooting animals in the face or in the gut, which is a horrifically painful way to die.

Several states allow a spring bear hunt during the months when bears emerge from hibernation. These bears are not only still lethargic, which makes them easy targets for hunters, but many of the females are either pregnant or lactating. Mother bears are often shot while out and about foraging, while hiding their cubs in trees or leaving them in their dens. When mother bears are killed, their nursing cubs have little to no chance of survival as they will either starve or be killed by predators.

The stress that hunting inflicts on animals — the noise, the fear and the constant chase — severely restricts their ability to eat adequately and store the fat and energy they need to survive the winter. Hunting also disrupts migration and hibernation and the campfires, recreational vehicles and trash adversely affect both wildlife and the environment. For animals like wolves, who mate for life and have close-knit family units, hunting can destroy entire communities.

Hunting is not Sport

Hunting is often called a "sport," to disguise a cruel, needless killing spree as a socially acceptable activity. However, the concept of sport involves competition between two consenting parties, adherence to rules and fairness ensured by an intervening referee and achieving highest scores but not death as the goal of the sporting events. In hunting, the animal is forced to "participate" in a live-or-die situation that always leads to the death of the animal, whereas the hunter leaves, their life never remotely at stake.

Hunting is not Fair Chase

Despite hunters' common claim of adhering to a "fair chase" code, there is no such thing. With an arsenal of rifles, shotguns, muzzleloaders, handguns, bows and arrows, hunters kill more than 200 million animals yearly – and likely crippling orphaning and harassing millions more. The annual death toll in the U.S. includes 42 million mourning doves, 30 million squirrels, 28 million quail, 25 million rabbits, 20 million pheasants, 14 million ducks, 6 million deer and thousands of geese, bears, moose, elk, antelope, swans, cougars, turkeys, wolves, foxes, coyotes, bobcats, boars and other woodland inhabitants. Hunters also frequently use food and electronic callers to lure unsuspecting animals in front of their weapons. The truth is, the animal, no matter how well-adapted to escaping natural predators she or he may be, has virtually no way to escape death once he or she is in the cross hairs of a scope mounted on a rifle or a crossbow.

Hunting Contributes to Species Extinction

Hunting has contributed to the historical extinction of animal species all over the world, including the Southern Appalachian birds, the passenger pigeon and the Carolina parakeet (the only member of the parrot family native to the eastern United States), the eastern elk, the eastern cougar, the Tasmanian tiger and the great auk.

Wild Animals are not Crops

Wildlife managers and hunters treat wild animals like a crop, of which a percentage can be "harvested" annually – to them; wild animals are no different than a field of wheat. This selective mis-management, with its exclusive focus on numbers to be killed, ignores the science that shows that nonhumans, just like humans, have similar capabilities to experience emotions and have families and other social associations built on multi-leveled relationships.

Natural Carnivores are the Real Ecosystem Managers

While hunters and so-called wildlife professionals pretend to have control over ecosystems and the animals they kill, natural predators such as wolves, mountain lions and bears are the real ecosystem managers, if allowed to survive naturally. For instance, the reintroduction of wolves to Yellowstone National Park caused ripple effects throughout the ecosystem, with an increase in biodiversity, including a higher occurrence of beavers, several bird and plant species and natural habitat and stream recovery.

References

- How-can-habitat-loss-affect-animal-welfare, knowledge-base: kb.rspca.org.au, Retrieved 26 January, 2019

- The-disturbed-habitat-and-its-effects-on-the-animal-population, online-first: intechopen.com, Retrieved 05 March, 2019

- Environmental-Challenge-and-Animal-Agency- 256294670: researchgate.net, Retrieved 28 April, 2019

- Stress-and-its-impact-on-farm-animals- 259331272: researchgate.net, Retrieved 08 July, 2019

- What-animal-testing, why-we-do-it: crueltyfreeinternational.org, Retrieved 05 August, 2019

- What-animal-cruelty, animal-cruelty: rspca.org.au, Retrieved 25 June, 2019

- Hunting, wild-animals-and-habitats: idausa.org, Retrieved 28 April, 2019

Animal Behavior, Rights and Ethics

Animal behavior deals with the study of interaction between animals and their environment. Animal ethics examine the human-animal relationships. Animal rights and ethics are the essential components of animal welfare. This chapter discusses about animal behavior, rights and ethics to provide an in-depth understanding of the subject.

Behavior in Animals

Animal behavior is the concept that is broadly considered referring to everything animals do, including movement and other activities and underlying mental processes. Human fascination with animal behavior probably extends back millions of years, perhaps even to times before the ancestors of the species became human in the modern sense. Initially, animals were probably observed for practical reasons because early human survival depended on knowledge of animal behavior. Whether hunting wild game, keeping domesticated animals or escaping an attacking predator, success required intimate knowledge of an animal's habits. Even today, information about animal behavior is of considerable importance. For example, in Britain, studies on the social organization and the ranging patterns of badgers (Meles meles) have helped reduce the spread of tuberculosis among cattle and studies of sociality in foxes (Vulpes vulpes) assist in the development of models that predict how quickly rabies would spread should it ever cross the English Channel. Likewise in Sweden, where collisions involving moose (Alces alces) are among the most common traffic accidents in rural areas, research on moose behavior has yielded ways of keeping them off roads and verges. In addition, investigations of the foraging of insect pollinators, such as honeybees, have led to impressive increases in agricultural crop yields throughout the world.

Even if there were no practical benefits to be gained from learning about animal behavior, the subject would still merit exploration. Humans (Homo sapiens) are animals themselves and most humans are deeply interested in the lives and minds of their fellow humans, their pets and other creatures. British ethologist Jane Goodall and American field biologist George Schaller, as well as British broadcaster David Attenborough and Australian wildlife conservationist Steve Irwin, have brought the wonders of animal behavior to the attention and appreciation of the general public. Books, television programs and movies on the subject of animal behavior abound.

Causation

Sensory-motor Mechanisms

At this level of analysis, questions concern the physiological machinery underlying an animal's behaviour. Behaviour is explained in terms of the firings of the neural circuits between reception of the stimuli (sensory input) and movements of the muscles (motor output). Consider, for example, a worker honeybee flying back to her hive from a field of flowers several kilometres away. The sensory processes the bee employs, the neural computations she performs and the patterns of muscular activity she uses to make her way home constitute some of the mechanisms underlying the insect's impressive feat of homing. In the course of exploring these mechanisms and those underlying other forms of animal behaviour, physiologists have learned an important lesson regarding the mechanisms underlying behaviour. They are special-purpose adaptations tailored to the particular problems faced by an animal, but they are not all-purpose solutions to general problems faced by all animals. Linked to this lesson is the realization that the physiology of a species will have limitations and biases that reflect individuals' need to deal only with certain behavioral problems and only in specific ecological contexts. In behaviour, as in morphology, an animal's capabilities are matched to its expected environmental requirements, because the process of natural selection shapes organisms as if it were always addressing the question of how much adaptation is enough.

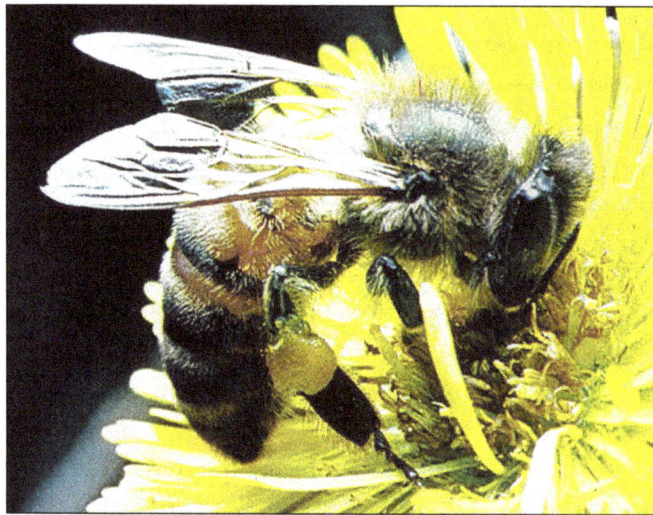

Honeybee (Apis mellifera).

Consider first the sensory abilities of animals. All actions (such as body movements, detection of objects of interest or learning from others in a social group) begin with the acquisition of information. Thus, an animal's sense organs are exceedingly important to its behaviour. They constitute a set of monitoring instruments with which the animal gathers information about itself and its environment. Each sense organ is selective, responding only to one particular form of energy; an instrument that responds indiscriminately to multiple forms of energy would be rather useless and similar to having none at all. The particular form of energy to which a sense organ responds determines its sensory modality. Three broad categories of sensory modalities are familiar to humans: Chemoreception (exemplified by the senses of taste and smell but also including specialized receptors for pheromones and other behaviorally important molecules), mechanoreception (the basis for touch, hearing, balance and many other senses, such as joint position) and photoreception (light sensitivity, including form and colour vision).

The capabilities of an animal's sense organs differ depending on the behavioral and ecological constraints of the species. In recognition of this fact and of the equally important fact that animals perceive their environments differently than do humans, ethologists have adopted the word Umwelt, a German word for environment, to denote an organism's unique sensory world. The umwelt of a male yellow fever mosquito (Aedes aegypti), for example, differs sharply from that of a human. Whereas the human auditory system hears sounds over a wide range of frequencies, from 20 to about 20,000 Hz, the male mosquito's hearing apparatus has been tuned narrowly to hear only sounds around 380 Hz. Despite its apparent limitations, a male mosquito's auditory system serves him perfectly well, for the only sound he must detect is the enchanting wing-tone whine of a female mosquito hovering nearby, a sound all too familiar to anyone who lingers outdoors on a midsummer's evening.

Pit vipers, colubrid snakes from the subfamily Crotalinae, which include the well-known rattle-snakes, provide another example of how the umwelt of a species serves its own ecological needs. Pit vipers possess directionally sensitive infrared detectors with which they can scan their envi-ronment while stalking mammalian prey, such as mice (Mus) and kangaroo rats (Dipodomys), in the dark. A forward-facing sensory pit, located on each side of the snake's head between the eye and the nostril, serves as the animal's heat-sensing organ. Each pit is about 1 to 5 mm (about 0.04 to 0.2 inch) deep. A thin membrane, which is extensively innervated and exquisitely sensitive to temperature increases, stretches from wall to wall inside the pit organ, where it functions like the film in a pinhole camera, registering any nearby source of infrared energy.

Human umwelt is not without its own limits and biases. Human eyes do not see the flashy adver-tisements to insects that flowers produce by reflecting ultraviolet light and human ears do not hear the infrasonic calls of elephants or the ultrasonic sounds of bats. Furthermore, human noses are limited relative to those of many other mammals. Moreover, humans completely lack the sense organs for the detection of electric fields or of Earth's geomagnetic field. Sense organs for the former occur in various species of electric fishes (such as electric eels and electric catfish), which use their sensitivity to electric fields for orientation, communication and prey detection in murky jungle streams, while the latter exist in certain birds and insects, including homing pigeons and honeybees, which use them to navigate back to the home loft or hive. At the same time, unlike most animals, humans are endowed with superb visual acuity and colour vision as a result of having evolved large, high-performance, single-lens eyes.

Each species' nervous system is an assemblage of special-purpose devices with species-specific and sometimes sex-specific capabilities. These capabilities become even more apparent when investi-gating how animals use their sense organs to acquire information for solving behavioral problems, such as territory defense or prey capture. Although an animal may possess diverse sensory organs that enable it to receive a great deal of information about the environment, in performing a partic-ular behavioral task, it often responds to a rather small portion of the stimuli perceived. Moreover, only a subset of available stimuli reliably provides the information needed to perform a particular task. Ethologists call the crucial stimuli in any particular behavioral context "sign stimuli."

A classic example of sign stimuli comes from the behaviour of male three-spined sticklebacks (Gasterosteus aculeatus) when these fish defend their mating territories in the springtime against intrusions from rival male sticklebacks. The males differ from all other objects and forms of life in their environment in a special way. They possess an intensely red throat and belly, which serve as signals to females and other males of their health and vigour. Experiments using models of other fish species have shown that the red colour is the paramount stimulus by which a territory-holding male detects an intruder. Models that accurately imitated sticklebacks but lacked the red markings were seldom attacked, whereas models that possessed a red belly but lacked many of the other characteristics of the sticklebacks or even of fish in general, were vigorously attacked.

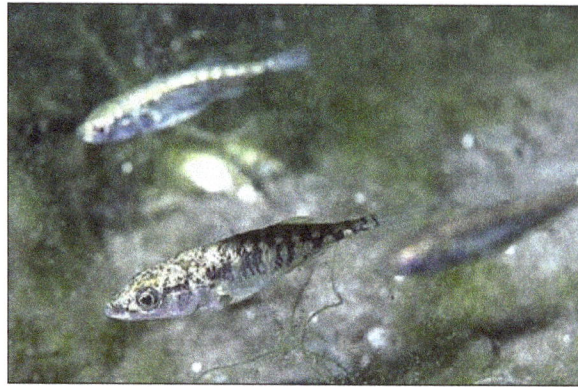
Stickleback: Three-spined stickleback (Gasterosteus aculeatus).

Similarly, the brain cells of some toads (Bufo) are tuned to pick out those features of the environment that reliably match the toads' natural prey items (such as earthworms). Experiments were conducted in which a hungry toad was presented with cardboard models moving horizontally around the individual at a constant distance and angular velocity. The research revealed that just two stimuli, the elongation of the object (that is, making the cardboard model longer to increase resemblance to prey) and movement in the direction of the elongation, were sufficient to initiate the toad's prey-catching behaviour. Subsequently, the toad jerked its head after the moving model in order to place it in its frontal visual field. Other stimuli, such as the colour of the model and its velocity of movement, did not influence the toad's ability to distinguish worms from non-worms, even though toads possess good colour and form vision. Even the broadly tuned human sensory system operates in a highly selective, yet adaptive, manner. For instance, a person hunting white-tailed deer seeks the prey almost exclusively by watching closely for deer-like movements amid the stationary trees of a forest, not by straining to sense the deer's shape, smell or sound.

As with sensory systems, the neural mechanisms by which animals compute solutions to behavioral problems have not evolved to function as general-purpose computers. Rather, the central nervous system (that is, the brain and spinal cord of a vertebrate or one of the segmental ganglia of an invertebrate) performs specific computations associated with the particular ecological challenges that individuals face in their environment. A helpful illustration of this point is the startle response of goldfish (Carassius auratus). If a hungry predatory fish strikes from the side, the goldfish executes a brisk swivelling movement that propels its body sideways by about one body length to dodge the predator's attack. How does the goldfish's central nervous system process information from the sense organs to instantaneously decide the correct direction (right or left) to move? The key neural element in the startle response of the goldfish is a single bilateral pair of neurons, called the Mauthner neurons, located in the goldfish's hindbrain. Each neuron on the left or right receives input from the lateral line system (a row of small pressure sensors that are triggered by the disturbances caused by nearby moving objects) located on the left or right side of the goldfish's body. Each neuron sends output to neurons that activate the musculature on the opposite side of the body. There is strong, mutual inhibition between the left and right Mauthner neurons; should the left one fire in response to a mechanical stimulus from the left side of the body, for example, the right one is inactivated. Inactivation prevents it from interfering with the crucial, initial contractions of the trunk muscles on the goldfish's right side. The net effect is that 20 milliseconds after sensing danger the goldfish assumes a C-like shape with the head and tail bent to the same side and away from the attacker. This reaction is followed 20 milliseconds later by muscle contractions on the other side of the body so that the tail straightens and the fish propels itself sideways, away from the danger. Thus, the two Mauthner neurons of the goldfish's nervous system function exquisitely for processing information regarding predator attacks and solving this crucial behavioral problem appears to be the only task that they perform.

Small-brained creatures, such as fishes, are not the only species whose nervous systems have evolved to solve tasks in a limited—but ecologically sufficient—way that turns difficult problems of computation into more tractable ones. For example, take the task of a human computing an interception course with a flying object, such as when a baseball player runs to catch a fly ball. In principle, the task could be solved with a set of differential equations based on the observed curvature and acceleration of the ball. What happens instead, evidently, is that the fielder finds a running path that maintains a linear optical trajectory for the ball. In other words, the player adjusts the speed and direction of his movement over the baseball field so that the trajectory of the ball appears to be straight. Unlike the more complicated differential equation approach, the linear trajectory approach does not tell the player when or where the ball will land. Consequently, the player cannot run to the point where the ball will fall and wait for it. If he did, complicating factors such as wind gusts diverting the ball might mean that he would end up in the wrong place. Instead, the player simply keeps his body on a course that will ensure interception.

Once an animal has received information about the world from its sense organs and has computed a solution to whatever behavioral problem it currently faces, it responds with a coordinated set of movements—that is, behaviour. Any particular movement reflects the patterned activity of a specific set of muscles that work on the skeletal structures to which they are attached. The activity of these muscles is controlled by a specific set of motor neurons that in turn are controlled by sets of interneurons connected to the animal's brain. Thus, a given behaviour is ultimately the result of a specific pattern of neural activity.

Sometimes neural control takes the form of a simple sensory reflex, in which the activity in the motor neurons is triggered by sensory neurons. This activity can be achieved directly or via one or two interneurons. Other times, as in the case of rhythmic behaviour (such as with birds flying or insects walking), a central pattern generator located in the central nervous system produces rhythms of activity in the motor neurons. Central pattern generators do not depend on sensory feedback. Feedback, however, commonly occurs to modulate and reset the rhythm of the motor output after a disturbance to the animal's behaviour, as in the case of air turbulence disrupting the wing movements of a flying bird.

Most commonly, the neural control of behaviour takes the form of a motor command in which the initiation and modulation of activity in the motor neurons is produced by interneurons descending from the animal's brain. The animal's brain is where inputs from multiple sensory modalities are integrated. In this way, a sophisticated tuning of the animal's behaviour in relation to its internal condition and its external circumstances can occur. Often the control of an animal's movements involves an intricate synthesis of all three forms of neural control: Patterned neural activity, simple sensory reflex and motor command. As in all aspects of behavioral physiology, an immense diversity exists among animal species and behaviour patterns in the way the components of behavioral machinery have been linked over time by natural selection.

Cognitive Mechanisms

Cognitive psychology proposes yet another way to study the causal mechanisms of animal behaviour. The aim of cognitive psychology is to explain an animal's behaviour in terms of its mental organization for information processing (that is, how the animal acquires, stores and acts on information present in its world). By studying cognitive mechanisms of an animal, one may study how the animal perceives, learns, memorizes and makes decisions.

Consider, for example, crows (Corvus brachyrhynchos) that crack walnuts open by dropping them from heights of 5 to 10 metres (about 16 to 33 feet) or more onto rocks, roads or sidewalks. The birds generally avoid dropping the nuts onto soil, where they would be unlikely to break open. Remarkably, the crows can discriminate between black and English walnuts, for they drop the harder black walnuts from greater heights. In addition, when a crow drops a nut, it takes into account the likelihood that a fellow crow might steal the contents before it can be retrieved. If fewer competing crows are perched nearby, the crow carries a nut higher into the air before releasing it. Thus, numerous processes of perception, learning and decision-making activity underlie the crows' nut-cracking behaviour.

Each of these processes may be analyzed. For example, how do crows judge the height from which to drop nuts? Do they have to learn to adjust the dropping height in relation to the type of walnut? When faced with the conflicting conditions of having a hard-shelled black walnut and seeing a number of other crows nearby, how do they decide what drop height to use?

It is possible, however, that the computational-representational approach exaggerates the richness and detail of animals' representations and the complexity of the brain processes operating on them. A good illustration comes from studies of the mechanisms by which ants (Cataglyphis fortis) living in the Sahara desert navigate home after conducting a circuitous search for food (mainly dead insects). Such a search can take these ants 100 metres (about 330 feet) or more (equivalent to 10,000 body lengths) from the entrance of their underground nest. To get back home, the ants rely on landmarks as visual signposts to show the way. Originally, it was assumed that these ants and other insects that orient using landmarks are able to store their knowledge of the nest environs in maplike internal representations called "cognitive maps." Doing so would give an ant tremendous flexibility in homing, equipped with a bird's-eye knowledge of the terrain over which it travels, an ant could return even from points where it had never before been. The mental representation used by these ants in landmark guidance is, however, actually somewhat simpler. Experiments have revealed that each ant stores a two-dimensional visual template—a kind of snapshot—of the landmark array it saw when it left its nest. When returning to its nest, the ant moves so as to match the current visual image as closely as possible with the memorized template. The snapshot-matching mechanism, unlike the cognitive-map one, enables an ant to steer its way home only from points it has recently visited, as opposed to novel sites to which it might be displaced by an experimenter. Although this mental mechanism provides a less complete and less flexible solution to the problem of finding home, it is entirely sufficient for the problems that desert ants routinely face.

An unseen and therefore largely unappreciated aspect of behaviour is the use of decision-making rules or "Darwinian algorithms." Organisms rely on these rules to process information from their physical and social environments and result in particular behavioral outputs that guide key behavioral and life-history decisions. Darwinian algorithms are made up of the sensory and cognitive processes that perceive and prioritize cues within an individual's perceptual range. These inputs are then translated into motor outputs. A Darwinian algorithm may involve a stimulus threshold (such as "when the day-length exceeds 10 hours, migrate north") or may depend on the occurrence of a cue that is normally associated with a fitness-enhancing outcome (such as "build nests in dense vegetation where chick survival is predictably high"). Darwinian algorithms are shaped through evolutionary time by the specific selective regime of each population. Which cues are relied upon depends on the certainty with which a cue can be recognized, the reliability of the relationship between the cue and the anticipated environmental outcome and the fitness benefits of making a correct decision versus the costs of making an incorrect decision. In general, Darwinian algorithms underlying behavioral and life-history decisions are only as complex as is necessary to yield adaptive outcomes under a species' normal environmental circumstances but not so complex as to cover all experimentally or anthropogenically induced contingencies.

An intriguing question in the study of animal cognition is the role of consciousness. Humans easily distinguish between merely responding to objects and being conscious of them. For example, while driving along a highway deep in thought or conversation, the driver may suddenly realize that he has not been conscious of the road for the past several miles. Indeed, it is well documented that humans can effectively perceive, memorize, process and even act on objects and events without the kind of awareness that underlies a verbal report of consciousness. It is possible, therefore, that the behaviour of animals occurs without conscious awareness. However, given that humans have consciousness, it seems reasonable to suppose that individuals in other species, especially social species (such as primates), also experience at least a rudimentary form of consciousness. To think otherwise would be to presume an evolutionary discontinuity between humans and all other forms of life. Thus, the possibility that at least some of the behaviour of animals is accompanied by conscious thinking seems reasonable.

Although most students of animal behaviour accept the idea that animal consciousness is a likely possibility, some argue that it is not yet possible to know whether any particular animal experiences consciousness because it is a private, subjective and, ultimately, unknowable state. In contrast, cognitive ethologists (a separate group of animal behaviourists), most notably American biophysicist and animal behaviourist Donald Griffin, argue that animals are undoubtedly conscious, since individuals from a wide variety of species behave with apparent intentions of achieving certain goals. For example, chimpanzees (Pan troglodytes) stalking a monkey high above them in the treetops will distribute themselves among the trees that would otherwise provide the monkey with an escape route and attack the creature simultaneously. Similarly, groups of female lions (Panthera leo) fan out widely and then coordinate their attacks on ungulate prey. In another example, a raven (Corvus corax), when presented with the novel situation of a meat morsel dangling from a long string tied to a perch, will study the situation briefly before it acts. Subsequently, the raven will quickly procure the meat by repeatedly pulling up a length of the string with its beak and clamping each length pulled up with its feet while sitting on the perch.

Ontogeny

Just as a thorough understanding of an animal's morphology requires knowledge of how it develops before it hatches from an egg or emerges from its mother's womb, a complete understanding of an animal's behaviour requires knowledge of the animal's development during its lifetime. To gain this knowledge, one asks how the individual's genes and its experiences cause it to behave as it does. The ontogeny of behaviour is a subject which arouses considerable interest, perhaps because of the seeming contrast between humans and other animals in how behavioral skills are acquired. Whereas humans extensively adjust their behaviour based on experience (that is, through the process of learning), the behaviour of many animal species seems to be automatic, as if it were pre-programmed. And yet, if there really were a difference between humans and other animals in how behaviour develops, it would certainly be one of degree, not of kind.

Behavioral development is a field of study in which there have been intense clashes of opinion. Prior to the 1960s there existed a profound disagreement between European (particularly German) ethologists and American psychologists regarding methods and interpretations of such studies. The ethologists described many examples of animals showing complex behaviour patterns in response to particular stimuli under circumstances that seemed to preclude the opportunity for learning. Indeed, learning (based on external influences) was contrasted with genetic control of behaviour (based on internal influences). Austrian zoologist Konrad Lorenz, who won a Nobel Prize for his ethological studies, went so far as to classify behaviour patterns into two distinct categories: Acquired and innate.

Regarding the latter, adult herring gulls (Larus argentatus) have a red spot on the lower tip of their bill. When these birds have food for their chicks, the adults point their bill downward while waving it slowly back and forth in front of the young. Newly hatched chicks will accurately peck at the red spot on the parent bird's bill, suggesting that a herring gull chick possesses innate (that is, genetically based) knowledge of where to peck for food. Ethologists termed pecking behaviour a "fixed action pattern" to indicate that it was performed automatically and correctly the first time it was elicited, apparently regardless of the animal's experience.

The psychologists, in contrast, assumed that experiences with the environment (that is, learning processes) were the main or even exclusive, determinants of ontogeny. Accordingly, they saw nothing in the pecking behaviour of herring gull chicks that could not be explained by learning while still in the egg, conditioning or by trial-and-error learning. For example, chicks might "learn" to peck before hatching as a result of the rhythmic beating of their heart or they might have a pecking reflex and simply learn to associate a food reward with pecking at the parent's bill. Moreover, a chick's pecking accuracy improves with age and after about two days it requires, in addition to the red spot, the complete configuration of an adult's head and bill to elicit pecking.

What the acquired-innate dichotomy obscured is that learning is possible only after the animal has already been steered by its genes to develop its behaviour in a certain way. An animal may well learn, but which experiences are important to the development of its behaviour depend on those that have promoted the genetic success of its ancestors. Reciprocally, whatever experiences an individual already has had can influence how its genes are activated and thus can affect their subsequent role in shaping its behaviour. Modern animal behaviourists see the stark dichotomy of acquired versus innate as far too simplistic; no behaviour is either strictly innate or entirely learned. Rather, all behaviours are the result of a complex interaction between genes and the environment.

Behavioral Genetics

The evidence is now compelling that genes influence behaviour in all animals, including humans. Indeed, an increasing share of biomedical research is devoted to the hunt for genes involved in human behavioral maladies such as alcoholism, obesity, schizophrenia and Alzheimer disease. Often these studies are pursued using animal models with subjects that include mice, rats and dogs with behavioral symptoms resembling those of humans. The principal point of confusion arises from equating genetic influence on behaviour with genetic determination of behaviour. To do so is to mistakenly believe that identifying genes "for" a behaviour implies that the gene controls, fully and inevitably, this behaviour. In actuality, to say that there are genes "for" a particular behaviour means only that within a population of individuals there exists genetic variation underlying some of the differences in this specific behaviour. To cite an example involving a morphological trait, the statement that there are genes for coat colour in guinea pigs (Cavia porcellus) or horses (Equus caballus) means that genetic variation in the guinea pig or horse population is responsible for some of the variation in coat colour.

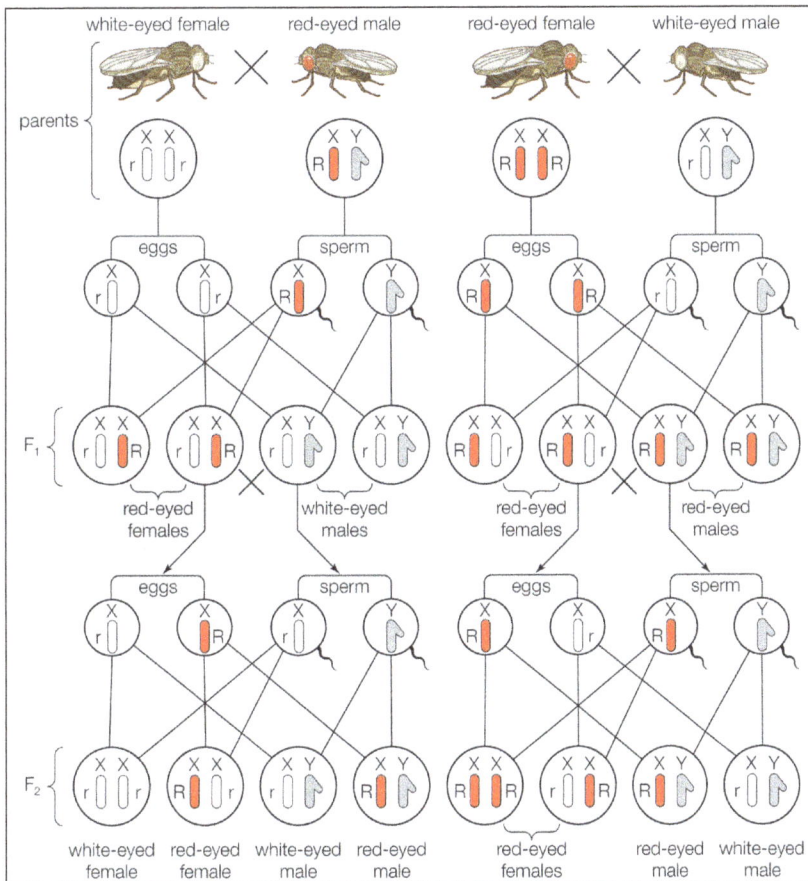

Sex-linked inheritance of white eyes in Drosophila flies.

Furthermore, identifying a gene that influences a behaviour does not imply that the behaviour is inevitable; there is considerable variation among behaviours in the relative importance of the individual's genetic constitution and its environment to the expression of the behaviour. Occasionally, the possession of a particular form of a gene does consistently result in the individual having a particular form of a behaviour; more frequently, however, the form of the behaviour is due to a complex interaction between genes and environment.

The strength of the influence of genes on a particular behaviour is quantified by a genetic measure called "heritability." Heritability is defined as the fraction of the total variation in a trait among individuals in a population that is attributable to the genetic variation among those individuals. The remaining source of the variation is, of course, the environment. Values of heritability range between zero and one. The smaller the environmental variation experienced by the individuals in a population, the greater will be the fraction of the total variation in the behaviour that is the result of genetic variation.

One way to measure the heritability of a behavioral trait is to determine the average values of the behaviour for the parents and offspring in a sample of families within a population and calculate the linear relationship between offspring values and parental values. The slope of this line reveals the heritability of the behavioral trait in that population. For example, the heritability of the calling behaviour that male crickets (Gryllus integer) use to attract females has been measured. In any one population, some males chirp away for many hours each night, others call for just a few hours and still others almost never call. The heritability of calling duration for one Canadian population that was studied was 0.53. The value indicates that slightly more than half of the variation in calling duration arose because males differed genetically and slightly less than half arose from environmental differences. (For example, the more parasites a cricket had acquired, the less food he had obtained and thus the less he might be able to call on a given night).

The degree of genetic influence on a particular behaviour is not a fixed characteristic. Rather, heritability can vary greatly depending on how much environmental variation is experienced by individuals in the specific population being studied. Thus, regarding the calling behaviour of male crickets, if every male fed well, thereby eliminating several environmental influences on calling, the numerical value of heritability would be considerably higher.

Numerous studies involving diverse species, including humans, have detected some level of heritability for every trait that has ever been examined. For example, the mean value of heritability for morphological traits, such as body and wing length, is 0.46; for life history traits, such as fecundity and life span, is 0.26; and for behavioral traits, such as calling duration and fighting stamina, is 0.30. Thus, the genetic influence on the characteristics of individual animals falls generally between 30 and 50 percent for most traits.

Instinctive Learning

An animal adjusts its behaviour based on experience—that is, it learns—when experience at one time provides information that will be useful at a later time. Viewed in this light, learning is seen as a tool for survival and reproduction because it helps an animal to adjust its behaviour to the particular state of its environment. An animal needs to know such things as what food is good to eat, when and where to find it, whom to avoid and approach, with whom to mate and how to find its way home. When these things are not genetically preprogrammed—because they depend on the particular circumstances of an individual's time and place—the animal must learn them.

Consider, for example, a female digger wasp called the bee wolf (Philanthus triangulum) who has finished excavating a tunnel in a sandy bank. She then digs a small outpocket where one of her young will develop and she stocks this cell with worker honeybees (Apis mellifera), which she has paralyzed by stinging and which will serve to provision her young. After laying an egg on one of the bees, she closes off the cell with sand and starts work on a new cell. To provision the cell, she must fly out to hunt more honeybees; however, after crawling out of her nest burrow, closing its entrance hole and launching into flight, she does not immediately depart the area. Instead, she hovers just over her nest site, inspecting the ground and flying in wider and wider arcs to scan an ever-increasing area. During this elaborate departure flight, the wasp memorizes the specific configuration of landmarks—sticks, tufts of grass and trees— around her burrow. Later, when she returns, she will use the information to pinpoint her nest's location. Her genes cannot provide her with knowledge of the landmark array around her nest, so she must learn it.

One of the clearest indications of the falseness of the old dichotomy between innate and learned behaviour is the fact that in most cases animals are genetically predisposed to acquire only specific information in developing their behaviour. One might say that most of the learning performed by animals is instinctive learning. This phenomenon is conspicuous in the flower-learning behaviour of honeybees (A. mellifera). Since at least the time of the Greek philosopher and scientist Aristotle, it has been known that worker bees show "flower constancy," a specialization by individual bees on a single species of flower. Flower constancy occurs in spite of the fact that honeybees are generalist foragers capable of exploiting many flower species. The flowers have much to gain from bees that remain faithful to them; specialist bees will be carrying the appropriate species of pollen. Therefore, the colours and odours of flowers probably evolved as conspicuous signals for the bees to learn. In turn, specialization benefits the bees by reducing flower-handling time and facilitating the collection of nectar.

Early in the 20th century, Austrian biologist Karl von Frisch demonstrated experimentally that honeybees are able to learn and distinguish a single floral odour from among at least 700 others. In addition, he found that they could distinguish colour from yellow into the ultraviolet across the electromagnetic spectrum. One striking feature of this type of colour and odour learning is the rigid programming of the timing. Research has revealed that a bee learns the flower's colour only during the final few seconds before beginning to feed and odour learning occurs during feeding. It is as if bees possess a set of switches that turn colour and odour learning on and off at specific times during the foraging process. The time course of this learning program is highly adaptive, being restricted to times when a bee is alighted on a rewarding flower. In this manner, its learning is focused on the colour and odour of the flowers of this rewarding species rather than on the hues and scents of any nearby flowers of unrewarding species.

Is this machinelike learning of bees fundamentally different from the learning processes in vertebrates? Until the mid-1960s, psychologists generally believed so. Studying mainly birds and mammals, they developed an approach known as "general process learning theory," which attempted to account for learning with a single set of principles, namely unconstrained "associative learning" as studied in instrumental (operant) conditioning and classical (Pavlovian) conditioning. Associative learning is said to occur when an animal changes its behaviour upon forming an association between an environmental event and its own response to the event. In operant conditioning, the animal learns to associate a voluntary activity with specific consequences. In classical conditioning, the animal learns to associate a novel (conditioned) stimulus with a familiar (unconditioned) one. For example, in his study of classical conditioning, Russian physiologist Ivan Petrovich Pavlov demonstrated that by consistently exposing a dog to a particular sound (novel stimulus) and simultaneously placing meat powder (familiar stimulus) in its mouth the dog could be made to salivate upon hearing the sound even without the meat stimulus. Initially, salivation was the unconditioned response, whereas the food stimulus was the unconditioned stimulus. Once the dog learned to associate the sound stimulus with the food stimulus, salivation became the conditioned stimulus to sound—that is, a stimulus that previously did not trigger a response.

The popularity of general process learning theory peaked in the 1940s and '50s. In the mid-1960s, however, American psychologist John Garcia discovered several puzzling phenomena that indicated adaptive limits on learning and contradicted the supposedly general principles of conditioning. One of the most important of these anomalies was flavour aversion learning. When rats (Rattus norvegicus) and many other vertebrates, including humans, sample a flavour and later become ill, they learn to avoid consuming that flavour in the future. This phenomenon has two remarkable properties. First, it occurs despite delays of several hours between experiencing the flavour (the conditioned stimulus or CS, in the Pavlovian conditioning paradigm) and experiencing the illness (the unconditioned stimulus or US); it does not require the brief delay specified by the general principles of conditioning. Second, in rats, learning with the US being illness is limited to flavours. This response was revealed in an experiment in which rats experienced a flash of light and the sound of a buzzer each time they took a drink from a tube of flavoured water (hence "bright noisy tasty water" became the CS). Some of the rats were made ill (nauseous) after drinking (hence illness became the US for them), whereas others were shocked through the feet shortly after they began drinking (hence pain became the US for them). After conditioning, the rats were tested with the noise plus the light alone or with the flavour alone. Those rats that had been made ill avoided drinking only the "tasty water," whereas the rats that had been shocked avoided drinking only the "bright noisy water." In other words, the rats could learn to associate a taste with an illness but not a visual and auditory stimulus. Conversely, the rats could learn to associate a visual and auditory stimulus, but not a taste, with pain.

These findings attracted tremendous skepticism when they were first reported because both the long delay between CS and US and the CS-US specificity contradicted the idea of general laws of learning. Both findings, however, make considerable sense in light of the problems faced by rats living in nature. If they consume a new food and become ill even hours later, they will not eat the food again and thus not suffer the illness associated with the food. Moreover, it is adaptive that rats learn to associate a taste cue, not an auditory or visual cue, with illness-causing food because rats discriminate foods best using chemical cues sensed by taste, olfaction or both. In contrast, something that causes pain is best recognized from a safe distance. Therefore, it is adaptive that rats learn to associate auditory and visual cues with painful experiences. Thus, these "anomalies" for general process learning theory can be understood by considering the functions that the rats' learning has evolved to serve.

There is now compelling evidence that human also possesses adaptive predispositions in learning abilities. Consider, for example, the curious anthropological discovery made in 1926 by Finnish sociologist Edward Westermarck that arranged marriages between children that grow up together (whether biological siblings or not) are far more likely to fail than arranged marriages between individuals not rose together. The failures most often result from sexual incompatibilities. Evidently, children are genetically guided to learn to treat as siblings all individuals with whom they are raised together. And because siblings tend to avoid sexual contact, presumably due to a long evolutionary history of detrimental consequences associated with inbreeding, marriages between these individuals tend to fail.

Today it is widely recognized that the general-purpose psychological approach to learning had overlooked its biological significance and that animals possess learning mechanisms that are specialized for solving the problems they face in the natural world. This view of learning explains the psychologists' observations of the limits of learning by animals in laboratory settings. It also makes sense of ethological reports of special forms of learning, such as imprinting (that is, the rapid identification of parents by newborn animals triggered by following the first object they see moving away from them), which have been studied in naturalistic settings. To a large extent, this picture of instinctive learning has brought a constructive end to the centuries-old debate about whether "nature" (genes) or "nurture" (experiences) is the source of adaptive behaviour of animals. Animals are shaped by their experiences; however, the interpretation of each experience is governed by a collection of rules (Darwinian algorithms) set by the genes in each species.

The general-purpose view of learning that prevailed during most of the 20th century was based on two assumptions: (1) the ability to learn is always beneficial and (2) animal learning abilities are like human learning abilities, which seem to be of completely general and unlimited applicability. Neither assumption is correct.

First, there are costs as well as benefits to learning, so learning abilities will be beneficial and favoured by natural selection, only when the benefits outweigh the costs. The costs include those involved in building and maintaining the required neural circuitry and also the time and mistakes involved in learning while the animal is fine-tuning its behaviour to the current or likely future state of its environment. When learning is a matter of life or death—as in geese (Anser and Branta), sheep (Ovis) and antelopes (family Antilopinae), where newborn young must keep up with mobile parents—the advantage of rapid learning (that is, staying together) and the danger of slow learning (that is, lagging behind) are both extremely high. By considering both the fitness costs and the benefits of different forms of learning, one can readily appreciate the reasons why imprinting occurs in these species, rather than the slower process of trial-and-error learning.

Second, the learning abilities of animals, including humans, are not completely general; learning abilities are adaptively specialized so that, in any particular context, animals take in only the most relevant information.

Function

In studying the function of a behavioral characteristic of an animal, a researcher seeks to understand how natural selection favours the behaviour. In other words, the researcher tries to identify the ecological challenges or "selection pressures," faced by a species and then investigates how a particular behavioral trait helps individuals surmount these obstacles so that they can survive and reproduce.

Until the mid-1960s, functional interpretations of animal behaviour were usually made in terms of how a behaviour was "good for the species." Social behaviours that excluded some individuals from reproducing (such as territorial defense and courtship displays) were seen as adaptations for regulating animal populations at levels that would prevent overpopulation, environmental destruction and extinction of the species. This view was based on the observation of ecological phenomena—such as the overgrazing of grassland by cattle, leading to the starvation of the animals. American evolutionary biologist George C. Williams and British ornithologist David Lack, however, revealed the underlying theoretical problem with the view that animals behave in ways that limit their reproduction for the good of their species. Williams noted that individuals who maximize their own reproduction will have greater genetic success than those who behave in ways that limit their reproduction. Thus, over time, in subsequent generations, reproduction-reducing behaviours will be replaced by reproduction-enhancing ones. Therefore, it has become evident that it is incorrect to interpret the behaviour of animals as having evolved to function "for the good of the species." Instead, the appropriate interpretation is how a behaviour has evolved for the "good of the individual."

Williams's theoretical argument was bolstered by Lack's long-term study of the reproductive behaviour of the European or common, swift (Apus apus). At first glance, swifts appear to voluntarily restrict their own reproduction. When Lack removed the eggs laid each day from a pair's nest he discovered that the female could lay up to 72 or more eggs in a season. Yet, surprisingly, she usually lays just two or three eggs. Are chimney swifts regulating their egg production to avoid overpopulation or does the number of eggs laid equal the number of young they can successfully rear each year? Lack answered this question by performing the experiment of adding one or two nestlings to the nests of certain pairs so that, instead of the normal two or three young, they would have to rear four or five. He then compared the reproductive success of these pairs to those that were left rearing the normal number. Lack found that the birds with four or five young were less successful (that is, rearing fewer young to fledging) than those in a control group who reared a normal-sized brood. Therefore, chimney swifts, in rearing just two or three offspring, are not withholding reproduction for the good of their species or local population; instead, they are producing as many young as they can successfully rear given a limited food supply, thereby maximizing their own reproduction.

Chimney swifts provide just one example of a pattern that has been found repeatedly by biologists studying the behaviour and reproduction of animals. They have found that individuals are "selfish," behaving in ways that benefit their own reproduction regardless of its long-term effect on the survival of their species. Sometimes, however, animals engage in apparent altruism (that is, they exhibit behaviour that increases the fitness of other individuals by engaging in activities that decrease their own reproductive success). For example, American zoologist Paul Sherman found that female Belding's ground squirrels (Spermophilus beldingi) give staccato whistles that warn nearby conspecifics of a predator's approach but also attract the predator's attention to the caller. Likewise, worker honeybees (Apis mellifera) perform suicidal attacks on intruders to defend their colony and female lions (Panthera leo) sometimes nurse cubs that are not their own (although some authorities note that such cubs suckle the lioness when she is asleep).

The key insight to understanding the evolution of such self-sacrificial behaviour was provided by British evolutionary biologist William D. Hamilton in the mid-1960s. He argued that natural selection favours genetic success, not reproductive success per se and that individuals can pass copies of their genes on to future generations. Genes are passed from direct parentage (the rearing of offspring and grand-offspring) and by assisting the reproduction of close relatives (such as nieces and nephews), a concept referred to as "inclusive fitness" or "kin selection."

Hamilton devised a formula—now called Hamilton's rule—that specifies the conditions under which reproductive altruism evolves:

$$r \times B > C$$

where B is the benefit (in number of offspring equivalents) gained by the recipient of the altruism, C is the cost (in number of offspring equivalents) suffered by the donor while undertaking the altruistic behaviour and r is the genetic relatedness of the altruist to the beneficiary. Relatedness is the probability that a gene in the potential altruist is shared by the potential recipient of the altruistic behaviour. Altruism can evolve in a population if a potential donor of assistance can more than make up for losing C offspring by adding to the population B offspring bearing a fraction r of its genes. For example, a female lion with a well-nourished cub gains inclusive fitness by nursing a starving cub of a full sister because the benefit to her sister (B = one offspring that would otherwise die) more than compensates for the loss to herself (C = approximately one quarter of an offspring), since the survival probability of her own, non-starving cub is only slightly reduced. Given that the average genetic relatedness (that is, r) between two full sisters is 0.5, then according to Hamilton's rule (0.5 × 1) > 0.25. In essence, genes for altruism spread by promoting aid to copies of themselves.

According to this view, which was popularized by British zoologist Richard Dawkins, the most appropriate way of viewing natural selection is from a gene-selection perspective, as embodied in Hamilton's rule. Genes those are best able to guide the organisms that bear them to propagate successfully will persist and proliferate over generations. Consequently, an explanation of the function of a particular behaviour should include how the behaviour promotes the success of the genes that underlie the behaviour. Of course, since an animal's behaviour almost always promotes genetic success by helping the animal survive and reproduce its genes, investigations of behavioral function typically address the survival and reproductive value of the behaviour.

Natural Selection in Action

The most straightforward way to study the function of a behaviour is to see how natural selection operates on it under current conditions by studying differential reproduction. Often this kind of investigation can be conducted by exploiting the naturally occurring variation among individuals, such as in a particular phenotypic (observable) trait in a population. Sometimes, however, the researcher must experimentally enhance behavioral variation where too little exists in nature. The experimental approach may have the disadvantage of involving unnatural variants, but it has the advantage of revealing how differences among individuals, even in a single trait, can cause variation in reproductive fitness. Either way, a study of natural selection acting on behaviour requires that the researcher be able to observe natural populations and obtain detailed information on each individual's survival, its ability to attract a mate, its fertility and so forth. All of this information is essential to assess an animal's success in passing on its genes.

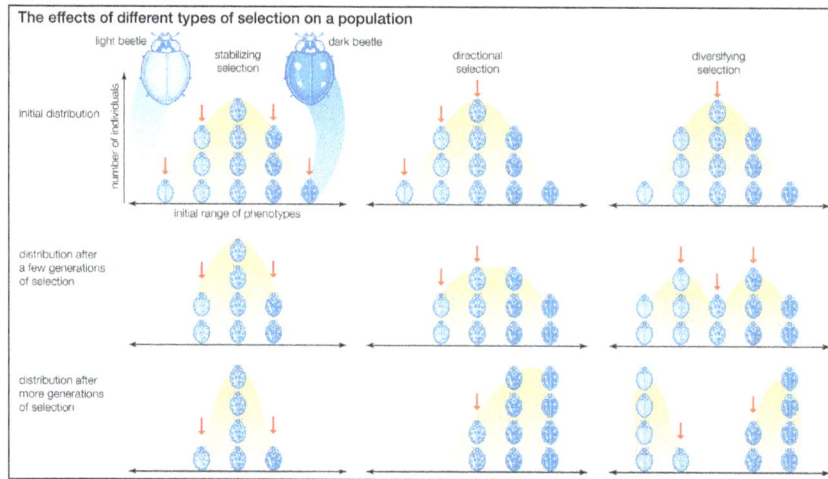

The effects of different types of selection on a population

Three types of natural selection, showing the effects of each on the distribution of phenotypes within a population. The downward arrows point to those phenotypes against which selection acts. Stabilizing selection (left column) acts against phenotypes at both extremes of the distribution, favouring the multiplication of intermediate phenotypes. Directional selection (centre column) acts against only one extreme of phenotypes, causing a shift in distribution toward the other extreme. Diversifying selection (right column) acts against intermediate phenotypes, creating a split in distribution toward each extreme.

An investigation of why male titmice or great tits (Parus major), woodland birds of Europe, sing multiple songs serves to illustrate how a behavioral function can be studied by exploiting naturally existing variation. Each great tit male has a repertoire of one to eight songs that he uses to advertise his presence on a territory. Investigators can acquire detailed information on the breeding biology of these birds because great tits are cavity nesters that readily accept man-made nest boxes. In one experiment on a wooded estate near Oxford, Eng., English zoologist John Krebs and his colleagues installed and regularly inspected nest boxes during the breeding season. The researchers recorded the singing behaviour of each breeding male in order to determine repertoire size. They also recorded the egg-laying date, the clutch size (number of eggs), the brood size (number of young) and the fledgling weight for the nests of numerous males. It was possible to monitor the survival of each male's young to the time of its own breeding, because all the young were banded before they fledged and most fledglings returned to the same woods to breed themselves.

The researchers found that individual tits had different repertoire sizes. Males with larger repertoires had chicks that were heavier at fledging and more of these chicks survived to breed than offspring of males with smaller repertoires. Thus male repertoire size and reproductive success were correlated. The underlying mechanism is that males with larger song repertoires were able to acquire superior territories—specifically, ones with better food. Previous studies had shown that size and survival of young tits depend on body weight at time of fledging: The bigger and heavier the fledgling, the greater its chances of survival to maturity. Thus, the function of a great tit male's singing multiple songs is to help him secure a top-quality breeding territory and mate. So why do all males not sing multiple songs? Perhaps songs are learned over time, so that only the oldest males can possess a large repertoire. Alternatively, perhaps there are costs (such as time away from foraging or increased vulnerability to predators) to singing multiple songs and only the biggest, strongest males can sing many songs and still survive.

Direct comparisons of individuals of the same species exhibiting natural variation in behaviour is a revealing way to study behavioral function. However, when appropriate natural variations do not exist, experimental manipulations can provide the needed variation in the behaviour. The variant forms are then studied in the field to determine how well extreme forms of the behaviour do in the face of natural selection. Using this method, American biologist Thomas Seeley investigated nest site choice in a species of Southeast Asian honeybee, Apis florea. Colonies build their nests of beeswax combs amid dense foliage, suspended from the branches of bushes and understory trees. Moreover, if a colony's nest loses its cover during the dry season when many trees shed their leaves, the colony will build its new nest in another leafy site. What is the function of this behaviour of nesting in dense vegetation? Is it to prevent the nest from overheating under the strong tropical sun or to conceal the nest from predators or both?

To test the antipredator hypothesis, pairs of naturally occurring colonies were identified. Within each pair the vegetation around the nest of one colony, which served as the experimental unit, was removed, leaving only enough to provide shade but rendering it conspicuous to predators. The vegetation surrounding the nest of the second colony, which served as the control, was not removed. Measurements of nest site temperatures one day later revealed no significant differences between the two nests. Within one week, however, four of the seven experimental colonies had been discovered and destroyed by predators (probably monkeys and tree shrews) whereas none of the control nests had suffered any damage. Thus, it appears that A. florea colonies choose dense vegetation as nesting sites primarily to conceal their nests from predators.

Another example of a well-controlled field experiment on the function of behaviour is Dutch-born British zoologist and ethologist Nikolaas Tinbergen's pioneering study of eggshell removal by black-headed gulls (Larus ridibundus). In a matter of hours after their eggs hatch, they pick up the empty eggshells, fly off and drop them well away from the nest. Why should a gull engage in this behaviour? One hypothesis was that the sharp edges of the shells might injure the chicks, a danger that is well known to poultry breeders. Another hypothesis was that the white insides of broken shells might attract predators, such as crows and herring gulls flying overhead and so endanger the brood. To test the latter hypothesis, Tinbergen and his colleagues distributed single gull decoy eggs around the dunes where the black-headed gulls nest and placed broken eggshells near some of the decoy eggs while leaving others isolated. The investigators found that the eggs near broken shells were preyed upon sooner than the isolated, less conspicuous eggs. Evidently, the removal of broken eggshells from the nest by gulls helps to maintain the camouflage of the brood, thereby reducing predation.

Many features of animal behaviour are so well suited to their function that it is impossible to imagine that they arose by chance. Echolocation by bats, the nest-building skills of weaver birds (family Ploceidae) and the alarm signals of ground squirrels all serve obvious purposes and the mechanisms that enable them are remarkably similar to what engineers would design to achieve those ends. However, such adaptive behaviours have no divine designer but instead have arisen through the process of natural selection.

Natural selection is an inherently optimizing process: It favours those versions of an organism's traits, including behavioral ones, which best enable the organism to propagate copies of its genes into future generations over alternative versions with lower fitness. Creating a formal optimality model is one way to infer the adaptive "design" or function of a behaviour. Using an engineering or economic model to work out the optimal behavioral solution for a given ecological problem is a way of specifying the best design out of a wide range of alternative possibilities. Therefore, if an optimality model embodies an accurate understanding of the function of a behaviour, it can predict the form of the behaviour that is observed in nature.

One of the attractions of using optimality models to test hypotheses about functional design is that these models yield quantitative predictions that can be easily tested. If a model's predictions regarding the form of a behaviour do not match reality, one knows immediately that the hypothesis expressed in the model is false. For example, foraging honeybees often return to the hive with less than a full load of nectar and biologists initially assumed this was because a bee maximizes its rate of energy delivery to the hive. The fuller the bee, however, the slower she can fly. As a result, the transportation of a full load was assumed to depress a bee's rate of nectar collection. On the other hand, when the bees were trained to forage from an array of artificial flowers in which each flower offered a fixed amount of nectar and the time spent flying between flowers was varied to alter the duration and cost of foraging, the size of the bee's load did not maximize her net rate of energy delivery to the hive. Further analysis revealed that a bee's decision of when she would return to the hive is based on the maximization of foraging efficiency. Evidently, bees behave so as to achieve the highest foraging efficiency rather than the highest food-delivery rate to the hive.

A classic example of application of the optimality approach to understanding the adaptive design of a behaviour is a study of copulation time in the yellow dung fly (Scatophaga stercoraria) by British evolutionary biologist Geoffrey A. Parker. Shortly after cow excrement is deposited in a meadow, it is invaded by female dung flies that come to lay their eggs on the dung and by males seeking to mate with the females. Competition among the males for females is fierce. Sometimes one male succeeds in kicking a rival off a female during copulation and mounts her himself. Unfortunately for the first male, this means that some of the female's eggs will be fertilized by the second male. The longer the first male copulates, the more eggs he fertilizes, but the returns for extra copulation time diminish rapidly. How much time should a male spend copulating with a female? Should he copulate for as long as is needed to fertilize all the eggs (about 100 minutes) or should he quit earlier (or permit himself to be displaced) so that he can go search for a new female? Parker hypothesized that a male dung fly chooses a copulation time that maximizes his overall rate of egg fertilizations. He tested his hypothesis using a graphical optimality model.

Before a male dung fly that has just finished copulating with a female can copulate with a new one, he must spend on average 156 minutes searching for her. Once he has found a new female, the proportion of her eggs fertilized by him as a function of copulation time is set by female physiology and this has been quantified as a curve based on experimentally measured values. The male cannot shorten the time necessary to find a new female or change the fertilization curve, but he can stop copulating at will. The optimal solution, assuming that his decision regarding copulation duration serves to maximize his rate of egg fertilizations, is to copulate for 41 minutes. Because the average observed copulation time, 38 minutes, is quite close to the predicted time of 41 minutes, it is clear that the Darwinian algorithm underlying a male dung fly's copulation behaviour serves to maximize his rate of egg fertilizations.

A second way of studying the adaptive design of a behaviour is what Darwin called the comparative method, which takes advantage of the thousands of "natural experiments" that have occurred over evolutionary time (that is, throughout the formation of new species and the evolution of their special characteristics). Here again, specific hypotheses regarding how natural selection has shaped a behaviour are tested. Rather than simply examining one species, behavioral researchers collect data from a number of species simultaneously. The idea is to compare the degree to which a particular behaviour occurs in each species with the degree to which the hypothesized selection pressure is part of the ecology of each species.

Australian zoologist Peter Jarman was one of the first to use the comparative method to study the diversity of mating systems, specifically among various species of African antelope. In some species, such as the dik-dik (Madoqua), individuals are solitary and cryptic; however, during mating season, they form conspicuous monogamous pairs. Others, such as the black wildebeest (Connochaetes taurinus), form enormous herds. During the breeding season, only a few males control sexual access to a group of females in a polygynous mating system. When Jarman compared these African ungulates, he found that body size, typical habitat, group size and mating system were interrelated. Specifically, smaller species with relatively high metabolic rates (such as the dik-dik) need to consume high-quality food—such as fruits and buds in the forests—while concealing themselves from predators. Because of the sparse distribution of food and the need to remain solitary and cryptic to avoid capture by predators, the smaller species are widely dispersed, leaving no opportunity for a single male to monopolize access to many females. Consequently, small-bodied species tend to be monogamous. In contrast, the larger species graze in open plains where food is generally abundant, although seasonally variable in its geographic distribution and they are highly visible to predators. Thus, species such as the wildebeest live in large herds that migrate with the seasons. Each individual may be hidden within the large number of other animals in the herd; however, group living creates the opportunity for one male to monopolize several females and polygyny tends to be found in the large-bodied species. This pattern, which holds true for birds and primates as well as ungulates, supports the hypothesis that the mating system of a species is derived from selection pressures associated with food and predation. Selection pressures determine the spatial distribution of females and thus their defensibility by individual males.

Not all comparative analyses of behaviour are so broad. Some focus on just one behaviour or a morphological correlate of behaviour. Consider the case of sexual dimorphism in body size where the males of some species tend to be considerably larger than the females. It had been hypothesized that size is a key advantage in species where males must fight to defend females from rival males. To test the hypothesis that sexual dimorphism was favoured by natural selection, American evolutionary biologist Richard Alexander and his colleagues compared social structure of the breeding group in primates, ungulates and pinnipeds with their degree of body-size dimorphism. They reported that body size is similar between males and females in species, including humans, where the breeding group typically consists of one male and one female or a few females. Male body size, however, increases compared with female body size in species that breed in groups made up of multiple males and females and it is highest in species where a single male defends a large group of females. Evidently, male size in primates is an adaptation related to the intensity of male-male physical competition for females.

The Moral Status of Animals

The Moral Considerability of Animals

A morally considerable being is a being who can be wronged. It is often thought that because only humans can recognize moral claims, it is only humans who are morally considerable. However, when we ask why we think humans are the only types of beings that can be morally wronged, we begin to see that the class of beings able to recognize moral claims and the class of beings who can suffer moral wrongs are not co-extensive.

Speciesism

The view that only humans are morally considered is sometimes referred to as "speciesism". In the 1970s, Richard Ryder coined this term while campaigning in Oxford to denote a ubiquitous type of human centered prejudice, which he thought was similar to racism. He objected to favoring one's own species, while exploiting or harming members of other species. Peter Singer popularized the term and focused on the way speciesism, without moral justification, favors the interests of humans:

> "The racist violates the principle of equality by giving greater weight to the interests of members of his own race, when there is a clash between their interests and the interests of those of another race. Similarly the speciesist allows the interests of his own species to override the greater interests of members of other species. The pattern is the same in each case".

Discrimination based on race, like discrimination based on species is thought to be prejudicial, because these are not characteristics that matter when it comes to making moral claims.

Speciesist actions and attitudes are prejudicial because there is no prima facie reason for preferring the interests of beings belonging to the species group to which one also belongs over the interests of those who don't. That humans are members of the species Homo sapiens is certainly a distinguishing feature of humans—humans share a genetic make-up and a distinctive physiology, we all emerge from a human pregnancy, but this is unimportant from the moral point of view. Species membership is a morally irrelevant characteristic, a bit of luck that is no more morally interesting than being born in Malaysia or Canada. As a morally irrelevant characteristic it cannot serve as the basis for a view that holds that our species deserves moral consideration that is not owed to members of other species.

One might respond that it is not membership in a biological category that matters morally, but rather the social meaning of those categories, meanings that structure not only the institutions we operate within, but how we conceptualize ourselves and our world. Humans have developed moral systems as well as a wide range of other valuable practices and by creating these systems, we separate the human from the rest of the animal kingdom. But the category "human" itself is morally contested. Some argue, for example, that racism is not simply or even primarily about discrimination and prejudice, but rather a mechanism of dehumanizing blackness so as to provide the conditions that makes humans white. According to this line of thought, speciesism isn't focused on discrimination or prejudice but is a central tool for creating human (and white) supremacy or exceptionalism.

Human Exceptionalism

Like speciesism, human exceptionalism can be understood in different ways. The most common way of understanding it is to suggest that there are distinctly human capacities and it is on the basis of these capacities that humans have moral status and other animals do not. But which capacities mark out all and only humans as the kinds of beings that can be wronged? A number of candidate capacities have been proposed—developing family ties, solving social problems, expressing emotions, starting wars, having sex for pleasure, using language or thinking abstractly, are just a few. As it turns out, none of these activities is uncontroversially unique to human. Both scholarly and popular work on animal behavior suggests that many of the activities that are thought to be distinct to humans occurs in non-humans. For example, many species of non-humans develop long lasting kinship ties—orangutan mothers stay with their young for eight to ten years and while they eventually part company, they continue to maintain their relationships. Less solitary animals, such as chimpanzees, baboons, wolves and elephants maintain extended family units built upon complex individual relationships, for long periods of time. Meerkats in the Kalahari Desert are known to sacrifice their own safety by staying with sick or injured family members so that the fatally ill will not die alone. All animals living in socially complex groups must solve various problems that inevitably arise in such groups. Canids and primates are particularly adept at it, yet even chickens and horses are known to recognize large numbers of individuals in their social hierarchies and to maneuver within them. One of the ways that non-human animals negotiate their social environments is by being particularly attentive to the emotional states of others around them. When a conspecific is angry, it is a good idea to get out of his way.

Animals that develop life-long bonds are known to suffer from the death of their partners. Some are even said to die of sorrow. Darwin reported this in The Descent of Man: "So intense is the grief of female monkeys for the loss of their young, that it invariably caused the death of certain kinds". Jane Goodall's report of the death of the healthy 8 year old chimpanzee Flint just three weeks after the death of his mother Flo also suggests that sorrow can have a devastating effect on non-human animals. Coyotes, elephants and killer whales are also among the species for which profound effects of grief have been reported and many dog owners can provide similar accounts. While the lives of many, perhaps most, non-humans in the wild are consumed with struggle for survival, aggression and battle, there are some non-humans whose lives are characterized by expressions of joy, playfulness and a great deal of sex. Recent studies in cognitive ethology have suggested that some non-humans engage in manipulative and deceptive activity, can construct "cognitive maps" for navigation and some non-humans appear to understand symbolic representation and are able to use language.

It appears that most of the capacities that are thought to distinguish humans as morally considerable beings, have been observed, often in less elaborate form, in the non-human world. Because human behavior and cognition share deep roots with the behavior and cognition of other animals, approaches that try to find sharp behavioral or cognitive boundaries between humans and other animals remain controversial. For this reason, attempts to establish human uniqueness by identifying certain capacities are not the most promising when it comes to thinking hard about the moral status of animals.

Personhood

Nonetheless, there is something important that is thought to distinguish humans from non-humans that is not reducible to the observation of behavior best explained by possessing a certain capacity and that is our "personhood". The notion of personhood identifies a category of morally considerable beings that is thought to be coextensive with humanity. Historically, Kant is the most noted defender of personhood as the quality that makes a being valuable and thus morally considerable. Kant writes:

> "Every rational being, exists as an end in himself and not merely as a means to be arbitrarily used by this or that will. Beings whose existence depends not on our will but on nature have, nevertheless, if they are not rational beings, only a relative value as means and are therefore called things. On the other hand, rational beings are called persons inasmuch as their nature already marks them out as ends in themselves".

And:

> "The fact that the human being can have the representation "I" raises him infinitely above all the other beings on earth. By this he is a person that is, a being altogether different in rank and dignity from things, such as irrational animals, with which one may deal and dispose at one's discretion".

More recent work in a Kantian vein develops this idea. Christine Korsgaard, for example, argues that humans "uniquely" face a problem, the problem of normativity. This problem emerges because of the reflective structure of human consciousness. Our reflective capacities allow us and require us to step back from our mere impulses in order to determine when and whether to act on them. In stepping back we gain a certain distance from which we can answer these questions and solve the problem of normativity. We decide whether to treat our desires as reasons for action based on our conceptions of ourselves, on our "practical identities". When we determine whether we should take a particular desire as a reason to act we are engaging in a further level of reflection, a level that requires an endorseable description of ourselves. This endorseable description of ourselves, this practical identity, is a necessary moral identity because without it we cannot view our lives as worth living or our actions as worth doing. Korsgaard suggests that humans face the problem of normativity in a way that non-humans apparently do not:

> "A lower animal's attention is fixed on the world. Its perceptions are its beliefs and its desires are its will. It is engaged in conscious activities, but it is not conscious of them. That is, they are not the objects of its attention. But we human animals turn our attention on to our perceptions and desire themselves, on to our own mental activities and we are conscious of them. That is why we can think about them. And this sets us a problem that no other animal has. It is the problem of the normative. The reflective mind cannot settle for perception and desire, not just as such. It needs a reason".

Here, Korsgaard understands "reason" as "a kind of reflective success" and given that non-humans are thought to be unable to reflect in a way that would allow them this sort of success, it appears that they do not act on reasons, at least reasons of this kind. Since non-humans do not act on reasons they do not have a practical identity from which they reflect and for which they act. So humans can be distinguished from non-humans because humans, we might say, are sources of normativity and non-humans are not.

Rational Persons

But arguably, Kant's view of personhood does not distinguish all and only humans as morally considerable. Personhood is not, in fact, coextensive with humanity when understood as a general description of the group to which human beings belong. And the serious part of this problem is not that there may be some extra-terrestrials or deities who have rational capacities. The serious problem is that many humans are not persons. Some humans—i.e., infants, children, people with advanced forms of autism or Alzheimer's disease or other cognitive disorders—do not have the rational, self-reflective capacities associated with personhood. This problem, unfortunately known in the literature as the problem of "marginal cases", poses serious difficulties for "personhood" as the criterion of moral considerability. Many beings whose positive moral value we have deeply held intuitions about and who we treat as morally considerable, will be excluded from consideration by this account.

There are three ways to respond to this counter-intuitive conclusion. One, which can be derived from one interpretation of Kant, is to suggest that non-persons are morally considerable indirectly. Though Kant believed that animals were mere things it appears he did not genuinely believe we could dispose of them any way we wanted. In the Lectures on Ethics he makes it clear that we have indirect duties to animals, duties that are not toward them, but in regard to them insofar as our treatment of them can affect our duties to persons.

> "If a man shoots his dog because the animal is no longer capable of service, he does not fail in his duty to the dog, for the dog cannot judge, but his act is inhuman and damages in himself that humanity which it is his duty to show towards mankind. If he is not to stifle his human feelings, he must practice kindness towards animals, for he who is cruel to animals becomes hard also in his dealings with men".

And one could argue the same would be true of those human beings who are not persons. We disrespect our humanity when we act in inhumane ways towards non-persons, whatever their species.

But this indirect view is unsatisfying—it fails to capture the independent wrong that is being done to the non-person. When someone rapes a woman in a coma or whips a severely brain damaged child or sets a cat on fire, they are not simply disrespecting humanity or themselves as representatives of it, they are wronging these non-persons. So, a second way to avoid the counter-intuitive conclusion is to argue that such non-persons stand in the proper relations to "rational nature" such that they should be thought of as morally considerable. Allen Wood argues in this way and suggests that all beings that potentially have a rational nature or who virtually have it or who have had it or who have part of it or who have the necessary conditions of it, what he calls "the infrastructure of rational nature", should be directly morally considerable. Insofar as a being stands in this relation to rational nature, they are the kinds of beings that can be wronged.

This response is not unlike that of noted animal rights proponent, Tom Regan, who argues that what is important for moral consideration are not the differences between humans and non-humans but the similarities. Regan argues that because persons share with certain non-persons (which includes those humans and non-humans who have a certain level of organized cognitive function) the ability to be experiencing subject of a life and to have an individual welfare that matters to them regardless of what others might think, both deserve moral consideration. Regan argues that subjects of a life:

> "Want and prefer things, believe and feel things, recall and expect things. And all these dimensions of our life, including our pleasure and pain, our enjoyment and suffering, our satisfaction and frustration, our continued existence or our untimely death—all make a difference to the

quality of our life as lived, as experienced, by us as individuals. As the same is true of animals they too must be viewed as the experiencing subjects of a life, with inherent value of their own".

A third way of addressing this problem has been taken up by Korsgaard who maintains that there is a big difference between those with normative, rational capacities and those without, but unlike Kant, believes both humans and non-humans are the proper objects of our moral concern. She argues that those without normative, rational capacities share certain "natural" capacities with persons and these natural capacities are often the content of the moral demands that persons make on each other. She writes,

> "What we demand, when we demand recognition, is that our natural concerns the objects of our natural desires and interests and affections be accorded the status of values, values that must be respected as far as possible by others. And many of those natural concerns the desire to avoid pain is an obvious example spring from our animal nature, not from our rational nature".

What moral agents construct as valuable and normatively binding is not only our rational or autonomous capacities, but the needs and desires we have as living, embodied beings. Insofar as these needs and desires are valuable for agents, the ability to experience similar needs and desires in patients should also be valued.

Legal Persons

In the courts, all humans and some corporations are considered persons in the legal sense. But all animals, infants and adults, are not legal persons, but rather, under the law they are considered property. There have been a few attempts to change the legal status of some nonhuman animals from property to persons. The Nonhuman Rights Project (NhRP) founded by Steven Wise, has filed a series of cases in the New York courts seeking to establish legal personhood for particular chimpanzees being held in the state, with the goal of protecting their rights to bodily integrity and liberty and allows them to seek remedy, through their proxies, when those rights are violated. Chimpanzees are a good test case for establishing nonhuman legal personhood as they are, according to the documents filed by NhRP, autonomous beings with sophisticated cognitive abilities including:

> "Episodic memory, self-consciousness, self-knowing, self-agency, referential and intentional communication, mental time-travel, numerosity, sequential learning, meditational learning, mental state modeling, visual perspective taking, understanding the experiences of others, intentional action, planning, imagination, empathy, metacognition, working memory, decision-making, imitation, deferred imitation, emulation, innovation, material, social and symbolic culture, cross-modal perception, tool-use, tool-making, cause-and-effect".

The legal arguments to extend personhood beyond the human parallel more general ethical arguments that extend ethical consideration outward from those who occupy the moral center. Turning to empirical work designed to show that other animals are really similar to those considered legal persons, primatologists submitted affidavits attesting to what they have learned working with chimpanzees. Mary Lee Jensvold suggests:

> "There are numerous parallels in the way chimpanzee and human communication skills develop over time, suggesting a similar unfolding cognitive process across the two species and an underlying neurobiological continuity".

James King notes:

> "Chimpanzees and humans resemble each other in terms of their ability to experience happiness and the way in which it relates to individual personality".

And Mathias Osvath makes remarkable claims about chimpanzee personhood:

> "Autonoetic consciousness gives an individual of any species an autobiographical sense of itself with a future and a past. Chimps and other great apes clearly possess an autobiographical self, as they are able to prepare themselves for future actions they likely can, just as humans, be in pain over an anticipated future event that has yet to occur. For instance, confining someone in a prison or cage for a set time or for life, would lose much of its power as punishment if that individual had no self-concept. Every moment would be a new moment with no conscious relation to the next. But, chimpanzees and other great apes have a concept of their personal past and future and therefore suffer the pain of not being able to fulfill one's goals or move around as one wants; like humans they experience the pain of anticipating a never-ending situation".

These claims, as well as those of others experts, identify the relevantly similar capacities that chimpanzees and other great apes share with humans and it is in virtue of these capacities that legal personhood is sought.

Sentience

Using rational nature or cognitive capacities as the touchstone of moral considerability misses an important fact about animals, human and nonhuman. Our lives can go better or worse for us. Utilitarians have traditionally argued that the truly morally important feature of beings is unappreciated when we focus on personhood or the rational, self-reflective nature of humans or the relation a being stands in to such nature or being the subject of a life or being legal persons. What is really important, utilitarians maintain, is the promotion of happiness or pleasure or the satisfaction of interests and the avoidance of pain or suffering or frustration of interests.

Contemporary utilitarians, such as Peter Singer, suggest that there is no morally justifiable way to exclude from moral consideration non-humans or non-persons who can clearly suffer. Any being that has an interest in not suffering deserves to have that interest taken into account. And a non-human who acts to avoid pain can be thought to have just such an interest. Even contemporary Kantians have acknowledged the moral force of the experience of pain. Korsgaard, for example, writes "it is a pain to be in pain. And that is not a trivial fact".

> "When you pity a suffering animal, it is because you perceive a reason. An animal's cries express pain and they mean that there is a reason, a reason to change its conditions. And you can no more hear the cries of an animal as mere noise than you can the words of a person. Another animal can obligate you in exactly the same way another person can."

When we encounter an animal in pain we recognize their claim on us and thus beings who can suffer are morally considerable.

The Moral Significance of Animals' Moral Claims

That non-human animals can make moral claims on us does not in itself indicate how such claims are to be assessed and conflicting claims adjudicated. Being morally considerable is like showing up on a moral radar screen—how strong the signal is or where it is located on the screen are separate questions. Of course, how one argues for the moral considerability of non-human animals will inform how we are to understand the force of an animal's claims.

According to the view that an animal's moral claim is equivalent to a moral right, any action that fails to treat the animal as a being with inherent worth would violate that animal's right and is thus morally objectionable. According to the animal rights position, to treat an animal as a means to some human end, as many humans do when they eat animals or experiment on them, is to violate that animal's right. As Tom Regan has written,

> "Animals are treated routinely, systematically as if their values were reducible to their usefulness to others, they are routinely, systematically treated with a lack of respect and thus are their rights routinely, systematically violated".

The animal rights position is an absolutist position. Any being that is a subject of a life has inherent worth and the rights that protect such worth and all subjects of a life have these rights equally. Thus any practice that fails to respect the rights of those animals who have them, e.g., eating animals, hunting animals, experimenting on animals, using animals for entertainment, is wrong, irrespective of human need, context or culture.

The utilitarian position on animals, most commonly associated with Peter Singer and popularly, though erroneously, referred to as an animal rights position, is actually quite distinct. Here the moral significance of the claims of animals depends on what other morally significant competing claims might be in play in any given situation. While the equal interests of all morally considerable beings are considered equally, the practices in question may end up violating or frustrating some interests but would not be considered morally wrong if, when all equal interests are considered, more of these interests are satisfied than frustrated. For utilitarians like Singer, what matters are the strength and nature of interests, not whose interests these are. So, if the only options available in order to save the life of one morally considerable being is to cause harm, but not death, to another morally considerable being, then according to a utilitarian position, causing this harm may be morally justifiable. Similarly, if there are two courses of action, one which causes extreme amounts of suffering and ultimate death and one which causes much less suffering and painless death, then the latter would be morally preferable to the former.

Consider factory farming, the most common method used to convert animal bodies into relatively inexpensive food in industrialized societies today. An estimated 8 billion animals in the United States are born, confined, biologically manipulated, transported and ultimately slaughtered each year so that humans can consume them. The conditions in which these animals are raised and the method of slaughter causes vast amounts of suffering. Given that animals suffer under such conditions and assuming that suffering is not in their interests, then the practice of factory farming would only be morally justifiable if its abolition were to cause greater suffering or a greater amount of interest frustration. Certainly humans who take pleasure in eating animals will find it harder to satisfy these interests in the absence of factory farms; it may cost more and require more effort to obtain animal products. The factory farmers and the industries that support factory farming, will also have certain interests frustrated if factory farming were to be abolished. How much interest frustration and interest satisfaction would be associated with the end to factory farming is largely an empirical question. But utilitarians are not making unreasonable predictions when they argue that on balance the suffering and interest frustration that animals experience in modern day meat production is greater than the suffering that humans would endure if they had to alter their current practices.

Importantly, the utilitarian argument for the moral significance of animal suffering in meat production is not an argument for vegetarianism. If an animal lived a happy life and was painlessly killed and then eaten by people who would otherwise suffer hunger or malnutrition by not eating the animal, then painlessly killing and eating the animal would be the morally justified thing to do. In many parts of the world where economic, cultural or climate conditions make it virtually impossible for people to sustain themselves on plant based diets, killing and eating animals that previously led relatively unconstrained lives and are painlessly killed, would not be morally objectionable. The utilitarian position can thus avoid certain charges of cultural chauvinism and moralism, charges that the animal rights position apparently cannot avoid.

It might be objected that to suggest that it is morally acceptable to hunt and eat animals for those people living in arctic regions or for nomadic cultures or for poor rural peoples, for example, is to potentially condone painlessly killing other morally considerable beings, like humans, for food consumption in similar situations. If violating the rights of an animal can be morally tolerated, especially a right to life, then similar rights violations can be morally tolerated. In failing to recognize the inviolability of the moral claims of all morally considerable beings, utilitarianism cannot accommodate one of our most basic prima facie principles, namely that killing a morally considerable being is wrong.

There are at least two replies to this sort of objection. The first appeals to the negative side effects that killing may promote. If, to draw on an overused and sadly sophomoric counter-example, one person can be kidnapped and painlessly killed in order to provide body parts for four individuals who will die without them, there will inevitably be negative side-effects that all things considered would make the kidnapping wrong. Healthy people, knowing they could be used for spare parts, might make themselves unhealthy to avoid such a fate or they may have so much stress and fear that the overall state of affairs would be worse than that in which four people died. Appealing to side-effects when it comes to the wrong of killing is certainly plausible, but it fails to capture what is directly wrong with killing.

A more satisfying reply would have us adopt what might be called a multi-factor perspective, one that takes into account the kinds of interest that are possible for certain kinds of morally considerable beings, the content of interests of the beings in question, their relative weight and the context of those who have them. Consider a seal who has spent his life freely roaming the oceans and ice flats and who is suddenly and painlessly killed to provide food for a human family struggling to survive a bitter winter in far northern climes. While it is probably true that the seal had an immediate interest in avoiding suffering, it is less clear that the seal has a future directed interest in continued existence. If the seal lacks this future directed interest, then painlessly killing him does not violate this interest. The same cannot be said for the human explorer who finds himself face to face with a hungry Inuit family. Persons generally have interests in continued existence, interests that, arguably, non-persons do not have. So one factor that can be appealed to is that non-persons may not have the range of interests that persons do.

An additional factor is the type of interest in question. We can think of interests as scalar; crucial interests are weightier than important interests, important interests are weightier than replaceable interests and all are weightier than trivial interests or mere whims. When there is a conflict of interests, crucial interests will always override important interests, important interests will always override replaceable interests, etc. So if an animal has an interest in not suffering, which is arguably a crucial interest or at least an important one and a person has an interest in eating that animal when there are other things to eat, meaning that interest is replaceable, then the animal has the stronger interest and it would be wrong to violate that interest by killing the animal for food if there is another source of food available.

Often, however, conflicts of interests are within the same category. The Inuit's interest in food is crucial and the explorer's interest in life is crucial. If we assume that the explorer cannot otherwise provide food for the hunter, then it looks as if there is a conflict within the same category. If you take the interests of an indigenous hunter's whole family into account, then their combined interest in their own survival appears to outweigh the hapless explorer's interest in continued existence. Indeed, if painlessly killing and eating the explorer were the only way for the family to survive and then perhaps this action would be morally condoned. But this is a rather extreme sort of example, one in which even our deepest held convictions are strained. So it is quite hard to know what to make of the clash between what a utilitarian would condone and what our intuitions tell us we should believe here. Our most basic prima facie principles arise and are accepted under ordinary circumstances. Extraordinary circumstances are precisely those in which such principles or precepts give way.

The multi-factor utilitarian perspective is particularly helpful when considering the use of animals in medical research. According to the animal rights position, the use of animals in experimental procedures is a clear violation of their rights—they are being used as a mere means to some possible end—and thus animal rights proponents are in favor of the abolition of all laboratory research. The utilitarian position, particularly one that incorporates some kind of multi-factor perspective, might allow some research on animals under very specific conditions. Before exploring what a utilitarian might condone in the way of animal experimentation, let us first quickly consider what would be morally prohibited. All research that involves invasive procedures, constant confinement and ultimate death can be said to violate the animal's crucial interests. Thus any experiments that are designed to enhance the important, replaceable or trivial interests of humans or other animals would be prohibited. That would mean that experiments for cosmetics or household products are prohibited, as there are non-animal tested alternatives and many options already available for consumers. Certain psychological experiments, such as those in which infant primates are separated from their mothers and exposed to frightening stimuli in an effort to understand problems teenagers have when they enter high school, would also come into question. There are many examples of experiments that violate an animal's crucial interests in the hopes of satisfying the lesser interests of some other morally considerable being, all of which would be objectionable from this perspective.

There are some laboratory experiments, however, that from a multi-factor utilitarian perspective may be permitted. These are experiments in which the probability of satisfying crucial or important interests for many who suffer from some debilitating or fatal disease is high and the numbers of non-human animals whose crucial interests are violated is low. The psychological complexity of the non-humans may also be significant in determining whether the experiment is morally justified. In the case of experimenting in these limited numbers of cases, presumably a parallel argument could be made about experimenting on humans. If the chances are very high that experimenting on one human, who is a far superior experimental animal when it comes to human disease, can prevent great suffering or death in many humans, then the utilitarian may, if side effects are minimal, condone such an experiment. Of course, it is easier to imagine this sort of extreme case in the abstract, what a utilitarian would think actually morally justified, again depends on the specific empirical data.

In sum, the animal rights position takes the significance of morally considerable claims to be absolute. Thus, any use of animals that involves a disregard for their moral claims is problematic. The significance of an animal's morally considerable interests according to a utilitarian is variable. Whether an action is morally justified or permissible will depend on a number of factors. The utilitarian position on animals would condemn a large number of practices that involve the suffering and death of billions of animals, but there are cases in which some use of non-human animals and perhaps even human animals, may be morally justified.

Alternative Perspectives on Human Relations to other Animals

Given the long-standing view that non-humans are mere things, there are still many who reject the arguments presented here for the moral considerability of non-humans and the significance of their interests. Nonetheless, most now realize that the task of arguing that humans have a unique and exclusive moral status is rather difficult. Yet even amongst those who do view animals as within the sphere of moral concern, there is disagreement about the nature and usefulness of the arguments presented on behalf of the moral status of animals.

Increasingly, philosophers are arguing that while our behavior towards animals is indeed subject to moral scrutiny, the kinds of ethical arguments that are usually presented frame the issues in the wrong way. Some philosophers suggest that rational argumentation fails to capture those features of moral experience that allow us to really see why treating animals badly are wrong. The point, according to commentators such as Stephen R.L. Clark and Cora Diamond, for example, is that members of our communities, however we conceive of them, pull on us and it is in virtue of this pull that we recognize what is wrong with cruelty. Animals are individuals with whom we share a common life and this recognition allows us to see them as they are. Eating animals is wrong not because it is a violation of the animal's rights or because on balance such an act creates more suffering than other acts, but rather because in eating animals or using them in other harmful, violent ways, we do not display the traits of character that kind, sensitive, compassionate, mature and thoughtful members of a moral community should display.

According to some in the virtue ethics tradition, carefully worked out arguments in which the moral considerability and moral significance of animals are laid out will have little if any grip on our thoughts and actions. Rather, by perceiving the attitudes that underlie the use and abuse of non-human animals as shallow or cruel, one interested in living a virtuous life will change their attitudes and come to reject treating animals as food or tools for research.

Alice Crary argues that shifting perceptions of our moral landscapes occur because these landscapes and more precisely the rich worlds of those who inhabit them, are not morally neutral. The characteristics that philosophers tend to look for in other animals to determine whether or not they are morally considerable, according to Crary, are already infused with moral importance, "human beings and other animals have empirically discoverable moral characteristics" that are, as she puts it "inside ethics". These values often sneak in under a supposedly neutral gloss. By explicitly locating these characteristics inside ethics, the texture, quality and purposes of our ethical reflection on moral considerability changes. Arriving at an adequate empirical understanding requires non-neutral methods, identifying historical and cultural perspectives as shaping how we consider other animals morally. What ethical questions we think are important and how we frame and answer them, will be different if we see our lives and the lives of other animals as already imbued with moral values.

Other feminist philosophers have taken issue with the supposedly morally neutral methods of argumentation used to establish the moral status of animals. For many feminists the traditional methods of rational argumentation fail to take into account the feelings of sympathy or empathy that humans have towards non-humans, feelings they believe are central to a full account of what we owe non-humans and why.

Feminist philosophers have also challenged the individualism that is central in the arguments for the moral status of animals. Rather than identifying intrinsic or innate properties that non-humans share with humans, some feminists have argued instead that we ought to understand moral status in relational terms given that moral recognition is invariably a social practice. As Elizabeth Anderson has written:

> "Moral considerability is not an intrinsic property of any creature, nor is it supervenient on only its intrinsic properties, such as its capacities. It depends, deeply, on the kind of relations they can have with us".

And these relationships needn't be direct. The reach of human activity has expanded across the entire globe and humans are entangled with each other and other animals in myriad ways. We participate in activities and institutions that directly or indirectly harm others by creating negative experiences, depriving them of their well-being or denying them opportunities to be who they are and pursue what they care about. Philosophers Elisa Aaltola and Lori Gruen have argued for refining our empathetic imagination in order to improve our relationships with each other and other animals.

Even though it is challenging to understand what it is like to be another and even though we are limited by our inevitable anthropocentric perspectives, being in respectful ethical relation involves attempting to understand and respond to another's needs, interests, desires, vulnerabilities, hopes and perspectives. What Gruen calls, "entangled empathy" is a process that involves both affect and cognition. Individuals who are empathizing with others respond to the other's condition and reflectively imagine themselves in the distinct position of the other while staying attentive to both similarities and differences between herself and her situation and that of the fellow creature with whom she is empathizing. Entangled empathy involves paying critical attention to the broader conditions that may negatively affect the experiences and flourishing of those with whom one is empathizing and this requires those of us empathizing to attend to things we might not have otherwise. It therefore also enhances our own experiences, develops our moral imagination and helps us to become more sensitive perceivers.

Animal Rights

Animal rights means that animals deserve certain kinds of consideration—consideration of what is in their best interests, regardless of whether they are "cute," useful to humans or an endangered species and regardless of whether any human cares about them at all. It means recognizing that animals are not ours to use—for food, clothing, entertainment or experimentation.

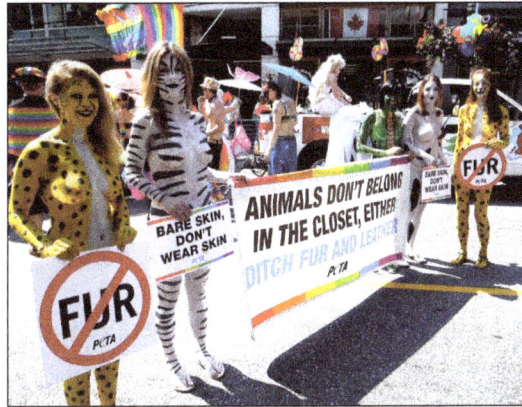

Animal rights are based on ethical and moral philosophy. It has been discussed by some of the world's most influential thinkers, from historical figures such as Pythagoras and Leonardo da Vinci – who embraced vegetarianism – to Jeremy Bentham, the founder of the utilitarian school of philosophy, who famously identified animals' capacity for suffering as the characteristic that gives them a right to equal consideration.

All animals have the ability to suffer in the same way and to the same degree that humans do. They feel pain, pleasure, fear, frustration, loneliness and familial love. Whenever we consider doing something that would interfere with their needs, we are morally obligated to take them into account.

The philosopher Peter Singer states that the basic principle of equality does not require equal treatment – it requires equal consideration. This is an important distinction when talking about animal rights. People often ask if animal rights mean that animals should have the right to vote or drive a car. Of course, that would be silly because those aren't rights that would benefit animals. But animals have the right not to suffer at the hands of humans and to live their lives free from suffering and exploitation because they have an interest in doing so. That is the difference between equal consideration and equal treatment.

It's Intuitive

You don't have to be a philosopher to know that hurting animals is wrong. At its core, animal rights are simple. It's about being kind to others – whether they're members of our own species or not.

Almost everyone cares about animals in some context, whether it's a beloved family companion, an irresistibly cute kitten or a majestic wild animal seen in a documentary. After all, we each have some built-in capacity for empathy and compassion, as can be seen from the lengths that children often go to in order to help animals.

Logically and morally, there's no reason to differentiate in the way we treat the animals we share our homes with and those who are farmed for food. They're all individuals, with the same capacity to feel pain and fear. Animal rights help us to look past the arbitrary distinctions between different species, to rediscover our innate compassion and to respect all animals equally.

It's a Way of Life

There's nothing abstract about animal rights and there are no barriers to getting involved. Anyone who cares about animals can start putting these principles into practice every single day with the food they eat, the clothes they wear and the products they buy. These choices are a form of nonviolent protest that makes a real difference both by reducing the profits of corporations that harm or kill animals and by creating a growing market for cruelty-free food, fashion, services and entertainment.

It's a Social Movement

Like other major social movements, animal rights bring people together from across political, religious and cultural boundaries to fight against injustice.

And like those movements, it's also about fairness. Only prejudice allows us to deny others the rights that we expect to have for ourselves. Whether it's based on race, gender, sexual orientation or species, prejudice is morally unacceptable. Alongside the struggles against racism, sexism and homophobia, there's the struggle against speciesism – discrimination against other beings on the basis of their species.

It's the Way Forward

Society is evolving and becoming fairer all the time. Despite all the people who say change will never happen, most countries in the world have outlawed human slavery and child labour Recognising the rights of animals is the next stage in our progress towards a fairer world.

As biologists and animal behaviourists learn more about animals' intelligence and the complexity of their lives, there's even less excuse for treating them as commodities rather than the sensitive individuals they are.

Most of us grew up eating meat, wearing leather and visiting zoos. Yet, just as we've made the mental shift towards a way of life that respects animals, so society as a whole must outgrow the unethical mindset that animals are here for us to use and kill as we please.

The Modern Animal Rights Movement

The fundamental principle of the modern animal rights movement is that many nonhuman animals have basic interests that deserve recognition, consideration and protection. In the view of animal rights advocates, these basic interests give the animals that have them both moral and legal rights.

It has been said that the modern animal rights movement is the first social reform movement initiated by philosophers. The Australian philosopher Peter Singer and the American philosopher

Tom Regan deserve special mention, not just because their work has been influential but because they represent two major currents of philosophical thought regarding the moral rights of animals. Singer, whose book Animal Liberation is considered one of the movement's foundational documents, argues that the interests of humans and the interests of animals should be given equal consideration. A utilitarian, Singer holds that actions are morally right to the extent that they maximize pleasure or minimize pain; the key consideration is whether an animal is sentient and can therefore suffer pain or experience pleasure. This point was emphasized by the founder of modern utilitarianism, Jeremy Bentham, who wrote of animals, "The question is not, Can they reason?, nor, Can they talk? but, Can they suffer?" Given that animals can suffer, Singer argues that humans have a moral obligation to minimize or avoid causing such suffering, just as they have an obligation to minimize or avoid causing the suffering of other humans. Regan, who is not a utilitarian, argues that at least some animals have basic moral rights because they possess the same advanced cognitive abilities that justify the attribution of basic moral rights to humans. By virtue of these abilities, these animals have not just instrumental but inherent value. In Regan's words, they are "the subject of a life."

Regan, Singer and other philosophical proponents of animal rights have encountered resistance. Some religious authors argue that animals are not as deserving of moral consideration as humans are because only humans possess an immortal soul. Others claim, as did the Stoics, that because animals are irrational, humans have no duties toward them. Still others locate the morally relevant difference between humans and animals in the ability to talk, the possession of free will or membership in a moral community (a community whose members are capable of acting morally or immorally). The problem with these counterarguments is that, with the exception of the theological argument—which cannot be demonstrated—none differentiates all humans from all animals.

While philosophers catalyzed the modern animal rights movement, they were soon joined by physicians, writers, scientists, academics, lawyers, theologians, psychologists, nurses, veterinarians and other professionals, who worked within their own fields to promote animal rights. Many professional organizations were established to educate colleagues and the general public regarding the exploitation of animals.

At the beginning of the 21st century, lawsuits in the interests of nonhuman animals, sometimes with nonhuman animals named as plaintiffs, became common. Given the key positions that lawyers hold in the creation of public policy and the protection of rights, their increasing interest in animal rights and animal-protection issues was significant. Legal scholars were devising and evaluating theories by which nonhuman animals would possess basic legal rights, often for the same reasons as humans do and on the basis of the same legal principles and values. These arguments were powerfully assisted by increasingly sophisticated scientific investigations into the cognitive, emotional and social capacities of animals and by advances in genetics, neuroscience, physiology, linguistics, psychology, evolution and ethology, many of which have demonstrated that humans and animals share a broad range of behaviours, capacities and genetic material.

Meanwhile, the increasingly systemic and brutal abuses of animals in modern society—by the billions on factory farms and by the tens of millions in biomedical-research laboratories—spawned thousands of animal rights groups. Some consisted of a mere handful of people interested in local and more traditional, animal-protection issues, such as animal shelters that care for stray dogs and cats. Others became large national and international organizations, such as PETA (People for the Ethical Treatment of Animals) and the Humane Society of the United States, which in the early 21st century had millions of members and a multimillion-dollar annual budget. In all their manifestations, animal rights groups began to inundate legislatures with demands for regulation and reform.

Slaves, human and nonhuman, may be indirectly protected through laws intended to protect others. But they remain invisible to civil law, for they have no rights to protect directly until their legal personhood is recognized. This recognition can occur in a variety of ways. British slavery was abolished by judicial decision in the 18th century and slavery in the British colonies was ended by statute early in the 19th century. By constitutional amendment, the United States ended slavery three decades later. Legal personhood for some animals may be obtained through any of these routes.

In 2013 the Nonhuman Rights Project (NhRP) filed petitions in three trial courts in the state of New York demanding that common law writs of habeas corpus be issued on behalf of four captive chimpanzees—Tommy, Kiko, Hercules and Leo. The petitions implicitly asked that the courts recognize that chimpanzees are legal persons who possess the fundamental legal right to bodily liberty. After all three petitions were denied, the cases moved to the New York state appellate courts, where two of the petitions were rejected on differing grounds and the third (on behalf of Hercules and Leo) was thrown out for lack of the right to appeal. The NhRP then indicated its intention to appeal Tommy's and Kiko's cases to New York's highest court, the Court of Appeals and to refile Hercules and Leo's petition in another jurisdiction. Meanwhile, the organization prepared to file additional lawsuits on behalf of other chimpanzees and elephants.

Abolitionist Animal Rights

The abolitionist nonhuman animal rights movement, a movement distinct in its explicit rejection of welfare reform and violent advocacy, established following the emergence of Gary Francione's Abolitionist Approach, an internet blog and information website. While nonhuman advocates have long called for a complete cessation of nonhuman use, the modern nonhuman movement, since its inception in the 19th century, has relied heavily on welfare reform. Thus, while the abolitionist goal is certainly not new, the tactics and repertoires utilized in the Francionian approach are distinctly so. Indeed, the abolitionist movement, comprised of grassroots and often localized individuals and small groups self-identifying according to Francione's theory, is less than a decade old.

Despite considerable productivity prior to the launch of Abolitionist Approach, Francione's work was largely unknown. Rather than advocating an incremental regulatory approach to reformed nonhuman animal use, Francione's abolitionist approach requires incremental cessation of use that culminates in the altogether elimination of nonhuman animal use. Though Francione had been arguing for an end to nonhuman animal use with ethical veganism as the moral baseline for two decades, it was not until his entry into the internet community that his theory found a sizeable audience.

Francione's theory improves on that of Tom Regan's notion of inherent value. Here, Regan argues that beings that are subjects of life possess worth, regardless of their capacity for suffering. However, Regan's life-boat scenario (the thought experiment whereby a boat could only stay afloat if either a human or a nonhuman was thrown overboard) posits that regardless of inherent value, the interests of human animals can override that of nonhumans because of their greater potential for and appreciation of, future satisfaction. Francione departs with Regan here and argues that any being that is sentient should not have their interests overridden and that both humans and nonhumans alike have an interest in continuing to live with an equal potential for future satisfaction. Regardless of Regan's problematic moral hierarchy, he does explicitly recognize the need to abolish use, rather than modify it. Thus, Regan's work stands as the foundation of abolitionist theory from which Francione and others build.

The primary concepts and stances held by abolitionism will be explored followed by a comparison to the humane product trend and welfarism. Finally, a critical examination of the current state of the abolitionist movement and existing challenges will be presented. It is argued that taking our moral obligation to nonhuman animals seriously necessitates the adoption of an abolitionist vegan approach to animal rights.

Finally, it is suggested that the relative newness of the abolitionist movement and strong countering from the mainstream nonhuman animal welfare movement has prevented abolitionism from obtaining a large presence within the nonhuman animal rights movement.

Because the literature on abolitionist nonhuman animal rights theory and the debate is relatively scant, there is a heavy reliance on the works of Gary Francione and Bob Torres. There is also a substantial use of unpublished works of influential abolitionist academics and those critical to the debates surrounding abolitionist theory. It is suggested that these sources provide an important insight into emerging discourse within the nonhuman animal rights movement. Furthermore, the terms "nonhuman animal" and "human animals" will be utilized in this writing as a rejection of speciesist language in recognizing the potential for language to demean, exclude and reinforce normative values.

Major Concepts and Stances

Despite a brief allusion to the intersections between the human abolitionist movement and the nonhuman abolitionist movement in Boyd's 1987 essay The New Abolitionists: Animal Rights and Human Liberation, in its application to nonhuman animal rights, abolition is indeed new. However, nonhuman rights abolitionism is based on the much older human abolitionist movement that preceded it. Francione highlights the parallel between the two movements in that the systems of human and nonhuman animal slavery both commodify sentient beings and respect their interests only insomuch as they are economically beneficial. Yet, Kim notes that while the comparison between the two systems of oppression is morally defensible, it could prove politically problematic for nonhuman animal rights activists in ignoring white normativity and thus challenging the potential for creating cross-group alliances. The nonhuman animal rights appropriation of these concepts also conflicts with other understandings of abolition. Certainly, the abolition of human slavery did not necessitate the abolition of racism and discrimination. Abolitionist work continued after the American Civil War. Of note, DuBois critiqued the failure of the reconstruction period and recognized that true abolition relies on representation and integration. Likewise, Davis highlights continued oppression of people of color in other structural systems of inequality, the prison system in particular. Neither of these applications of abolitionist thought is directly relevant to the nonhuman animal issue as yet. As such, the nonhuman animal rights understanding of abolition harkens to human abolitionist activities that specifically challenged the property status of human slaves and discriminatory ideology. Indeed, a popular human and nonhuman abolitionist website, Quotes on Slavery, juxtaposes excerpts from the human animal and the nonhuman animal abolitionist movements with no distinction between the two.

Drawing from the human animal abolitionist experience, abolitionist nonhuman animal rights is based on the premise that nonhuman animals are functionally and legally property in human animal society. So long as nonhuman animals are considered property, their interests can always be overridden by human animal interests in conflict situations. There is not a push for equal rights between nonhuman animals and human animals, as nonhuman animals have different natures than human animals, but rather a push for equal consideration based on the specific requirements of nonhuman animals based on their telos. Central to these specific requirements, it is recognized that nonhuman animals have the right not to be treated as property. Recognition of this right necessarily entails an abolition of institutionalized nonhuman animal use and exploitation which perpetuates the property status of nonhuman animals. Likewise, abolition recognizes and rejects societal speciesism. Speciesism is the prejudice against nonhuman animals that arbitrarily assigns varying values and levels of moral worth. Dunayer elaborates on Ryder's definition adding that it is, "a failure, in attitude or practice, to accord any nonhuman being equal consideration and respect". Speciesism manifests in differential treatment and discrimination based on species, notably in the human practice of exploiting nonhumans for flesh and labor. It is understood that there are no meaningful differences between nonhuman and human animals which would justify unequal consideration:

> "The species of a sentient being is no more reason to deny the protection of this basic right than race, sex, age or sexual orientation is a reason to deny membership in the human moral community to other humans".

Thus, the abolitionist nonhuman animal rights movement calls for a rejection of the property status held by nonhuman animals, a rejection of speciesism and a need for equal consideration.

Abolitionism, as defined by Francione, also entails a strict adherence to nonviolence. Violence entails any action that causes harm physically or emotionally, this would include bodily harm, threats and intimidation, property damage (as it has the latent effect of instilling fear and creating the potential for unintended harm). The definition of violence certainly fluctuates significantly in the nonhuman movement and many reject that certain tactics, particularly property damage, can constitute violence. However, any action that causes harm and, "treats others as means to ends rather than as ends in themselves" is considered antithetical to the peaceful society Francionian abolitionists hope to create.

Ahimsa, a rule of conduct borrowed from Jainism, Hinduism and Buddhism, is often used to describe this notion within the Francionian abolitionist movement: "Ahimsa is the principle that we should not act violently toward others in our thoughts, speech or action". A practicing Jain, Francione draws on the principle of ahimsa as the "highest religious duty". Thus, the Francionian abolitionist plan of action dismisses violence as a useful or acceptable manner to work towards ending nonhuman animal use:

> "Violence is the problem; it is not any part of the solution. Those who advocate violence against institutional users of animals fail to recognize the simple fact that these users are

only responding to a demand created by others. The real exploiters are those who create the demand. Therefore, violence against institutional users makes no sense".

Violence, which is often negatively associated with the nonhuman animal rights movement due to the activities of the Animal Liberation Front and the subsequent animal terrorist laws is seen as both detrimental and counterproductive to abolition by many abolitionists. State reaction to violent activism increases costs of all nonhuman activism, even that which is peaceful. Further, according to Francione, embracing nonviolence and adhering to ahimsa is essential to challenging the violence towards nonhuman animals which advocates seek to end. As such, ahimsa and veganism are "inseparable and presuppose each other" as "All animal products—including dairy and wool—involve inflicting suffering and death on mobile, five-sensed-beings". Other nonhuman animal rights theorists have alluded to the religious basis for respecting the rights of nonhumans as well. However, there are an increasing number of atheistic abolitionist activists who recognize the parallel between nonhuman animal rights and moral rationalism and reject the spiritual element entirely. Indeed, many abolitionists adopt the notion of nonviolence without any reference to the principle of ahimsa.

A rejection of violence, however, remains a commonality among abolitionists. It is a continuation of nonviolent collective action drawn from the human abolition movement as well as contemporary social movements. Nonviolent resistance is thought to impose less risk and thus increases movement participation. Abolitionist activists believe that it increases participation, which in turn, increases resources and movement power. What's more, the adherence to nonviolence is believed to increase credibility and is thought to be congruent with the nonviolent society abolitionists hope to create.

Subsequently, abolitionism adopts veganism as a necessary baseline. Veganism both challenges the property status of nonhuman animals and is consistent with nonviolence:

> "As a direct protest against the commodity form and property relations that animals are subject to, it is a great refusal of the system itself, a no-compromise position that does not seek reform, but which seeks abolition. For anyone who wants to end animal exploitation, living as a vegan is living the end that we wish to see—no one will exploit animals for mere choices of taste and convenience".

Abolitionism requires a complete rejection of nonhuman animal consumption and production both directly (as food or fashion) and indirectly (as entertainment, research subjects or companion and "pet" animals). It is understood that it is logically inconsistent to strive for an end to nonhuman animal use while continuing to consume them. Recognizing that there are no defensible grounds for excluding nonhuman animals from moral concern, human animals must extend equal consideration to nonhuman animals. The principle of equal consideration means taking nonhuman animal interests seriously. It recognizes that nonhuman animals, like human animals, have morally significant interests in not suffering and in not being used as resources. It follows, then, that respecting a moral obligation to nonhuman animals as objects of moral concern with interest in not suffering could not reasonably include consumption: "Veganism is the only way forward that does not trade off the interests of animals today in the vast hope of some bright future right down the road". The assumption here is that consumption necessarily entails harm. The use of nonhuman animals as resources, fatally or not, constitutes harm to the nonhuman animal whose interest lies in not experiencing use or suffering. Adherents to the abolitionist movement are expected to both adopt veganism and promote the growth of veganism necessary for effectiveness through education.

Critical Comparisons with Humane Products and Welfarism

The trend towards humane products and welfare reform are dominant approaches within the nonhuman animal rights movement. Abolitionists believe that neither of these approaches fully addresses the necessity of abolishing entirely the use of nonhuman animals. Rather, they focus on modifying use. The argument could be made that the humane product trend and welfare reform are at times one and the same. However, a distinction can be based on the economic focus of humane products as opposed to the welfarist movement's addressing of a wide array of nonhuman animal issues beyond food. Importantly, the humane product trend is comprised of nonhuman animal exploiters while the welfare movement is largely comprised of nonhuman animal advocates. The argument for these approaches will be explained, followed by an abolitionist critique that will be argued that both the humane products and welfare reform movements seriously fail to satisfy our moral obligations to nonhuman animals.

The Humane Products Trend

The humane product trend, representing the recent growth in humane product availability and discourse, is an approach to nonhuman animal use that does not challenge the property status of nonhuman animals, but does address the ways in which those animals are treated. Largely commercially driven, this approach recognizes a consumer concern with the humaneness of the nonhuman animal products and attempts to improve the welfare for the nonhuman animals involved. Labeling is used to highlight process and quality. Labels such as "free-range," "grass-fed," "organic," "humanely-raised," "cage-free," and so forth all contend with consumer concerns with the treatment of nonhuman animals. The humane product trend purports to respect the telos of nonhuman animals, adhering to what "nature intended" and farming in "harmony with nature" working with "animals' natural behaviors". They are also less likely to see death as a harm, as the actual killing of nonhuman animals is not considered in defining humaneness of production. If use of the nonhuman animals can be understood as in accordance with the telos of those nonhumans and the nonhuman animals are not harmed by death, the humane products approach is not likely to see any contradiction in the human moral obligation to nonhuman animals.

The humane product approach exists in opposition to abolitionism because it is not concerned with the possibility that human animal society will ever be willing to abolish nonhuman animal flesh and excretions from the diet. Here, there is recognition of continued demand for these products coupled with a growing conscious consumption. The humane trend is, at its heart, an economic enterprise which intends to profit from nonhuman animals. Tellingly, grocery stores such as Whole Foods are adopting labeling schemes to promote nonhuman animal products of higher welfare practices as beneficial to their business.

Unfortunately, it appears that this approach is not improving welfare for nonhuman animals as consistent with popular belief. Values-based labeling can often be misleading. Investigations initiated by mainstream nonhuman animal welfare organizations are uncovering evidence that humane products vary dramatically in levels of suffering imposed on nonhuman animals and are often substantively minimal in improvements. Regardless of any improvements, nonhuman animals raised for flesh will unavoidably lose their lives.

Additionally, direct death or indirect death following over-expenditure in egg, dairy, etc. production is inevitable. Furthermore, the move to humane products continues to support institutional exploiters with no goal of ever abolishing the exploitation. This is problematic if we wish to enact equal consideration: "The moment we use another being instrumentally, we have denied that being its right to exist on its own terms". Here, the use of nonhuman animals is not a relevant issue. Instead, supposedly more humane use becomes commodified. Consumers can pay extra for peace of mind and nonhuman animal agriculture, as a business, is happy to oblige: "Though some producers will be slow to come along, the industry operates on thin enough margins that it will recognize a market opportunity when it sees it and happily provide alternatives for people of conscience, provided it can reasonably profit from those alternatives". The industry of humane products, then, fails to challenge nonhuman animal use and instead exploits public concern with nonhuman animal suffering and death. There is no expectation that use will decrease or cease. Certainly, as those involved with this movement profit from nonhuman animal use and have no desire to see it end, not much in the way of abolition is to be expected here. It remains problematic, however, in that much of the public and many major nonhuman animal rights organizations believe that this movement towards higher welfare could lead to abolition.

Another concern with this approach is the inherent contradiction created by managing values-based labeling of products within a capitalist framework. The genuineness of the producers' commitment to nonhuman animal welfare will necessarily come into question when profits are involved. Likewise, as the niche market for more responsible products increases, adherence to the initial moral vision will necessarily be challenged. Furthermore, the use of the term "humane" is questionable. It is difficult to argue that exploitation and death could ever be defined as humane. Based on this misleading terminology and minimal improvements in rearing nonhuman animals, it is probable that consumers would be left with a confused understanding of the reality behind the products. Likewise, it can be questioned as to what psychological impact the humane products trend is having on a public concerned with the use of nonhuman animals. Humane labels must certainly assure consumers that the interests of nonhuman animals are being adequately addressed and create a social comfort with nonhuman animal use. With labeling and governmental reform, consumers can unquestioningly assume necessary changes have been made. This can create complacency with concern over moral obligation and even increase consumption: "Such promotion [of humane nonhuman animal products] may actually increase consumption by people who had stopped eating animal products because of concerns about treatment and will certainly provide as a general matter an incentive for continued consumption of animal products". Ultimately, the reality of humane products remains contrary to the perpetuated popular myth.

Equally unsettling, the humane product approach and the welfarist movement often overlap. Several welfarist organizations work directly with the labeling of humane products. The American Society for the Prevention of Cruelty to Animals (ASPCA) and the Humane Society of the United States (HSUS), for example, are partners of Humane Farm Animal Care, an organization which certifies humane treatment. Compassion over Killing operates a long-standing campaign for the reformation of Animal Care Certified labeling.

The Welfarist Movement

Welfarism will be treated as a distinct movement from the humane products trend as it does, for the most part, seriously consider our moral obligations to nonhuman animals and is more expansive in its involvement with nonhuman animal use. Furthermore, the humane product trend is generally run by institutional exploitative producers, whereas welfarism is generally not-forprofit. Welfarism is the dominant ideology within the animal rights movement and is distinguished from abolition in its strategy of regulation and reform: "The ethic which has emerged in mainstream society does not say we should not use animals or animal products. It does say that the animals we use should live happy lives where they can meet the fundamental set of needs dictated by their natures and where they do not suffer at our hands". That is, welfarism focuses on suffering, not use.

Welfarism may or may not expect an eventual end in nonhuman animal use based on ideological differences. Francione distinguishes between traditional welfarism and new welfarism. Traditional welfarism adopts instrumentalism and is concerned with humane treatment and prevention of unnecessary suffering. There is no long term goal of reduction in use: "Animal welfare is seen as important enough, so long as it does not interfere too much with farming and economic concerns". New welfarism differs in that it recognizes a goal of abolition, but utilizes welfarist tactics in an effort to achieve that goal. Abolitionist tactics are assumed to be ineffective in the immediate future. In the meantime, the short-term tactic of welfare reform is adopted: "It represents a realistic appraisal of what can be achieved now and in the short term, given the present vulnerable and arrogant state of the human condition". Therefore, while those in the new welfarist movement espouse an abolitionist end, welfarist reform is assumed to be efficacious and morally acceptable as a means to achieve that end.

Welfarists criticize abolitionism on two major points: We must work to reduce suffering in the here and now and total abolition of nonhuman animal use is an unachievable goal. Those arguing that total abolitionism will never be attained maintain that resources spent towards an unrealistic goal of abolition are wasted. That is, if abolitionism is wasting resources, the suffering of presently exploited nonhuman animals remains unaddressed. Alternatively, it is sometimes suggested that the uncontrolled suffering of nonhuman animals is somehow beneficial to the abolitionist cause. Here, it is presumed that abolitionists advocate extreme suffering under the assumption that the public will become so disgusted that an eventual backlash will develop in favor of abolition.

Importantly, these critiques do not give much weight to veganism as direct and immediate action. Abolitionism, which endorses veganism as a necessary baseline, can be argued as reducing suffering in the here and now by reducing consumer demand through a consistent promotion of and adherence to veganism:

> "Abolitionists identify the promotion of veganism as the one essential tool for bringing an end to the exploitation of animals. Instead of pursuing legislation or litigation intended to reduce the suffering of animals, Abolitionists educate people about veganism in order to make veganism more prevalent and thereby eventually eliminate the exploitation of animals".

Furthermore, according to abolitionists, welfarism itself is not reducing suffering in any significant way. While the modification of confinement, for example, might make life for nonhuman animals slightly less sufferable, the suffering reduced is generally trivial in relation to the immense anguish and eventual death that remains unaddressed by reform. Furthermore, regulation of nonhuman animal use might have the psychological effect of making human animal consumers more comfortable with the exploitation. Thereby, the actual use of the nonhuman animal is not addressed and use will invariably continue: "we cannot hope to produce a world that is free of animal suffering and exploitation by promoting gentler forms of suffering". Lastly, it has been the case that most regulation has been imposed only when economically beneficial to the institutional exploiters.

Francione points to the Humane Slaughter Act and the campaign to adopt controlled atmosphere killing of chickens as to key examples of the marriage of nonhuman animal welfare reform and increased profitability and efficiency of exploitative institutions. The passage of the Humane Slaughter Act of 1958 proceeded with the support of producers, as it improved efficiency by reducing carcass damage and worker injury. The vice president of the American Meat Institute reported that his organization was urging the approval of this legislation: "The experience of our members has been that humane slaughter methods are efficient methods. They result in improved productivity". Likewise, People for the Ethical Treatment of Animals (PETA) and HSUS have promoted the controlled atmosphere killing of chickens as profitable to producers through increased production capacity, affordability of gases, improved working conditions, improved food quality, shelf-life, safety and reduced carcass damage and labor costs. The push to end castration, too, is marketed as a profitable move for ranchers. It is argued that failing to castrate will result in faster growth, shaving approximately three months from the raising process at an increased profit to ranchers. How could the increased efficiency of exploitative institutions be much good to the nonhuman animals whose continued suffering remains unchallenged? Here then, the concern of welfarists with our moral obligation to nonhuman animals becomes enmeshed with the desires of profit-driven institutional exploiters:

> "While we may be able to make that commodification "nicer" through "compassionate" or "happy" meat or measures like eliminating gestation crates, commodification will never simply fade away on its own, as it is the foundational logic of the system itself. Provided it can continue to commodify animals as property, the system will adapt, even to the most stringent regulations. What's more, if those regulations become too onerous domestically, it seems likely that the industry will simply increase the already substantial offshore production taking place to skirt around these domestic regulations. For these reasons, our activism must fight the system at its roots, targeting property and the imposition of the commodity form on animals, rather than hoping that an ethically bankrupt system will do the impossible task of reforming itself given demands to do so".

The insistence of mainstream nonhuman animal organizations to continue to support such reforms is resulting in questionable alliances and counterproductive results. The abolitionist nonhuman animal rights movement is largely defined by its rejection of this aspect of welfarism: "We recognize that we will not abolish overnight the property status of nonhumans, but we will support only those campaigns and positions that explicitly promote the abolitionist agenda. We will not support positions that call for supposedly "improved" regulation of animal exploitation".

The Abolitionist Agenda and Subsequent Challenges

Abolitionism seeks to reach its goal of ending nonhuman animal use through consumer-based resistance. Consumption-based resistance is a political strategy adopted by many social movements in response to injustices involved with product content and preparation. Consumers are seen as active holders of responsibility with the ability to change both market capitalism and society. Personal consumption, in other words, can become a political action.

Abolitionism seeks to reduce and eventually eliminate consumer demand for nonhuman animal use as consistent with a serious consideration of our moral obligations: "Essentially the demand is the demand of speciesism: The view that human beings can legitimately use and override the rights of nonhuman animals for a whole variety of purposes". Central to consumption-based resistance is abolitionism's vegan baseline. It is presumed that through the implementation of vegan education programs, a critical mass of vegans will materialize. With this critical mass should come political power and social influence. However, resistance that continues to function within capitalism might not be sufficient in adequately challenging the problems with an economic system that is built on consumption and exploitation. What's more, capitalist-based resistance could potentially delude social responsibility and obligations in reducing participation to purchases in the checkout lane. It might also run into problems of access with minorities and lower income individuals as fresh and whole food products can often be more expensive or difficult to find. In addition to these potential problems, abolitionism is a relatively new movement and is subsequently quite small with limited power. DeCoux suggests that abolitionism's overreliance on the property status of nonhuman animals and its failure to adopt depictions of suffering has stunted its success.

Furthermore, abolitionism has been heavily criticized as utopian, as depicted in welfarist critiques that find goals of ending nonhuman animal use to be unobtainable. However, it is important to recognize the newness of the abolitionist movement as it pertains to nonhuman animal rights. And, given DeCoux's critiques, abolition may still have room to grow so far as putting theory into practice. Further, many mainstream groups that are decidedly not rights based, such as PETA, lay claim to the term "rights," further confusing our moral obligation to nonhuman animals: "People for the Ethical Treatment of Animals (PETA), with more than 2 million members and supporters, is the largest animal rights organization in the world". Yet, PETA does not explicitly campaign for veganism or the end of nonhuman animal use, but rather the modification of use (promotion of controlled atmosphere killing, vegetarianism and single issue campaigns such as fur bans). Nonetheless, the organization has become the face of "animal rights." This misuse of the term "rights" can only further complicate the sluggish path to abolition.

Importantly, abolitionism has been effectively shut out of mainstream nonhuman animal welfare organizational claims-making. Ending use entirely is downplayed in the mainstream agenda. Veganism, too, is only weakly supported, if at all: "Unfortunately, the current groups making up the mainstream animal rights movement have a rather spotty record promoting veganism as a viable alternative and very few groups have made it a primary focus of their outreach and activism. Furthermore, the momentum of abolitionism is quickly slowed as counter movements are constructed by institutional exploiters of nonhuman animals and welfarist organizations alike. As Francione notes, "Abolition has not taken center stage because the welfarist organizations do not want it as center stage. It is easier to fundraise when you promote welfare reforms and do not seek to persuade people to make changes in their lives". Indeed, abolitionists are often labeled as extremist or fanatical. Building on Francione's observations, two reasons might be given for this exclusion. One, it might be assumed that the radical nature of such an absolute goal might deter participants and potential participants in the nonhuman animal movement. Secondly, as previously noted, the abolitionist goal is often seen as utopian.

Abolitionism, unlike the approaches, is asking human animals to completely reconfigure their understanding of nonhuman animals to one that recognizes nonhumans as persons requiring moral obligations. This is a much larger task than simply asking human animals to modify use, as this does not touch deeply rooted speciesism. Thus, the abolitionist movement will necessarily be slow moving, as it must undertake an enormous societal shift in the gestalt: "Social change is happening, but social change is slow". Unlike any other nonhuman animal social movement, the abolitionist movement is addressing rampant inequalities that invade nearly every aspect of human animal existence. Human animals have been effectively exploiting nonhuman animals for thousands of years. Furthermore, nonhuman animals are largely voiceless and lack the capacity to effectively communicate in the human animal arena. While Hribal documents a rich history of nonhuman animals engaging in individual resistance to their oppression (retaliations, escapes, etc.), it remains the case that nonhuman animals will likely never be able to become a class for itself in the Marxian sense and be able to collectively act on their own behalf. Hence, the movement to end speciesism and nonhuman animal use is facing unique and difficult challenges.

Furthermore, the nonhuman animal welfare movement dominates nonhuman animal rights discourse and is consequently able to influence nonhuman animal rights ideology. Control over ideology is maintained through framing and the active construction of meaning. Within a paradigm dominated by welfarism, abolitionism must struggle for recognition. Further, abolitionism is often framed negatively and what it means to recognize our moral obligation to nonhuman animals is constructed according to the dominant ideology. Abolitionism faces the challenge of channeling enough power and resources to adequately challenge this ideology, reframe the abolitionist representation and begin reshaping societal understandings of our moral obligation to nonhuman animals.

In changing deeply held societal views, the end goal of abolition may appear distant. Abolitionism is still in the process of gaining momentum and is still establishing itself as a viable movement. On the contrary, welfarist reform has been operating for several centuries and nonhuman animal use has been increasing exponentially. Abolitionism remains locked out of mainstream advocacy: "The problem is that the mainstream animal rights movement has never really tried such activism in earnest. Instead, it relies on a weak system of reforms, with the hope that these gradual changes will someday, in some way, in some distant and far-off future, lead to the complete abolition of animal exploitation". Furthermore, criticisms that label abolitionism as utopian, may be representative of fizzling motivation: "This kind of pessimism dressed up as realism reveals a poverty of ambition and probably indicates a degree of 'burn-out' that many social movement participants experience". Because abolitionism as a clear and distinct movement is quite new, it is too early, Yates argues, to become pessimistic. Only with increased acceptance and adherence will real social change emerge.

DeCoux suggests that abolitionist success has stagnated because the movement fails to create a critical mass of vegans because of its reluctance to utilize descriptions of suffering. The welfarist movement, she argues, has been able to tap into the empathy and concern that is resultant from descriptions of suffering. Welfarists have thus been able to dominate mainstream nonhuman animal rights and channel those emotional reactions into ineffectual tactics. Jasper and Poulsen also point to the importance of incorporating this strategy to increase recruitment. Others, however, question effectiveness. Moral shocks can be off-putting rather than engaging or entirely ineffectual for peripheral groups such as vegetarians. Regardless, the context of social movement tactics can influence their effectiveness. The abolitionist movement might find it difficult to direct emotional reactions towards abolishing use in a society heavily influenced by welfarism where reactions are generally directed towards reform. So long as welfarism remains the dominant paradigm, there is a strong potential that moral shocks might pull recruits towards a desire to reform use, rather than abolish it.

Animal Ethics

Over the course of the last two centuries, traditional forms of the treatment of animals have been turned upside down by industrialized farming, genetic experimentation, artificial insemination and other techniques (hormones, crossbreeding, cloning and so forth). These techniques transform animals into "biomachines" which have to produce the highest possible yield at the lowest possible cost. The depiction of this reduction of animals "not only to production and overactive reproduction of meat for consumption, but also of all sorts of other end products," as Derrida says in The Animal That Therefore I Am, was the starting point of the animal movement in the 1970s. "The unprecedented proportions of this subjection of animals" raised for food due to the increase of the global meat production since 1970; the confinement of chickens, cows and pigs that make it impossible for them to fulfill their nature, as seen with pregnant sows in gestation crates; the slaughtering of animals at such high speeds that some are cut apart while still alive; and the number of species endangered because of man's activities drove some thinkers into taking part in the public debate to make such cruelty to other living beings a pressing ethical issue.

Although his utilitarian approach, which comes from Jeremy Bentham, is put into question and even rejected by other leading figures of animal ethics such as Tom Regan, it provides some guidelines to denounce abuses of animals, which exceed, in sheer number of affected individuals, any other mistreatment, as seen with the meat industry. Moreover, the key concepts of Singer's animal ethics are worth examining since they revolve around the principle of equality of interests, which does not imply the equality of treatment but the taking into account of the suffering of a sentient being.

One can discuss the way Singer equates sentience with a capacity or a power to experience pleasure, pain and suffering and his reinstating the human/animal, mind/body dichotomies he first considered as responsible for the cruelty to animals. By the same token, Regan's vocabulary of rights, which grants any subject of a life inherent value, may pertain, in spite of the abolitionist implications of this approach, to a liberal framework that falls into a metaphysical tradition grounding ethics on the capacities argument and determines the human/animal difference on the basis of some animal deprivations.

However, the founding fathers of animal ethics in the Western tradition have contributed to two major changes in ethics. First, the criteria for ethics change once one considers that membership in the Homo sapiens species and the faculties of discourse are not some sufficient measures for moral worth. The word speciesism, which was coined in 1971 by the Oxford psychologist Richard Ryder, suggests that such discrimination is as unjust as sexism and racism. In other words, there is a need for a nondiscriminatory approach of ethics. Animal ethics, which for Singer and Regan goes hand in hand with the rejection of speciesism, is part of such effort to overcome the human-centered or anthropocentric traditional ethics. To be sure, animal ethics shares with environmental ethics a common effort to provide an alternative to anthropocentrism. Both denounce the posture of man as a tyrant prone to dominate nature and reduce other living beings to their instrumental value. By focusing on the individuals, animal ethics however distinguishes itself from environmental ethics, especially from ecocentrism for which the species is all-important.

The second major change in ethics that occurs thanks to animal ethics is due to the focus on the animal viewed as a sentient being, whose uniqueness and own biography are taken into account. This insistence upon the richness of animal life and the acknowledgment of the subjectivity of animals, although they do not have the same cognitive capacities as humans, explain why animal ethics is currently turning into a more critical interdisciplinary study. The animal question, far from being "one question among others," is "the limit upon which all the great questions are framed and determined," as Derrida puts it. The status and the meaning of ethics are at stake in the way some ethicists from various countries envisage the animal question. Their goal is actually to displace the moral boundaries and dichotomies we inherited from the humanist tradition. The latter has excluded the animal from the sphere of our moral consideration and advocates a position of dominion over the other beings, which explains and sometimes justifies violence and mistreatment to animals.

The feminist contribution to animal studies and Derrida's approach indicate that animal ethics is no longer a specialized ethics. Making our relations with animals the point of departure of an inquiry into the framework of our ethics, politics and ontology lead us to adopt a new way of thinking, which is post-humanist or implies another humanism. Whereas animal ethics dealt with the moral status of animals and sometimes advocated the extension of rights to animals, as seen in the Great Ape Project, many philosophers and ethicists deeply committed to the defense of animals and promoted a nonviolent, vegan lifestyle, showing that the animal question drives us into making responsibility and vulnerability the major concepts of ethics and politics, which concern both humans and animals. The way we understand justice toward animals, be they domesticated, wild or liminal, is at stake in the animal question, which is part of a broader, holistic approach encompassing the reflection upon our inhabiting the earth and sharing resources with other species.

Singer's Principle of the Equal Consideration of Interests

Singer's approach to ethics involves the calculation or counting of interests: A good action is an action that maximizes the expected satisfaction of interests. As in Bentham, all the parties affected by my possible action count, including animals. Acting morally is choosing the action those results in the greatest net satisfaction of interests.

Utilitarianism is a type of situation ethics that rests upon a case-by-case basis and implies the calculation of net interests in each case. Along with the idea that various mental capacities make a difference in the anticipation of death, for instance, such an approach to ethics leads Singer to assess that, under certain circumstances, animal experimentation is morally acceptable, whereas a carnivorous diet imposing upon billions of animals a life of suffering and a painful death is not. To be sure, a deontological approach such as the rights-based approach we find in Regan has abolitionist consequences. However, the point that makes Singer's ethics break up with the tradition is his reference to the principle of the equality of interests.

As Bentham wrote in The Principles of Morals and Legislation, the question was not whether a being can think or talk, but whether he/she can suffer. Sentience is thus a sufficient measure for moral worth. A sentient being has interests: He/she wants to be free from suffering and is looking for enjoyment and pleasure. No matter what the species of the being, the principle of equality requires that its suffering be counted equally with the like suffering of any other being. Singer's animal ethics revolves around the principle of the equal consideration of interests. It is not the faculty of reason or discourse that should be decisive when the moral worth of animals is concerned, but the capacity to suffer is sufficient to grant or ascribe a moral status to a being.

Therefore, animals and humans who have the capacity to suffer have interests. More precisely, the cognitive capacities that make the anticipation of a painful experience or a pleasure more intense are taken into account in Singer's calculation. Such argument drives Singer into justifying some comparisons between an encephalic baby or a comatose patient and a chimpanzee or a horse, which are more conversable than the "defective persons." The standard capacities upon which Singer's ethics is based are questionable. However, the impact of Singer's animal ethics has been stressed worldwide, not only does it show that speciesist prejudices are arbitrary and in conflict with the values we cherish in our life or the possessions we consider as essential in order to enjoy life, but it also provides guidelines to make some drastic changes in our lifestyles. According to Singer, when we are eating, we are brought on into direct touch with the most extensive exploitation of animals that has ever existed. Our food choices are political and they have consequences on other beings, including other human beings experiencing hunger in part because the cereals produced by local farmers in Africa are sold to Europe and the USA to feed their cattle. The principle of the equality of interests does not imply that animals and humans will receive the same treatment. Singer's capacities argument therefore has some drawbacks since it pertains to a cognitive ontology that goes hand in hand with hierarchical and elitist representations drawn from an archetype or a model of normality, which explains that the beings who are "most like us" will have more interests, whereas the persons suffering from cognitive impairments and some animals with whom we do not have any relation have less to lose. However, it highlights something essential, moral consideration and thus respect toward animals does not necessarily mean that they will be granted some rights.

Furthermore, the relevance of Singer's approach to ethics lies in the assertion that once we place some beings outside the sphere of our moral consideration, cruelty to these beings is predictable. There is no way of speaking of animal welfare since we continue to draw a line between the members of our species, who deserve respect and the others, who do not count. Moral progress lies in the extension of our moral consideration to other sentient beings, whose life is as important for them as ours is for each of us. When we come to include animals in the sphere of our moral consideration, we can no longer accept to rear them for food, since meat is nowadays a substitutable pleasure and, as Plutarch said, it is neither necessary nor natural to people who can eat fruits and vegetables and find other sources of protein than the flesh of another living being.

Animal ethics therefore means that the starting point for some changes in our lifestyles as well as in the production of food is the individual, since he/she becomes aware of the moral status of animals. Although the chances of persuading all the persons worldwide to abandon animal products may be remote, as Singer himself acknowledges, the animal question has entered the public debate. Many philosophers involved in grounding a less anthropocentric or chauvinist ethics but also consumers, even when they are not prone to adopt a vegan lifestyle, want to know the origin of the animal products they buy and some of them try to replace meat, because animal welfare has become an ethical issue for them or because they understand that industrialized factories have an environmental cost and generate hazards to human health (epizootic diseases, cancer and so forth).

Regan's Rights-based Approach: The Subject of a Life

Regan stands for the abolitionist approach to animal ethics. However, his contribution to such field is not only due to his refusal of any reformism. To be sure, he rejects any strategy trying to improve the welfare of animals used in farming: "animal rights require empty cages, not larger cages," as he says. Individuals who experience life and have perception, memory, desire, belief, self-esteem, intention and a sense of the future are holders of fundamental rights. To be the subject of a life is the criterion for moral worth in such a non-speciesist theory, which also advocates the inclusion of any individual as possessing fundamental rights.

Thus, for Regan, some nonhuman animals and only some human beings are holders of such rights that are considered, as Dworkin said, as trump cards, that is to say, their basic rights are to be protected. The utilitarian approach, which leads to tolerate animal experimentation for the benefit of a large number of human beings or even animals, is no longer relevant in Regan's animal ethics. Good ends do not justify the exploitation of animals, whose inherent value is assessed.

Any subject of a life has the prima facie right of individuals not to be harmed and killed. Regan's theory, which implies that some animals have negative rights and that we have the obligation to guarantee their inviolability, is interesting because it deeply puts into question some traditional beliefs and cultural habits that draw a line between those whom "thou shall not kill" and the others. Once individual rights rest upon the capacity of an individual to be the subject of a life, killing an animal can no longer be so easily distinguished from murder. Regan's approach invites us to ground human rights on the individual sentient being who has a subjective experience of life, even if he/she does not have a philosophy and cannot take part in deliberative democracy as framed in Rawls or Habermas. This makes a difference in the human rights theory that will lead to more comprehensive developments, as seen in Zoopolis by Kymlicka and Donaldson.

To be sure, there is no consensus that the use of animals for food or research is morally reprehensible. The controversy is particularly important when we opposed the rights-based approach in animal ethics and those who assess that the pro-animal use does not raise any ethical issues. However, even if one accepts Stephen Schiffer's view that biological evolutionary offers a sound explanation for the validity of animal modeling in human disease, it is necessary to provide a metaphysical foundation in order to justify that some sentient beings be sacrificed for the good of other beings and for the sake of science. We then come back to a utilitarian approach of the animal question and the answer depends on our speciesist or anti-speciesist convictions.

Moreover, the theological ordering of animal and human that can be mentioned to ground man's superiority upon animals and enable us to use the latter for food and research is fragile. Not only does the Genesis advocate the image of man as a steward of the creation or even as a member of a biotic citizenship he shares with the other beings and with nature, as B. Callicott put it, but there is also Francis of Assisi for whom God's glory requires the respect for all creatures. Be that as it may, it seems that any attempt to ground animal experimentation upon metaphysical reasons does not succeed. The only justification for animal experimentation is that men and even animals may benefit from the progress of science that it makes possible. The point, for those who refuse the rights-based approach and its absolute anti-speciesism, is then to show respect toward animals during the experimentation. This leads to the guidelines that are at the core of the ethics of animal experimentation: Reduce, refine and replace.

It is because there is no way of overcoming such opposition between anti-speciesism and the pro-animal use that the animal ethics has entered another stage of its history, drawing a path that travels from ethics to justice toward animals. This shift implies a further inquiry into the animal-rights debate, but it also suggests that the focus be less on the legal status of animals than on the foundations of our ethics and politics that the animal question helps us to critically examine.

Justice Toward Animals

The authors of Zoopolis: A Political Theory of Animal Rights contends that animals have negative rights, but they abandon the capacities arguments and the cognitive ontology underpinning them. Whereas the interpretation of subjectivity as a capacity or a power drives into excluding some animals and also the human beings who are suffering from severe cognitive impairments, they equate selfhood with vulnerability. This reinterpreting of Bentham's criteria for ethics goes hand in hand with their effort to sort out political theory and even political liberalism from the intellectualist framework that explained why disabled persons were the recipients of justice but could not take part in collective decisions. Following the insights of some researchers who have reconfigured autonomy to make it relevant in the case of dependent agents, they provide a political theory in which the interests of animals can be included in our policies.

Moreover, they give content to the concrete obligations we have toward them. These obligations, which enable them to speak of positive rights for animals, are drawn from the relations we have with them. Wild animals that have their own societies and do not want to live with us do not have the same needs or the same rights as domesticated animals that are dependent on us. Lastly, we do not have the same obligations toward liminal animals, such as mice or foxes, which colonized our gardens without our inviting them at home, but it does not enable us to deny them the right to exist.

The core notion of such theory is the notion of zoopolis, which was first coined by Jennifer Wolch to design the coexistence of human beings and animals in urban areas. In Kymlicka and Donaldson, this word suggests that the interests of nonhuman animals are to be integrated in the definition of the common good. This means that we have to take into account the interests of animals in our policies since we share with them the resources, the lands, the sky and so forth. Our politics is no longer to be considered as if it only concerned human beings and nations. Our politics is a cosmopolitics, because we are always dealing with nature and natural elements that make us live or breathe and it is also a zoopolis, a community in which the different interests of other beings have to be taken into account.

This way of highlighting the political dimension of the animal question implies that our relations with animals are a matter of justice and not only of morality. Far from reducing the justice toward animals to a rights-based approach, such inquiry requires our reassessing the main ethical, legal and ontological categories that are the framework of our relations to animals but also of our relations to the others in general. Animal ethics is no longer a specialized discipline: Although the animal question calls for an examination of all the pressing animal issues, the point of departure of the reflection is less the moral status of other living beings than our way of understanding them and our relations with them.

The question of who we are is at stake in such an approach, which inherits the reference to the key concept of sentience from animal ethics. The way we treat animals is a mirror in which human beings look at themselves. The awareness of the violence we impose upon other beings and which also refers to the lines we draw between humans and animals, excluding the latter from our moral community and operating on the basis of dichotomies (human/animal, mind/body, nature/culture, freedom/instinct), stresses the strategic role of the animal question. The philosophers who are currently writing another chapter of animal studies borrow from the founding fathers of this field a pathocentric ethics and the insistence upon sentience. However, the two major concepts that aim at displacing the traditional moral frontiers, that is to say, vulnerability and responsibility, request the overcoming of the capacities argument we find in Singer and Regan.

Thinking through the Animal Question

The animal question is an essential chapter of Derrida's deconstruction of the metaphysical tradition, which assimilates differences into sameness. Animal is a word that men have given themselves the right to give, in order to draw a line separating human and man and to ground the notion of the subject defined as an autonomous individual. The word "animot," which Derrida coined to show that ethics and politics are caught up in language, suggests that most philosophers, even those who advocate animal rights, reinstate the same hierarchy and reconstitute, in spite of their opposition to Descartes, a version of the rational Cartesian subject.

Animals, whose diversity is neglected, are deprived of the logos, even in Levinas, whose notion of the otherness of the other nonetheless inspired Derrida, who speaks of the individual animal as a wholly other. The description of his encounter with his cat in his bathroom, at the beginning of The Animal That Therefore I Am, aims at reversing the traditional trend. Whereas most philosophers continue to think that the subject is a first person who speaks and decides, Derrida, suggesting that there is somebody behind the fur and that the cat looking at him is not totally understandable, says that there is a call coming from the animal.

This comparison between sexism and speciesism we find in Bentham and at the beginning of the animal movement will be further analyzed by feminist ethicists. As in Derrida, the main point is to overcome the dichotomies human/animal, man/woman, mind/body, nature/culture and reason/affects, which characterize a dualist ontology. The insistence upon sensitivity is the starting point of such critique of dualism, but as in Derrida sentience ceases to be considered as a capacity or a power. It is rather viewed as a certain passivity that is constitutive of the self of any other. Vulnerability, which becomes the core category of such ethics and its underlying embodied ontology, means that human beings and animals are experiencing a "not being able," a non-power and this sense of one's vulnerability before another being is the entry to ethics.

Responsibility does not make any sense, except for a being who is suffering in his or her flesh, except for a vulnerable person, Levinas said. Today's animal ethics insist upon the responsibility we have toward all the vulnerable beings. Even nature, whose frailty and finitude are acknowledged, has become the object of our responsibility. This focus on vulnerability, which does not mean that animals are always frail creatures, pertains to an ontology wherein the corporality of the subject is all-important. The mortality that belongs to the finitude of life, the needs we have as embodied beings, calls for an ethics that exceeds any calculation and rules.

Virtue ethics is an approach that describes and encourages the moral traits that make us feel responsible in our daily life as well as in our social and political commitments and that enable us to be open to the other – including the wholly other which is the animal. It plays an important role in animal ethics in promoting a nondiscriminatory ethics and in reinstating compassion in justice. As both Carol Adams and Derrida said, our violence toward animals is a war on compassion. It calls for an examination of the place of compassion in justice. Thinking through the animal question is thus an opportunity to reinvigorate ethics and to move toward a more comprehensive, if not holistic, approach of justice toward both human beings and animals.

3Rs of Animal Ethics

The principles of the 3Rs (Replacement, Reduction and Refinement) were developed over 50 years ago providing a framework for performing more humane animal research. Since then they have been embedded in national and international legislation and regulations on the use of animals in scientific procedures, as well as in the policies of organisations that fund or conduct animal research.

Definitions of the 3Rs

	Standard	Contemporary
Replacement	Methods which avoid or replace the use of animals.	Accelerating the development and use of models and tools, based on the latest science and technologies, to address important scientific questions without the use of animals.
Reduction	Methods which minimise the number of animals used per experiment.	Appropriately designed and analysed animal experiments that are robust and reproducible and truly add to the knowledge base.
Refinement	Methods which minimise animal suffering and improve welfare.	Advancing research into animal welfare by exploiting the latest in vivo technologies and by improving understanding of the impact of welfare on scientific outcomes.

Replacement

Replacement refers to technologies or approaches which directly replace or avoid the use of animals in experiments where they would otherwise have been used.

For many years research animals have been used to answer important scientific questions including those related to human health. Animal models are often costly and time-consuming and depending on the research question present scientific limitations, such as poor relevance to human biology. Alternative models can address some of these concerns. In the last decade or so, advances in science and technology have meant that there are now realistic opportunities to replace the use of animals.

We divide replacement into two key categories, full and partial replacement.

- Full replacement avoids the use of any research animals. It includes the use of human volunteers, tissues and cells, mathematical and computer models and established cell lines.

- Partial replacement includes the use of some animals that, based on current scientific thinking, are not considered capable of experiencing suffering. This includes invertebrates1 such as Drosophila, nematode worms and social amoebae and immature forms of vertebrates2. Partial replacement also includes the use of primary cells (and tissues) taken from animals killed solely for this purpose (i.e. not having been used in a scientific procedure that causes suffering).

Reduction

Reduction refers to methods that minimise the number of animals used per experiment or study consistent with the scientific aims. It is essential for reduction that studies with animals are appropriately designed and analysed to ensure robust and reproducible findings.

Reduction also includes methods which allow the information gathered per animal in an experiment to be maximised in order to reduce the use of additional animals. Examples of this include the use of some imaging modalities which allow longitudinal measurements in the same animal to be taken (rather than for example culling cohorts of animals at specific time points) or micro-sampling of blood, where small volumes enable repeat sampling in the same animal. In these scenarios, it is important to ensure that reducing the number of animals used is balanced against any additional suffering that might be caused by their repeated use.

Sharing data and resources (e.g. animals, tissues and equipment) between research groups and organisations can also contribute to reduction.

Refinement

Refinement refers to methods that minimise the pain, suffering, distress or lasting harm that may be experienced by research animals and which improve their welfare. Refinement applies to all aspects of animal use, from their housing and husbandry to the scientific procedures performed on them. Examples of refinement include ensuring the animals are provided with housing that allows the expression of species-specific behaviours, using appropriate anaesthesia and analgesia to minimise pain and training animals to cooperate with procedures to minimise any distress.

Evidence suggests that pain and suffering can alter an animal's behaviour, physiology and immunology. Such changes can lead to variation in experimental results that impairs both the reliability and repeatability of studies.

References

- Animal-behavior, science: britannica.com, Retrieved 16 May, 2019

- Moral-animal, entries: plato.stanford.edu, Retrieved 19 August, 2019

- What-do-you-mean-by-animal-rights: peta.org, Retrieved 23 April, 2019

- What-is-animal-rights: peta.org.uk, Retrieved 31 March, 2019

- The-modern-animal-rights-movement, animal-rights: britannica.com, Retrieved 15 May, 2019

4

The Welfare of Farming Animals

The welfare of farming animals is important for animals to live a longer, healthier and active life. Welfare of goats, pigs, hens, cows, horse, etc. have been studied under it. This chapter closely examines the aspects associated with the welfare of farming animals to provide an extensive understanding of the subject.

The Welfare of Goats

Goats are intelligent and inquisitive and are quick to learn new things. A quiet approach when handling goats is important. The amount of stress experienced by the goats and the risk of injury to both goats and their handlers is decreased when good handling facilities are available, as this will reduce the need to apply pressure to move the goats.

Human-animal interactions can be enhanced by improving handling procedures and facilities, selecting appropriate animals for the husbandry system, getting them used to human contact and attending to the skill and training of the handlers.

Knowledge of goats' flight (or safety) zone and the point of balance (the line through the animal's shoulder which determines whether it will move forwards or backwards in the presence of a handler) will help with moving animals and in reducing fear. Animals with large flight zones, such as feral goats, become fearful and agitated when people invade this zone and when they are confined or unable to move away. The size of the flight zone depends on an animal's genotype, its previous contact with people and whether this contact was negative or positive.

Goats that are not accustomed to yarding can become stressed and those that feel pressured are more likely to bully their herd-mates. Goats with horns present additional risk of injury. These goats require patient handling and plenty of space.

Smothering of goats when yarding is a risk, especially when the goats are not accustomed to routine handling (e.g. feral goats). Goats are also at a particular risk of smothering when contained in groups in confined spaces, when backing boards are used, at pressure points such as gateways and yard corners or when adults and kids are in the same mob. The risk can be minimized by quiet and patient handling, managing animals in small groups and by appropriate yard design.

Minimum Standard

- Goats must be handled at all times in such a way as to minimize the risk of pain, injury or distress.
- Goats must not be struck or prodded with a goad in the udder, anus, genitals or eyes.

- Goats must not be prodded in sensitive areas.

- Electric prodders must not be used.

- Only the minimum force required must be used when moving goats.

Example Indicators for Minimum Standard of Animal Handling

- Stock handlers' behavior towards goats is always patient.

- Stock handlers have knowledge of the easiest ways to move goats and do not need to resort to prodding or hitting to make goats move.

- Goats are not lifted by the horns.

- Stock handlers appreciate how goats may react to and interact with other goats, other animals, humans, strange noises, sights and smells.

- Yards and handling systems are designed with knowledge of goat behavior to ensure that goats will readily move through facilities.

- Stock handlers are trained in the use of handling equipment.

Recommended Best Practice

- Goats have a strong instinct to herd and individuals should not be unnecessarily isolated. The amount of time that individual goats are kept alone or out of sight of other goats should be minimized.

- Stock handlers should understand and recognise stress factors for goats and take steps to minimize them.

- Aids to facilitate handling of goats, such as vehicles, dogs, sticks and flags (when used as an extension of the arm) should all be used minimally and carefully so as not to distress or injure the goats.

- Tails should not be lifted or twisted when moving goats.

- If it is necessary to use dogs, they should be under control at all times and muzzled where appropriate.

- When performing husbandry procedures on aggressive animals, they should be separated, given additional space and kept in yards for the minimum time necessary to complete the tasks.

Restraint and Tethering

The facilities that are available for restraining goats on farm will depend on the farming system used but may include races, backing gates, crushes, cradles and head bails. This equipment can be used to guide a goat in a required direction or to hold it in position to enable efficient examination and treatment. Stock handlers need to be aware that head bails and crushes can cause injury to goats and people if they are not managed properly.

Goats are sometimes tethered or restrained in order to keep areas of land grazed and free of weeds. Goats tethered in this way are usually restrained by a collar or halter and chain or rope. Tethered goats have some particular requirements that must be met in order to ensure that their needs are satisfied.

Goats are social animals and need to be provided with one or more companions. While interaction with humans (in the case of pet goats) may provide a substitute for some of their social and behavioral needs, the welfare of goats that are tethered on their own is compromised. Providing a goat with the company of other goats is preferable, however, goats can also live with companions such as sheep, cows or horses. If it is not possible to keep a goat in a herd with social companions, providing goats with the opportunity to see or hear other goats (or other animals) can provide some welfare benefits.

When tethering goats in close proximity to other tethered goats, they need to be a sufficient distance away from each other so that the tethers cannot become entangled. When tethering goats, the use of an aerial running line, in which the chain of the tether is attached to an aerial wire or rope so that the goat can move along the line, can be beneficial and provide a goat with additional space in which to exercise and access feed.

Minimum Standard

- Equipment used for restraining goats must be fit for purpose and applied in such a manner that stress and risk of injury to the goat are avoided.

- Methods of mechanical restraint must allow for the animal to be released quickly.

- Goats that are restrained by tethering must be:

  - Placid and trained to the conditions.

  - Provided with access at all times to food, water and fully shaded and dry shelter that provides protection from extremes of heat and cold.

  - Able to walk and move around without undue hindrance.

  - Inspected at least once every 12 hours.

- Kids, sick goats, pregnant or nursing does or goats physiologically compromised in any other way must not be tethered.

- Tethers used on goats on roadside verges must prevent goats from getting into the path of vehicles.

Example Indicators for Minimum Standard of Restraint and Tethering

- Maintenance of goat restraint equipment is up-to-date and recorded and there are no protruding parts or sharp-edged parts on the equipment that might injure goats.

- If any difficulty is encountered when restraining a goat (e.g. the goat panics, is distressed or is at risk of sustaining injury to itself), it is released quickly.

- Collar is made of leather, nylon or other pliable and durable material.

- Goats that are tethered are calm and have been trained as kids to accept approach and handling by humans and have been trained to accept tethering after weaning, but before one year of age.

- Where a goat is on a roadside verge, the placement of the anchor and length of tether is such that the goat cannot get into the path of vehicles but the tether is of sufficient length that the goat is able to exercise and access sufficient amounts of feed.

- Sites that are to be used for tethering goats are examined beforehand for potentially harmful objects that a goat could eat such as toxic plants or litter and for objects or vegetation that might snag or catch on the tether or collar and prevent the animal's movement.

- Tethered goats have access to suitable shelter and are not showing signs of cold stress.

- Food and water requirements of restrained (including tethered) goats are met according to food and water minimum standards and indicators.

- Tethered goats have the ability to walk and move around within the constraints of the tethered range.

Recommended Best Practice

- Goats should be kept in herds or at least with one social companion. If this is not possible, goats should be kept where they can see or hear other goats (or other animals).

- Stock handlers should be trained in the safe operation and rapid release of goats from restraints and facilities.

- Backing gates should be used carefully and should not be used in a manner likely to result in pain, injury or distress.

- Goats should not be tethered as they are social animals.

- Chains should not be used as a collar for goats.

- Tripod collars or hobbles should not be used to limit a goat's ability to move.

Mustering and Droving

The mustering and droving of extensively managed or feral goats has the potential to significantly affect their welfare. The handler's skill lies in understanding the behavior of the animals and adapting their own behavior (and that of any dogs) in a way that facilitates mustering while minimising stress to the animals. Mustering is best undertaken as slowly and as quietly as possible, although it is recognised that certain categories of goats, e.g. feral goats, will require more encouragement than those more familiar with human contact. Knowledge of camping (resting) areas, grazing patterns and movement routes and times will facilitate the mustering of feral goats. Goat farmers/handlers need to be aware of their responsibilities and liabilities with regard to council regulations and road rules when undertaking stock movement activities.

Minimum Standard

- Goats being moved on foot must not be forced to proceed at a pace likely to cause exhaustion, heat stress or injury.

Example Indicators for Minimum Standard for Mustering and Droving

- Goats are calm and move steadily when mustered.

- The pace of mustering or droving is that of the slowest animals in the mob, with particular attention given to kids, goats that are pregnant and those with illness or injury.

- If any goat being mustered or driven is seen to have difficulty breathing (mouth open and tongue hanging out) then it is allowed to rest and recover.

- Goats are settled and calm when they reach the destination yard, with little bullying.

- When injuries occur while mustering, goats receive immediate care and attention.

Recommended Best Practice

After mustering or droving, animals should be provided with suitable conditions and time to settle down, mother up or find shelter before further handling takes place or before the onset of darkness.

Mixing Goats

Goats like to live in groups in which they establish social hierarchies. Whenever animals are introduced into a herd, they will be challenged as newcomers and will have to establish their place in the group. These challenges can be aggressive and lead to injury and distress, especially where goats have horns. Such behavior needs to be managed and this is particularly important when introducing young goats into a herd for the first time. Bucks are potentially dangerous at all times and especially during the mating season. Bucks need to be handled with special care to ensure their own safety and that of other animals.

Goats with horns are at a distinct advantage during social challenges and can inflict serious injuries. This is more likely to happen when animals are being yarded or space is restricted. It is preferable that dairy goats are disbudded to limit the opportunity for injury from horns. Running goats together in mobs of similar ages will also reduce the impact of social bullying on younger goats.

Minimum Standard

- Where goats are mixed, they must be managed to minimize the effects of aggression.

Example Indicators for Minimum Standard for Mixing Goats

- Sufficient space is provided to enable bullied goats to move away from their aggressor.

- Goats subjected to persistent bullying are removed from the herd.

- Particular care is taken when mixing horned goats.

Recommended Best Practice

- The introduction of new animals to the herd should not occur more frequently than necessary, because of the social distress involved while the introduced and resident goats re-establish a hierarchy.

- Goats should be provided with sufficient space so that newcomers can move into free space if pushed or bunted by other animals.

Feed and Water

Food

When considering the amount of food, nutrients and water that a goat requires, a number of different factors need to be taken into account e.g. age, physiological state (growing, pregnant, lactating) and weather conditions. Feed requirements vary throughout the year, but are generally greatest during lactation, late pregnancy, growth, during periods of excessive cold and following shearing. Pregnant does are especially vulnerable following winter shearing, as are cashmere goats with limited opportunity for hair regrowth and may require increased feeding for up to six weeks following shearing. Nutritional requirements are best determined by monitoring body condition and live weight.

Plants, including pasture and browse, are the main source of feed for goats in farming systems. There is considerable variation in pastoral management systems associated with seasonal and climatic differences, land and soil types and whether the system is extensive or intensive. Regular body condition scoring is an important management tool. Body condition scoring is a useful method of assessment to determine whether animals are receiving adequate nutrition (Schedule II – Body Condition Scoring (BCS)). Hair and fleece may hide body contours, especially in fibre goats, so goats must be handled and the bony points of the ribs, backbone and pelvis palpated for accurate assessment of body condition. Where animals are housed or fed supplements, herd hierarchy and bullying can limit access of individual goats to feed. This can be dealt with by appropriate design and management (e.g. by segregating animals or providing extra feeder space). Human intervention may be required to ensure all goats have access to feed.

Goats can gain significant condition (1.0 - 1.5 points) on spring and early summer grass and so individuals with access to large amounts of grazing at this time need to be monitored to ensure they do not become obese. Pregnant does may lose body condition during late pregnancy and early lactation and so care needs to be taken to ensure that they are receiving adequate nutrition at this time. Goats have a high requirement for minerals, especially selenium and iodine. Goats may be reluctant to leave shelter for extended periods during wet weather so it may be necessary to provide additional supplement feed that the goats can obtain without leaving their shelter. Goats will also not eat muddy or contaminated feed or pasture and so care needs to be taken to ensure that the available feed is clean. Many feedstuffs can constitute a danger to animal health. Goats prefer to browse and this may reduce their internal parasite burden, but they will readily eat many toxic plants. Stock handlers need to be aware of the possible dangers such as frothy bloat, nitrate poisoning, effects of toxic plants (including garden prunings), rumen acidosis, choke and the effects of fungal or bacterial contamination of feed.

Minimum Standard

- Goats of all ages must receive sufficient quantities of food and nutrients to enable each animal to:

  - Maintain good health.

  - Meet their physiological requirements.

  - Minimize metabolic and nutritional disorders.

- If any goat shows signs of emaciation or if the body condition score of any individual goat (other than kids or yearlings) falls below 2 (on a scale of 0–5), urgent remedial action must be taken to improve condition or the animal must be destroyed humanely.

- Automated feeding systems must be checked at least once every 24 hours to ensure they are in working order and any problems rectified promptly.

Example Indicators for Minimum Standard for Food

- Goats are given sufficient daily feed to maintain appropriate body condition.

- Any goat at a body condition score less than 2 is identified and receives appropriate remedial action through improved nutrition, husbandry practice, veterinary attention or is culled from the herd.

- Recently shorn goats are provided with additional feed.

- Staff understand and ensure that they quickly identify, seek advice on and remedy: Nutritional deficiencies and metabolic diseases – Conditions that might arise from faulty feeding such as poisoning, rumen acidosis or metabolic disturbance and have the resources to prevent or manage these conditions.

- Any automated feeding system supplies the correct amount of feed when tested.

Recommended Best Practice

- Body condition score at kidding should be at least 3 but not obese (BCS 5), to minimize kidding and metabolic problems.

- Goats should be maintained within the range of body condition scores 2 to 4 inclusive.

- Female goats should be well fed to meet pregnancy requirements and in summer and autumn to meet lactational and fibre growth demands and to ensure that they are in good body condition prior to winter.

- Growing goats should be well fed in all seasons to realise their growth and future production potential.

- When browse and pasture growth are not adequate, alternative or supplementary feed should be provided.

- Changes in diet should be introduced gradually over several days, especially if feeding grain and other readily fermentable carbohydrates. This will allow rumen bacteria to adjust and thus prevent digestive problems and reduce the risk of death through grain poisoning (acidosis).

- Feeding methods should be designed to reduce fouling and wastage.

- Measures should be taken to minimize access of goats and particularly pregnant does, to toxic plants and noxious or harmful materials including:
    - Most ornamental garden plants.
    - Toxic weeds such as ragwort and tutu (although these may be tolerated in small quantities, meaning that goats may be used in weed control programmes provided they have choice and are not forced to consume excessive amounts.
    - Lead-based paints and toxic timber preservatives.
    - Electrical fittings and materials used in buildings such as plastics and papers.
    - Loose fencing wire.
    - Twine and plastic wrap, such as baleage wrapping.

- When feeding brassicas and concentrates, a supplementary source of roughage such as hay, barley straw, silage or baleage should be added to the diet to aid proper digestion.

- Goats maintained for long periods of time on diets containing a high proportion of grain should receive appropriate dietary supplementation to ensure they maintain levels of essential vitamins and minerals.

- Supplementary feeds should be conserved and stored in a way that feed quality is preserved, mould-growth is inhibited and contamination by rodents, birds and cats is prevented.

- Mould-contaminated or excessively dusty supplementary feeds should not be fed to goats.

- Animals in ill-health, poor condition, late pregnancy or early lactation should not be deprived of food for longer than 12 hours.

Water

The provision of an adequate supply of water is critical for maintaining goat health and welfare. Water needs for different classes of goats vary widely and there is seasonal variation as well. If water needs are not met then animal health and welfare both deteriorate.

Water and shade needs increase when goats are grazing dry summer pastures and during drought, especially for young and light-weight goats. Appropriate water allowance varies with animal size, diet and lactational state. When planning water for dairy goats, ensure that the reticulation system can provide nine litres/head/day. Goats drink less water than sheep when shade is provided, but in the absence of shade they will drink more.

Young goats and kids will often mistakenly jump into troughs during play. Deep troughs may be covered to prevent such accidents. Concrete blocks or bricks can be placed in the trough to enable any goat that falls in to escape.

Minimum Standard

- All goats must have access daily to a reliable supply of drinking water that is palatable, sufficient for their needs and not harmful to their health.

- In the event of a water delivery system failure, remedial action must be taken to ensure that daily water requirements are met.

- Any goats retained in yards or barns for longer than 12 hours must have access to drinking water.

- The water delivery system must be at a height that is accessible to all goats being supplied.

Example Indicators for Water

- Goats are provided with sufficient water.

- Water quality is monitored and does not contain any contaminants at a level harmful to the health of goats.

- The water reticulation system provides a sufficient volume of water to meet the daily needs of the goats, is monitored and maintained efficiently and any failure is rectified immediately.

- Yards and barns where goats are retained for periods of 12 hours or longer have an adequate water supply to meet the goat's requirements.

- The height of troughs and drinkers ensure that goats do not suffer any injuries or distress and the smallest goat in any herd can reach the water supply.

Recommended Best Practice

- Watering facilities should be designed to reduce fouling and wastage.

- Troughs should be cleaned regularly and often to ensure that water is available and uncontaminated.

- Goats held in yards and barns for longer than six hours should have access to drinking water.

Shelter and Housing Facilities

Shelter

Goats do not possess the ability to withstand cold conditions to the same extent as other species of livestock due to a different distribution of fat and consistency of their coat. Goat farmers in New Zealand therefore need to be aware of the animal welfare implications of inadequate shelter and develop management plans to provide shelter in adverse weather and after shearing to prevent heat and cold stress.

While goats are resilient to cold temperatures when conditions are dry, occasions arise when weather extremes can cause stress and goats are particularly prone to hypothermia when conditions are wet. Shelter can also be important when environmental conditions are not extreme. Goats seek shelter for kidding and to hide their young and a goat that is ill may separate itself from its group to seek protection in a sheltered area.

Signs of Cold and Heat Exposure in Goats

Early signs of significant cold exposure in goats include behavioral changes such as seeking shelter, facing away from the wind or rain with the back hunched, heads down, not eating, shivering and huddling together. Where animals are exposed to cold conditions with which they cannot cope, their core body temperature drops below the normal range (hypothermia). As hypothermia progresses, animals become depressed and listless and may die. Such depression and listlessness indicates the need for urgent remedial action.

When goats are exposed to conditions that cause heat stress, they will try to find relief in a number of ways. These include increased respiration rate, reduced grazing activity, seeking shade and increased water consumption. If the heat load continues to rise, animals will progress to open mouth panting with tongues extended when severe. Fibre goats in heavy fleece are more susceptible to heat exposure. Effective shelter at stock level may be provided in a number of ways including the use of topographical features such as caves and overhangs, gullies or hollows of adequate depth, natural features such as stands of trees or scrub, hedges, shelter belts or thickets of plants like pampas and gorse.

Alternatively, artificial structures such as field shelters, buildings or hay stacks can be used. Shelter needs to have the effect of providing goats with the ability to stay dry, to get off wet ground and to get out of the wind. Management plans for dealing with stressful climatic events include ensuring that goats are in good physical condition to withstand periods of stress and by providing additional feed of appropriate type, e.g. increased roughage to help generate rumen heat and relieve cold stress.

Unweaned kids that are being hand-reared can usually be protected from the effects of adverse weather by housing with dry bedding in a well ventilated building without draughts. Where kids are suckling from a doe, shelter should be provided so that the doe can ensure that the kid is situated in a sheltered area.

While hypothermia is generally not a problem for a well fed doe with normal hair and fleece cover, it may be a problem for both does and kids when kidding occurs in cold, wet or windy weather. Newborn, wet or sick kids and those that have been transported or deprived of food, are particularly vulnerable and need to be managed accordingly. Goats up to yearling age are more susceptible to cold than adults. Adult goats can also experience hypothermic stress during cold or wet weather, especially after shearing or if they are thin or unhealthy.

Caution is required where bad weather is prolonged over a number of days, as animals will remain in shelter for extended periods and may not eat, thus increasing the risk of hypothermia. Subordinate goats may be evicted from housing or shelter by dominant goats. All goats need access to sufficient shelter.

Protection can be provided by the appropriate use of covers, especially for sick animals and kids. Covered animals may be bullied and will need to be monitored. Horned goats may get their horns tangled in covers and so will need to be monitored and separated if necessary. When covering kids, stock handlers need to ensure that the doe recognises and accepts the kids for feeding. While ambient temperature and humidity are important factors contributing to heat stress, solar radiation is a major factor contributing to heat loading, especially in dark-coated animals. This is effectively reduced by shade. A substantial increase in body temperature may occur during mustering or when walking long distances on hot days. When goats are yarded in conditions that are hot and dusty there is an increased risk of an outbreak of enzootic pneumonia (a specific pneumonia condition that is linked to handling/management, especially associated with mustering). Shade is especially important to help mitigate this risk. Information on preparing for emergencies and adverse events can be obtained from Federated Farmers, industry organisations, MPI, local or national goat associations, farm management professionals or veterinarians.

Special attention is needed for:

- Newborn kids.

- Newly-shorn goats especially cashmere-bearing goats.

- Does close to kidding and at kidding.

- Lactating does.

- Animals in ill-health or stressed from other causes.

- Goats in areas subject to extreme weather.

Minimum Standard

- All goats must have access to shelter to reduce the risks to health and welfare caused by exposure to cold or heat.

- Goats close to kidding must be provided with effective shelter to shield the dam and newborn kid from weather conditions.

- Very young kids that have been removed from their mothers for hand rearing must be provided with shelter at all times.

- Newly shorn goats must be provided with extra feed and effective shelter until their fleece has regrown sufficiently to provide some protection.

- Where animals develop problems associated with exposure to adverse weather conditions (including adverse heat or cold), priority must be given to remedial action that will minimize the consequences of such exposure.

Example Indicators for Shelter

- There is sufficient accessible shelter available for all goats in the event of adverse weather.

- Newborn kids being hand-reared are provided with shelter and additional warmth (e.g. with a heat lamp) where conditions are cold.

- Sick goats, kids being hand-reared and goats after shearing have access to shelter during inclement weather.

- Where environmental conditions are such that goats start to develop signs of cold stress (e.g. shivering and huddling), immediate action is taken to move goats to effective shelter and provide additional feed and their condition is monitored until it improves.

- Where environmental conditions are such that goats start to develop signs of heat stress (e.g. open mouth panting with tongues extended), immediate action is taken to provide goats with more appropriate shade and their condition is monitored until it improves.

- Planning for shearing includes planning the feed supply and shelter required to meet the goat's additional energy requirements and to ensure that all goats can maintain their body temperature until their fleece has sufficiently regrown.

- Goats receive additional inspections when adverse weather occurs after shearing.

Recommended Best Practice

- Activities such as mustering, prolonged yarding and transportation should be avoided in hot, sunny and humid conditions likely to result in heat stress.

- Timing of shearing should be managed to minimize the risks associated with bad weather.

- To reduce the animal welfare impact of drought, floods and storms farmers should have an emergency response plan in place that will ensure that they can continue to meet their obligations under this Code should any of these environmental extremes eventuate.

Farm Facilities

Farm facilities include fences, gates, holding pens, internal yards and additional areas such as a milking parlour or shearing facility, depending upon the nature of the goat production system. The proper construction, maintenance and operation of farm facilities are important to facilitate management and provide a safe and hygienic environment for procedures such as milking and shearing. Careful planning and design will assist movement of animals and minimize stress of both animals and handlers.

Minimum Standard

- All facilities must be designed, constructed, maintained and operated in a manner that minimizes the likelihood of distress or injury to animals.

- All electrical fittings and attachments to mains voltage must be out of reach of goats or protected from interference or damage by goats.

- Floors must be constructed of a non-slip material.

Example Indicators for Farm Facilities

- The design and construction of facilities encourages the free movement of goats, enables them to walk comfortably and prevents injury, crowding or smothering.

- Stock handlers are trained and familiar with the operation of farm facilities and understand how incorrect operation may affect the goats in their care.

- Floor surfaces are not slippery.

- The farm maintenance programme ensures that problems such as damaged flooring, protrusions and sharp objects are removed or repaired in a timely manner.

- Where injuries related to facilities occur, the reason is determined and the problem rectified.

- There are no toxic health remedies, toxic materials, power cables or fittings in areas to which goats have access.

- If sheep and cattle facilities are used, they are adapted to suit goats.

Recommended Best Practice

- Loading ramps should be constructed with non-slip footing and have side-boards or rails to prevent animals falling off or getting their legs trapped.

- Netting fences that allow goats with horns to become trapped should not be used.

- Excrement should not be permitted to accumulate to an extent that it poses a threat to the health and welfare of goats.

- Toxic paint and timber preservatives should not be used on surfaces or floors that are accessible to goats.

- Any mechanical equipment used in the handling and management of goats should be maintained in sound working order.

- Goat shearing facilities should be designed, constructed, maintained and located in a way that ensures shearing can be conducted in an environment that maximizes safety and minimizes stress for the animals, shearers and staff.

Housing for Goats

While barns provide shelter from inclement weather, the main reason for this practice is to control internal parasites. In these situations animals are totally dependent on their handlers for all their daily requirements, welfare and safety and farmers need to be aware there are additional responsibilities of care. The well-being of the animals needs to be a key consideration when goat housing systems are designed and constructed. Does and kids require accommodation that is dry, well ventilated and draught-free. The optimal space allowances for housed animals vary depending on whether goats receive some or all of their feed supply in the housing area. The important factor is to allow enough area per goat to ensure that they all have the opportunity for adequate rest.

Goats prefer to lie on soft surfaces and are reluctant to lie down when the surface is slippery or wet. If the surface type and area per goat are not adequate there will be reduced lying times, underfeeding and an increased incidence of disease.

As a guide, a level of 10–15 ppm of ammonia in the air can be detected by smell and an ammonia level over 25 ppm may cause eye and nasal irritation in people. In general, if the level of noxious gases within a housing facility is uncomfortable for people, it will be uncomfortable for goats. Such levels compromise animal welfare and may predispose goats to respiratory disease and reduced performance.

The material used as bedding or on surfaces and flooring, for goats needs to be chosen with the aim of minimising the presence of toxic chemicals that could be poisonous to goats (e.g. timber preservatives, some paint) or materials that could cause irritation of the skin (e.g. rimu sawdust). As a guide, 50 lux is sufficient light to read a newspaper at arm's length. Signs of bullying include bite marks on ears and hocks, bare skin patches and ill-thrift. These are also an indication that goats do not have good access to feed. Excessively bullied goats will tend to remain outside of the main group.

Care is required where hand-reared kids are group housed as they often crowd together, which can result in smothering of the kids. To help prevent this, corners need to be screened from the pen and if providing an external source of heat, e.g. a heat lamp, measures need to be taken to ensure that kids cannot crowd below the heat source.

Minimum Standard

- Goats must be able to lie down and rest comfortably for a sufficient time each day to meet their behavioral needs.

- Group housed goats must be able to stand, move about and lie down without undue interference from each other.

- Bedding must be of good quality material, friable and with minimal risk of toxic agent contamination.

- Goats must be inspected at least once a day in the housing area for signs of discomfort or distress.

- Ventilation control or other measures must ensure that housed goats do not become overheated or cold stressed and prevent a build up of harmful concentrations of gases such as ammonia and carbon dioxide.

- Immediate and appropriate action must be taken to reduce ammonia levels if they exceed 25 ppm at goat level.

- Goats must be managed in groups of suitable size and age and with regard to whether they have horns, to minimize injuries resulting from aggressive behavior.

- Goats must not be released from prolonged periods indoors without ready access to shelter and shade.

- Goats must be provided with natural or artificial light of appropriate intensity for a minimum of nine hours each day.

Example Indicators for Housing for Goats

- Goats are all able to lie down and rest simultaneously.

- At least 2 m2 of space is provided per individual mature housed goat.

- Bedding materials are dry and comfortable for goats to lie on.

- Humidity, dust, temperature or ammonia (as detected by smell) are kept within acceptable levels.

- Immediate corrective action is taken where ammonia levels are 25 ppm or greater (by increasing ventilation, reducing litter moisture or reducing stocking density) and instances where this has occurred are documented.

- Waste food and contaminated bedding material does not accumulate to an extent that it poses a threat to the health and welfare of the animals (e.g. wet, mouldy or noxious).

- Where thermal stress occurs it is immediately remedied.

- Goats do not show signs of excessive bullying such as bite marks on ears and hocks, bare skin patches or ill-thrift.

- Group composition and size is organised to avoid excessive bullying.

- Inspections of goats show minimal signs of discomfort, distress or disease (e.g. sneezing, coughing, heavy breathing, runny noses or eyes).

- When goats that have been housed indoors for long periods of time are released, they are provided with shelter in weather conditions that are likely to result in heat stress, cold stress or sunburn.

- Contingency plans are in place for dealing with any hazards or emergencies and incorporate the ability to rapidly release goats into a secure environment.

Recommended Best Practice

- Emergency response plans should be in place for potential hazards and all stock handlers should be aware of these plans and the routines required to ensure the safety and welfare of goats and handlers in an emergency, e.g. evacuation plans.

- Feeding and watering systems should be constructed to be readily accessible, prevent competition and take into account the feed, stock type and size of the enclosure.

- The bedding area should be dry and covered with material to provide a comfortable resting surface.

- A minimum space allowance of 3 m² per mature goat should be provided to reduce the chance that underfoot conditions become wet.

- Ammonia levels should not exceed levels of 10 ppm at ground level.

- During inspection periods, natural or artificial light of at least 50 lux should be available at the level of resting goats in loafing barns and houses.

- A feeding space/trough width of 40 cm per adult goat should be allowed when all goats need access to feed. If food is continually available then space may be less.

- A separate pen should be provided to hold and treat unwell or injured goats until recovery or to house goats that persistently bully other goats or are persistently bullied by other goats.

- Environmental enrichment should be used by making 'toys' available such as boxes or rocks on which the goats can climb or by providing positive human contact or a radio to accustom goats to a range of noises and voices.

- Goats that are unfamiliar to each other should be monitored when mixed, to ensure that fighting is kept to a minimum.

Husbandry Practices: Kidding Does

Kidding is a critical period for the welfare of both doe and kid. Potential compromises to animal welfare at this time are diverse and include feeding levels during pregnancy, disturbance from other animals and humans, predisposition to dystocia (difficulties during birthing), the weather and available shelter. The appropriate level of supervision will differ depending whether does are intensively or extensively managed.

Domestication of the goat has meant that stock handlers have to balance the natural tendencies of goats to give birth undisturbed and often in isolation, with any requirements to assist with difficult births. The requirements of does during kidding may also vary between breeds with some breeds being more likely to exhibit problems during kidding than others. Disturbing or providing assistance to does that are farmed extensively or with minimal intervention may lead to the doe deserting the offspring. Nutrition around the kidding period is especially important. Trace element and mineral status need to be considered, as well as feed quality and quantity. The important features to be taken into consideration when deciding to assist a doe to kid are:

- An assessment of the size and number of kids and whether they are alive and in the correct orientation for delivery.

- An assessment of doe health and condition.

- The amount and direction of traction, which alters as the kid enters and passes through the pelvic canal.

Minimum Standard

- Intensively farmed goats must be inspected frequently before and after kidding to ensure that they are not experiencing difficulties.

- If any doe is having difficulty kidding and the stock handler is unable to resolve the problem, expert advice must be sought as soon as possible or the animal humanely destroyed.

- Excessive traction must not be used to kid any doe.

Example Indicators for Kidding Does

- Mortality rates (kids and does) are documented and minimized.

- Sufficient staff with appropriate training are available to inspect animals around the time of kidding.

- Farm routines show that inspections occur at least twice every 24 hours in intensive farming situations, that inspection results are analysed and necessary changes are incorporated into future planning.

- Stock handlers have knowledge of kidding problems and how to correct them and have appropriate equipment to assist kidding does.

- Stock handlers have knowledge of how to access expert advice and such advice is available and is sought when required.

Recommended Best Practice

- Where animals are unaccustomed to daily supervision such as in extensive systems, breeds or strains suited to easy births and good maternal care should be used. In more intensive systems, where animals are habituated to the presence of humans and management activities, assistance should be provided to animals experiencing difficulties without unduly disturbing others giving birth in the vicinity.

- Easy-kidding sires should be selected for goatling mating as large kids can cause significant injuries to small does.

- Goats close to kidding should be inspected frequently; preferably at least every 6 hours.

- Kidding paddocks should provide dry ground, shelter and protection from adverse weather.

- Does that have been trying to kid for more than 1 hour without progress should be given assistance or veterinary help (kidding in this context means vigorous abdominal straining).

- To minimize the potential for damage to either doe or kid, controlled traction should only be used if the operator has diagnosed an unrestricted birth canal and the kid is in the normal position for delivery and should be conducted with plenty of lubrication. The amount of traction used should be no more than a single person can apply.

Hand Rearing and Fostering Kids

Newborn and young animals are particularly vulnerable to negative welfare outcomes resulting from adverse environmental conditions and poor management. Consequently, all kids require special attention to ensure they are healthy and to allow their individual needs to be assessed. In dairying systems, kids are removed from their mothers at a young age.

Good management of young kids is essential for their welfare. Some are destined to only live a few days before they are killed, but that does not remove the obligation to manage them to the same standard as every other animal on the farm. Kids from meat or fibre goats that are rejected by their mothers or orphaned may be fostered onto nurse does, hand fed or humanely destroyed.

Colostrum is the first milk produced by the doe after kidding and contains special nutrients and antibodies that are essential to protect the kid from disease. The newborn kid absorbs antibodies from colostrum, but begins to lose this ability from about six hours after birth. In addition, the concentration of antibodies in the colostrum diminishes rapidly after the doe has kidded and is reduced markedly after two milkings. A newborn kid does not have a functional rumen and therefore needs to be given liquid feeds until the rumen has developed sufficiently to allow it to utilise solids as its sole source of nutrition.

Colostrum, either fresh or stored, can provide local immunity in the gut and is a highly digestible, high quality food. Note that antibodies cannot be absorbed by the kid beyond 24–36 hours after birth and so colostrum needs to be fed as soon as possible after birth. Cow colostrum, ewe colostrum or commercial dried whole colostrum may be used if goat colostrum is unavailable or where a disease management programme is in place. Doe vaccination programmes, e.g. clostridial vaccines to boost the level of antibodies in colostrum, may be considered. These practices can be discussed with a veterinarian.

Hygienic practices are required for the maintenance of feeding equipment, bedding material and toileting areas to keep kids healthy. When kids are fed in groups, care is needed to ensure that all kids, even the slowest drinkers, are consuming what they need.

Minimum Standard

- Premature kids that are unlikely to survive and kids that have debilitating congenital defects, must be humanely destroyed immediately.

- Kids must be handled and moved in a manner that minimizes distress and avoids injury or suffering.

- Newborn kids must receive sufficient colostrum or a good quality commercial colostrum substitute.

- Hand-reared kids must be given suitable liquid feeds until the rumen has developed sufficiently to allow it to use solids as the sole feed source.

Example Indicators for Hand Rearing and Fostering Kids

- Planning for kidding includes ensuring that stocks of colostrum or a suitable substitute are on hand to supplement kids if necessary.

- Stock handlers' behavior towards kids is patient.

- Stock handlers understand the importance of colostrum and are trained to provide it when a kid has not received it in sufficient amounts, e.g. by stomach tube.

- Farm staff are trained in the humane destruction of kids.

- Stock handlers are trained to recognise if a kid is not receiving adequate feed and remedy the situation.

- Kid-rearing programmes provide kids with their specific nutritional needs as a preruminant.

- Kids are not weaned until they are receiving at least 75% of their daily feed requirements from solid feed.

Recommended Best Practice

- Every kid should receive colostrum as soon as possible after birth, preferably within the first six hours. If it is suspected that a kid has not received colostrum, then colostrum or a suitable substitute should be given to the kid within 24 hours of birth.

- Colostrum, milk or milk replacer should be fed at the rate of 10-12% of bodyweight per day, preferably in four or more feeds per day.

- Kids should not be weaned until they are at least six weeks old and preferably not until they are 8-10 weeks of age.

- Any technique used to foster a kid onto a doe should not compromise the welfare of either doe or kid, should cause minimal stress to both the doe and the kid and should be closely supervised.

- When two or more kids are fostered onto a nurse doe they should be of a similar size and age.

- Nurse does with kids at foot should be inspected at least once every 24 hours to ensure that both does and kids are in good health.

- During the first 48 hours of life, liquid feeds should be warm, but not above the kid's normal body temperature (39°C).

- Colostrum should not be overheated or micro-waved as this will destroy antibodies.

- Kids should also have access to solid feeds (appropriate concentrates, hay, silage or pasture) from their first week of life. Consumption of these solids will enhance rumen development and will contribute increasingly to satisfying the kid's nutrient requirements.

- Kids should have adequate access to fresh water.

Lactating Does and Milking Systems

In dairying systems, efficient milking is essential for the good health, welfare and productivity of the doe. The modern dairy goat may produce more milk than its kids can consume and needs to be milked regularly for good udder health; farmers traditionally milk goats twice a day. The milking process needs to be carried out calmly and with regular routines to create a stress-free environment for the doe. This will ensure that complete milk let-down occurs in the doe before or during milking. Gathering goats from the paddock or housing facility, driving along the race, holding them in the yard and entering and exiting from the milking bail are all part of this process.

Milk removal, conducted in good environmental conditions and with an efficient milking machine, is complete after about 6-8 minutes for most does, depending on milk yield and rate of milk flow. Signs of discomfort (kicking the cups off and constant movement by the doe while milking) and an increased incidence of sores on the teats can indicate faults in the vacuum level or pulsation system or the presence of stray electrical voltages (electrical shorts) in the farm dairy.

Signs of poor teat condition include redness and chapping. This is more likely to occur during wet and windy weather.

Minimum Standard

- All does must be milked or suckle kids frequently enough during lactation to minimize discomfort and maintain udder health.

- Milking equipment must be well maintained to minimize the risk of damage and infection of the teats and udder.

Example Indicators for Milking

- Any goat with an over-extended udder or other signs of discomfort (e.g. restlessness, heat or pain on palpation) is examined immediately, the cause determined and remedial action taken.

- Upon inspection of teats and udders, minimal damage from milking equipment is observed.

- Stock handlers have knowledge of udder health and have procedures in place to recognise and treat problems.

- Records show that the milking plant has passed its routine inspection and audit.

Recommended Best Practice

- Regular routines for milking should be established, in order to minimize or avoid distress.

- Does in dairying systems should be milked within 12 hours of separation from their kids.

- All lactating does, including those being sold or exhibited, should be milked or suckle kids at least once every 24 hours unless good management practices dictate otherwise.

- To minimize the risk of discomfort or damage to the teats, the partial vacuum in the milking machine should not be higher than 40 kPa and the teat-cup liners and the pulsation system should function properly.

- Care should be taken to avoid over-milking.

- Milking machines should be tested at least once a year and more frequently if the milking process is compromised, as indicated by milking speed, teat damage and doe behavior. All faults should be corrected immediately.

- The risk of teat and udder infections should be minimized by practising good hygiene.

- The teat condition of does in dairying systems should be monitored and an appropriate remedy used if condition deteriorates.

- Goatlings that are to be managed in dairying systems should be familiarised with the milking facility prior to kidding.

- Where there is a risk of an extended failure of the electricity supply, provision should be made for an independent generator to operate the milking machine and ancillary equipment.

Drying-off Dairy Does

To prepare for their next kidding, does in dairying systems generally go through a drying-off process to end their lactation. Individual animals may be dried-off earlier for other farm management reasons (e.g. feed shortages). The aim is to shut down milk secretion and allow the teat canal to seal as rapidly as possible.

Does may be milked less frequently before drying off to assist with discomfort at drying off. Although lower feeding levels seem to reduce discomfort after dry-off, does fed less are likely to experience hunger. Investigation of alternative dry-off procedures, such as feeding low-quality diets ad libitum, is recommended as these methods can maximize the benefits of lower milk yields before dry-off, without causing hunger.

Recommended Best Practice

- The drying-off process should be done in a manner that minimizes discomfort.

- For at least three weeks after dry-off, does should be monitored weekly for signs of udder pain or swelling.

- Dairy does that are being dried off should be kept in a clean area to minimize the risk of udder infection.

Shearing and Dagging Fibre Goats

Shearing is an important part of fibre goat farming and goats need to be handled carefully during the procedure and managed well afterwards to prevent hypothermia. The timing of shearing needs to be carefully considered, heed taken of warnings of approaching storms or inclement weather and planning needs to include provision of shelter from unexpected storms. The most appropriate type of shelter varies between farms and may be natural or artificial. The appropriate frequency of shearing varies according to the type of goat, with Angora goats (mohairproducing) generally shorn every six months. For Angora goats, separate parts of the fleece may also be removed to promote their welfare. Dag removal from around the breech helps reduce the risk of fly-strike as well as reducing discomfort and inflammation of the underlying skin. Fibre growing from the face may be removed to prevent vision being obscured and from the belly to facilitate suckling. When shearing

Cashmere goats, "patch shearing" can be used. This technique involves shearing only the areas which are growing harvestable cashmere, thus helping to prevent hypothermia. Cashmere goats require special consideration at shearing time for several reasons. They are generally only shorn during the winter or early spring when weather conditions are cool and may be stormy. Their fibre production is seasonal and they may have very little regrowth and their increased feed and shelter requirements following shearing may persist for many weeks to prevent the occurrence of hypothermia. Cashmere goats are often kept in extensive situations with little regular contact with humans so mustering and penning for shearing add to the stress they experience at shearing. Goats may also experience additional stress if shorn with a full rumen so a short time off feed prior to shearing will be beneficial in this case.

Newly shorn fibre goats are especially vulnerable to adverse weather conditions and require more feed than normal for six weeks after shearing to sustain body temperature and to maintain body condition and immune function. In addition to using patch shearing to help prevent hypothermia in Cashmere goats, there are also major benefits from using combs that retain some of the coat. Goats with a residual coat length of 4 mm need additional feed to maintain body warmth at ambient temperatures below 15 °C, whereas an 8 mm coat means that additional feed will be required below 11 °C.

Minimum Standard

- Fibre goats must be shorn as frequently as is necessary to mitigate animal health and welfare concerns from long fleeces.

- In winter and in districts subject to cold or wet weather, fibre goats must be shorn in a way that ensures that they retain an insulating layer of fibre e.g. patch shearing or by using snow or cover combs, lifters or blade shears.

- Goats must not be shorn if the forecast is for cold wet weather, unless the animals are provided with adequate shelter to minimize the risk of hypothermia.

- Goats must be provided with sufficient shelter and additional feed (especially hay or other suitable fibre) after shearing to minimize the risk of hypothermia.

- All severe cuts or injuries must be treated immediately.

Example Indicators for Shearing and Dagging Fibre Goats

- Planning for shearing includes careful consideration of weather forecasts, provision of shelter and adequate feed, including making food and water available for animals immediately after shearing.

- No fibre goat has an excessively long coat that is either soiled, impedes the goat's movement or causes skin or other disease, especially in hot weather conditions.

- Shearing is timed to coincide with forecast of good weather. Where weather forecasts are for cold or wet conditions, shearing does not proceed unless adequate shelter is provided.

- In winter and when there is risk of hypothermia, an insulating layer of fibre remains after shearing.

Recommended Best Practice

- Shearing and dagging should be carried out skilfully and carefully by competent operators to ensure that shearing cuts, especially those to the teats, vulva and prepuce are kept to a minimum.

- Angora goats should be shorn at least every eight months.

- Freshly shorn goats should not be put into dusty yards for longer than necessary to reduce risk of infection in shearing cuts.

Reproductive Technologies and Selection of Animals for Mating

Breeding management techniques and programmes that optimise genetic potential have been adopted in all sectors of the goat industry in New Zealand. In addition to selecting animals with desirable genotypes for breeding, there are a number of established and developing technologies being used to facilitate genetic gains and better manage animals.

Multiple births are common with goats, especially the dairy breeds where three or four kids per pregnancy are common. Does carrying multiple pregnancies require more feed during the latter stages of pregnancy. Gestation length may be shorter and there may be more malpresentations or difficult births and poorer bonding between doe and offspring. These factors mean increased supervision is necessary when multiple births occur to ensure newborn animals survive and receive colostrum.

Minimum Standard

- Electroejaculation and laparoscopic artificial insemination must be carried out only by veterinarians or by trained and competent operators under veterinary supervision, using appropriate pain relief, sedatives or anaesthesia.

- Cervical artificial insemination and pregnancy diagnosis must only be carried out by persons trained and competent with the techniques.

NAWAC has recommended that surgical embryo transfer be listed as a significant surgical procedure, as defined by the Act.

Recommended Best Practice

- Less invasive procedures (e.g. semen collection using an artificial vagina) should be used in preference to more invasive ones (e.g. semen collection by electro-ejaculation).

- Any procedure used to alter the pattern of seasonal breeding or to increase litter size, should only be used where the extra requirements to ensure good welfare (feed, farm labour, shelter and other inputs required before and after the animal gives birth) have been thoroughly assessed and can be provided.

- When selecting goats for breeding, attention should be given to selecting animals of appropriate physical size (both buck and doe), kidding experience and previous management history to match the system in which they will be farmed (i.e. previously kept extensively or intensively).

Painful Husbandry Procedures

Farming goats involves a number of husbandry procedures such as disbudding, castration and occasionally dehorning which have been identified as causing pain and distress. These procedures are covered in a separate Code of Welfare and readers are directed to Code of Welfare: Painful Husbandry Procedures for information and requirements.

Minimising the stress, pain or discomfort of these procedures requires attention to the suitability of the area in which the operation is performed, the catching facilities, the type and amount of restraint, the selection and maintenance of appropriate instruments, good hygiene, the subsequent care of the animals and the skill of the stock handlers carrying out the procedures.

The skull of a goat kid is much thinner than that of a calf. Thermal cautery disbudding techniques need to be carried out carefully to avoid damaging the underlying tissues, including the brain.

Recommended Best Practice

- Pain relief should be provided when performing any painful husbandry procedure.

- Male goats that are castrated before puberty should be monitored for joint abnormalities and arthritis as they age as, in some cases, they can experience abnormal continued growth of the long bones causing their legs to become distorted.

Animal Identification

Ear tags are commonly used to identify individual goats. Permanent identification such as ear notching, marking and tattooing and branding may also be used. These procedures cause pain and the general principles outlined in the Code of Welfare: Painful Husbandry Procedures apply.

Permanent identification of individual goats is required by various legislation and laws; goat industry organisations can provide further information. Neck bands may be useful for temporary identification of young kids but their use requires supervision to prevent entanglement.

Minimum Standard

- All identification procedures must be applied by a competent operator.

- Pain relief must be used with hot or freeze branding.

Example Indicators for Identification

- No ear injuries or infections are apparent.

Recommended Best Practice

- Goats should not be branded.

- Permanent tags should be inserted using the applicators designed for the purpose and according to the manufacturer's specifications and with good hygiene.

- Goats' ears are very sensitive and care should be taken when inserting ear tags to avoid hitting cartilage ridges or major blood vessels.

- Any infection resulting from tag application should be treated promptly.

- The size and number of tags required should be kept to a minimum.

- Where tattooing is used, it should be carried out by a competent operator.

- The use of ear punches for identification purposes should be restricted to those situations where tagging is not feasible. As little as possible and no more than 10% of ear tissue should be removed using an instrument that is clean and sharp.

- When goats are vaccinated for Johne's disease they are required to have an ear notched and this should be done using the appropriate triangular ear punch tool according to the manufacturer's instructions and with good hygiene.

Pre-transport Selection

When selecting animals for transport, other industry standards and codes for transport need to be considered. In cases of doubt about the condition of an animal, a veterinarian needs to be consulted. A veterinarian can certify an animal as fit for transport, in which case the appropriate documentation must accompany the animal on its journey.

Transporting goats can cause them significant stress. This is particularly the case for feral goats and goats that are not used to human contact. The presence of horned goats in the group will also exacerbate stress. Good stockmanship is essential to minimize anxiety and distress during transportation.

The preparation of mature animals for transport, especially pregnant does, will depend on the method, the distance and the time involved. In particular the suitability of the truck for transport should be considered – some sheep trucks are not appropriate for dairy does. For guidelines on preparation for long-haul journeys, a veterinarian or suitably experienced transport operator should be consulted. Providing sheds and holding facilities that are darkened and minimize noise will assist in settling goats being held for transport.

Minimum Standard

- All goats selected for transport must be examined by the person in charge prior to loading to ensure that they are fit for transport and are able to withstand the journey without suffering unreasonable or unnecessary pain or distress.

- Any animal likely to give birth during transport must not be selected.

- Every unweaned kid to be transported off the farm must have been fed at least half of that day's ration of colostrum or milk, not more than two hours before transportation.

- Lame goats must not be selected for transport.

Example Indicators for Pre-transport Selection

- All goats transported are fit and healthy and can support their weight on all four limbs.

- Unweaned kids to be transported off the farm are given a feed no more than two hours before they are loaded.

- No goat gives birth during transport.

Recommended Best Practice

- The design of holding facilities at loading areas should offer adequate shelter and comfort for all goats, easy access for the stock handler and transport operator and facilitate efficient handling of the animals.

- In the absence of ramps, when goats have to be lifted onto a transporter, their whole body should be supported in the lift.

- Pregnant goats should not be selected for transport in the last three weeks before the expected date of kidding.

- Goats should not be mustered for long distances the day before transport.

- Every effort should be made to ensure kids and cull goats are transported for the shortest possible time.

- Goats that will not be acceptable to the processing plant should not be loaded for transport.

- During preparation for transport, prolonged deprivation of food and water should be avoided. Yearling and adult goats should be held off green-feed for a minimum of four to six hours before transportation but for no more than 12 hours. Clean water should be available during this time.

- When undertaking long journeys, goats should be nutritionally prepared beforehand by supplying them with the type of feed that they will receive at rest stops during the journey and upon its completion.

- Dogs should be under control at all times and should not be used to move young kids.

Health

Owners and persons in charge of goats have an obligation to ensure that the health needs of their animals are met. Stock handlers need to be familiar with the more common health problems of goats and observe their stock frequently and carefully for early signs of disease. Any potential problems need to be noted as early as possible and steps taken to rectify the problem.

Diseases that can be particularly problematic for the goat farmer include gastro-intestinal parasitism, Johne's disease, outbreaks of pneumonia, scabby mouth (orf), periodontal disease, CLA (caseous lymphadenitis) and CAE (caprine arthritis-encephalitis). When these diseases are suspected, an expert should be consulted to confirm the diagnosis and to advise on appropriate disease control measures to be included in the animal health programme. Organic production systems may present special challenges to goat health and welfare and require particular attention to management and disease prevention strategies to avoid health and welfare compromise.

Parasitic Diseases

Farmed goats are relatively susceptible to worms and, unlike sheep and cattle, do not develop agerelated resistance to worms. Management systems therefore need to be structured to combat internal parasites throughout the life of the goat. Drench resistance has developed in some worm species and this can limit the treatment options available to the goat farmer. There are a greater number of options for worm control in fibre producing goats as with-holding times on anthelmintics (meaning that milk and meat from treated goats cannot be sold within that period) can limit the available options for dairy and meat goats. Long-acting drugs can, however, be useful in fibre goats where residues are of minimal importance.

Goats are known to metabolise anthelmintics faster than sheep and so dose recommendations need to be tailored specifically for goats.

Diseases of the Hoof

Lameness is a painful condition and warrants immediate and effective treatment. Hoof growth is rapid in goats and if the environment (including housing) does not allow the hoof to wear away naturally, then routine trimming may be required to prevent the horn from curling underneath the foot. Goats are prone to developing foot scald and foot rot when conditions are wet because of the deep interdigital cleft between the toes.

Regular foot care including foot-bathing where necessary will assist with maintaining good hoof health and minimising lameness. In many animals, judicious hoof trimming and foot baths of zinc or copper sulphate will achieve the desired result.

Skin Acclimatisation

Goats need time to acclimatise to changing conditions when they are moved from indoors to outdoors. White haired and pink skinned goats that are not accustomed to being in direct sunlight may become sunburnt if moved outside their housing area, e.g. when barns are being cleaned out.

Minimum Standard

- Those responsible for the welfare of goats must be competent at recognising ill health or injury and take prompt remedial action as appropriate.

- Any injured or ailing goat must be immediately treated by a knowledgeable and competent stock handler or be destroyed humanely.

- A veterinarian must be consulted if there is any significant disease or injury or if an animal health problem persists in spite of treatment.

Example Indicators for Health

- Stock handlers are trained and competent to recognise ill-health and injury and to undertake prompt action and treatment as necessary.

- All sick or injured goats are treated immediately by a competent stock handler or destroyed humanely.

- There is a documented herd health plan that includes prophylactic treatments such as vaccination schedules and parasite management.

- Animal health records show that all animal remedies have been used appropriately.

- A veterinarian is consulted when a significant animal health problem persists.

Recommended Best Practice

- Goats should be inspected as frequently as necessary to detect any problem at an early stage.

- Stock handlers should be familiar with the more common health problems of goats and observe their stock carefully for early signs of disease including pain, discomfort and weight loss. They should take early action to prevent worsening of any condition and organise prompt expert attention should this occur.

- If appropriate, goats showing signs of ill-health should be separated from herd-mates to prevent bullying and to facilitate treatment.

- Any goat that is unable to stand should receive veterinary attention within 48 hours of becoming recumbent or be destroyed humanely. These recumbent goats should be inspected frequently, kept in an upright position (i.e. lying on their sternum with legs tucked under the body) on a soft dry surface and shifted from side to side as often as possible.

- On commercial farms, animal health records should be kept, including details and timing of parasite control measures, foot care procedures, appropriate vaccinations, supplementation of nutrients that are deficient in the diet, culling strategies and cross-grazing with other species as appropriate.

- Goats should be given regular and effective treatments to prevent internal and external parasite burdens, as recommended by veterinarians or product manufacturers.

- Animal remedies should only be used in accordance with registration conditions, manufacturer's instructions and professional advice.

- Goats should be managed with the aim of minimising the incidence of lameness.

- All staff should be trained in the prevention, identification and treatment of lameness and where it is observed, the affected foot is carefully examined and treated immediately.

- Veterinary advice should be sought when there is: i) persistent ill-thrift, lameness, pain or poor performance that does not respond to treatment ii) concern about the welfare of the animal.

Emergency Humane Destruction

The overriding consideration during emergency humane destruction is to prevent the animal from suffering further pain or distress. Humane killing depends on rapidly inducing failure of brain function. This can be achieved by causing sufficient brain damage to render the animal insensible and then cutting the major blood vessels of the neck to cause heart failure and death. There are a number of methods that may be used for the humane and effective killing of goats on farm.

Whenever a firearm is used, it is very important that the operator is competent to use it and takes care in ensuring the safety of themselves and other animals. There are two types of captive bolt firearm – penetrating and non-penetrating. A penetrating captive bolt enters the skull and comes into contact with brain tissue; a non-penetrative captive bolt employs a "mushroom" percussive head. Both methods provide a concussive blow to the skull, resulting in insensibility because of brain tissue damage, although the damage caused by the penetrating captive bolt will result in less chance of the animal regaining sensibility. The correct position and direction of aim are critical for the humane and effective killing of goats and kids.

Minimum Standard

- Goats must be rapidly rendered insensible and remain in that state, until death.

- Persons undertaking emergency destruction must be competent in the handling and killing of goats.

- The spinal cord must not be severed or broken in any goat, until after death.

Example Indicators for Emergency Humane Destruction

- Written farm procedures identify the appropriate methods used for humane destruction of unwanted animals.

- Stock handlers who carry out the humane destruction of goats are trained in appropriate routines.

- Stunned goats do not recover consciousness and death occurs rapidly after any stunning procedure.

Recommended Best Practice

- Free-bullet firearms should never be used at point blank range. Shotguns and rifles should be at least 10 cm from the head when aimed.

- Captive bolt firearms, of a suitable design and calibre, should be used to render animals insensible.

- Wherever possible, emergency slaughter of goats should be conducted discreetly and at a site distant from other animals so as not to cause anxiety to other goats.

Hornless Goats

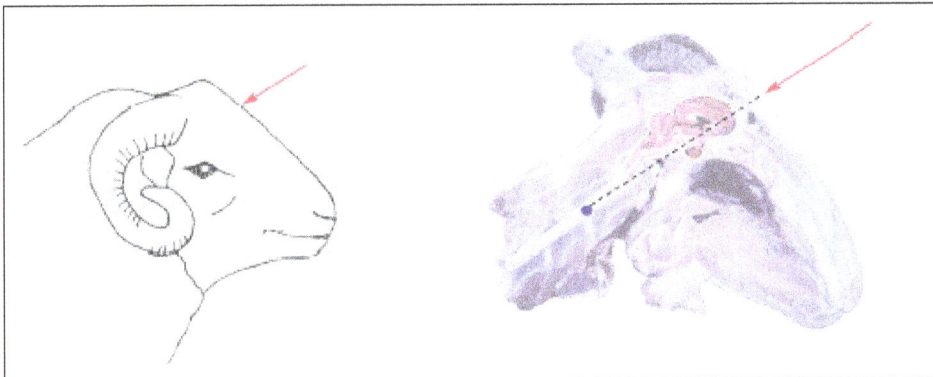

The optimum position for hornless goats is on the midline.

Horned Goats

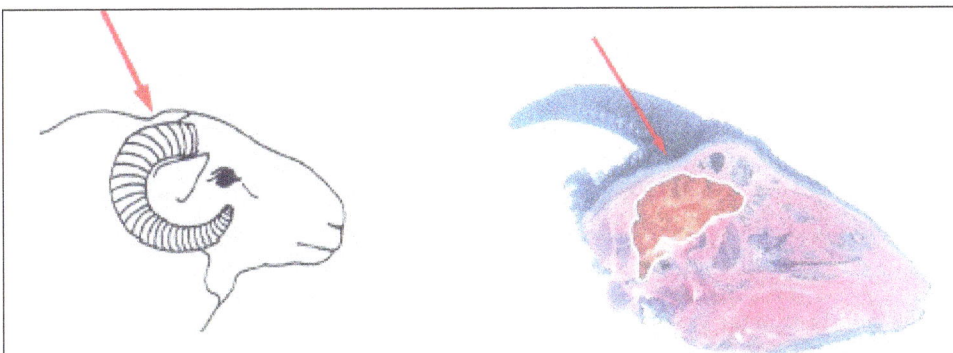

The optimum position for horned goats is behind the poll, aiming towards the angle of the jaw.

Quality Management

A quality assurance programme that provides written procedures is a useful tool to ensure that standards of animal welfare and husbandry are maintained, especially on commercial farms of all types.

Recommended Best Practice

- To ensure that standards of animal welfare and husbandry are maintained, each farm should have a quality assurance programme that provides documented animal health and welfare procedures.

- The elements of the quality assurance programme should provide for the minimum standards and, where possible, the recommendations for best practice of this Code.

- The quality assurance programme should enable all incidents resulting in significant sickness, injury or death of animals to be investigated and documented.

- The quality assurance programme should incorporate continual review of existing systems, procedures and training schedules that could enhance the welfare of goats.

- The quality assurance programme should include a record of problem issues identified and the remedial action taken.

The Welfare of Pigs

In intensive pig farms all three of these are compromised by periods of confinement in cages, barren environments and mutilations. Pigs also suffer during long distance transport for further fattening and slaughter.

Welfare Issues for Pigs

Housing of Breeding Sows: Sow Stalls

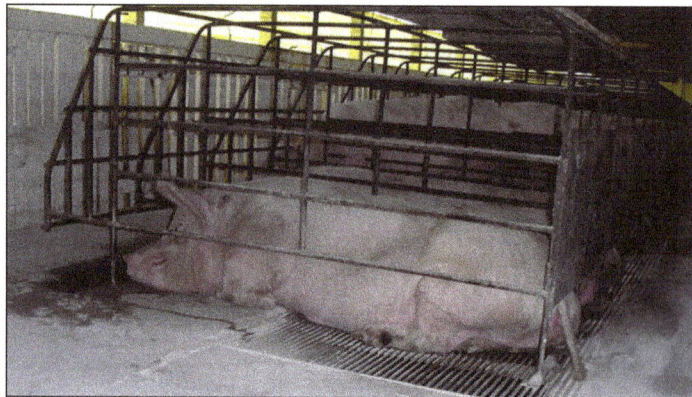

In much of the world it is common for a pregnant sow to be kept in a sow stall (also called a gestation crate) for the whole of her 16-week pregnancy. A sow stall is a metal cage – usually with a bare concrete/slatted floor – which is so narrow that the sow cannot turn around and she can only stand up and lie down with difficulty.

Sow stalls deprive pregnant sows of almost all natural behaviors; they cannot explore, exercise, forage or socialise. Most will never go outside in their lives. Pigs are naturally curious animals who spend much time exploring their environment and searching for food. Keeping sows in cages means they suffer from boredom and frustration; they do not have a life worth living.

Sow Stall Conditions

Potentially upsetting scenes of animal suffering. Sow stalls also increase abnormal behavior such as sham chewing and bar-biting, indicating severe frustration and stress and sows in crates can exhibit behavior likened to clinical depression. Feed is often restricted during pregnancy, causing chronic hunger and increasing the level of frustration.

Sow stalls are illegal in Sweden and the UK. Their use is limited in the EU, with a partial ban enforced from 2013. However it is still permitted for sows to be kept in sow stalls from weaning of the previous litter until the end of the first 4 weeks of pregnancy. They are being phased out in certain states in the US and in New Zealand and there is a voluntary industry agreement to phase out their use in Australia. A number of food producing companies are starting to phase them out voluntarily on animal welfare grounds, due to consumer pressure.

Farrowing Crates

Shortly before she is due to give birth (referred to as 'farrowing'), a sow is typically moved to a farrowing crate. This is similar to a sow stall except that there is space to the side for the piglets. Bars keep the sow out of the piglets' lying area to prevent crushing.

Like sow stalls, farrowing crates also severely restrict the sow's movement and frustrate her strong motivation to build a nest before giving birth. They prevent the sow from being able to get away from her piglets, for example if they bite her teats. It is common for piglets to have their teeth ground down or clipped, without anaesthetic, to minimize biting injuries.

Piglets are weaned and taken away from their mother when they are 3 to 4 weeks old and even earlier in some countries. In the wild, sows would continue to feed their piglets until they were around 13-17 weeks old but the females would often stay together as adults. Male pigs disperse to find a mate and start their own family group.

Within a couple of weeks of weaning, the sow is inseminated again (often artificially) and starts her next pregnancy. Commercial sows normally produce just over 2 litters a year with around 10-12 piglets per litter. She has a breeding lifetime of about 3 years before being sold for slaughter and replaced.

Farrowing crates have been banned in Sweden, Norway and Switzerland. In the rest of the world they are widely used.

Housing of Fattening Pigs

Fattening pigs are bred for meat and often kept in barren, crowded conditions. This can be on slatted concrete floors without straw for bedding or rooting. These pigs have no access to outdoors and will never experience fresh air or daylight. They are unable to behave naturally and become bored and frustrated. They tend to fight and to bite each other, sometimes causing severe injury, particularly to their tails.

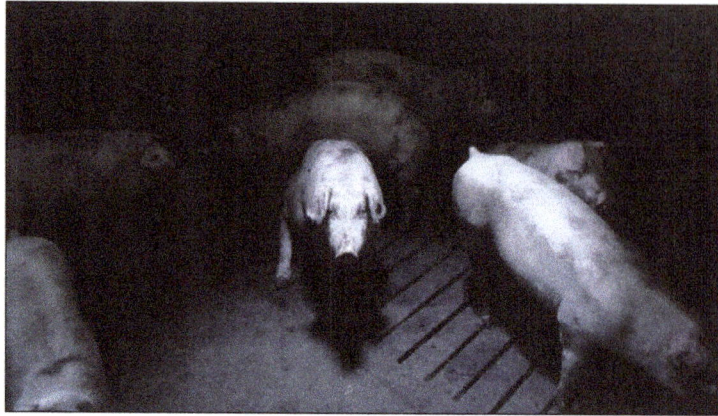

In addition to tooth cutting, most piglets have their tails docked to discourage tail biting. Both of these procedures are painful and performed without pain relief. Stress, illness and conflict often result when piglets are abruptly weaned and mixed with unfamiliar young pigs.

Most male piglets in Europe (but not in the UK and Ireland) are castrated. Public pressure has led to a voluntary declaration aimed at ending the surgical castration of pigs in Europe by 2018. As a first step, signatories will ensure that prolonged pain relief is used for surgical castration of pigs from 2012.

Mutilations

Tooth Clipping

Soon after they are born, the teeth of piglets are often clipped. The purpose of teeth clipping is to reduce injuries caused by piglets to each other and to their mother as they fight for the best teats.

Sows don't always have enough milk to feed all their piglets, especially if they have large litters or their bodies are in poor conditions. To ensure that at least some of the piglets survive, the strongest get preferential treatment.

The teats nearest the front of her body get the most milk. The teats towards the back of the body get progressively less. Once a piglet has established ownership of a teat, he or she will vigorously defend it.

Castration

Within a week of being born, many male piglets are surgically castrated, usually without anaesthetic or pain relief. This is done by cutting the scrotum with a scalpel, pulling out the piglet's testes and cutting them off. In Europe, this is around 70% of all males, the equivalent to around 90 million piglets every year. This is a painful procedure and major welfare concern.

The main reason piglets are castrated is to prevent "boar taint". This is a smell or taste of pork, caused by the sex hormones testosterone and androstenone. Males that are not castrated may also be aggressive and show more sexual behavior. This may cause injury to others if they fight or mount each other and can be dangerous to farm workers if they are aggressive during handling.

Welfare Issues of Castration

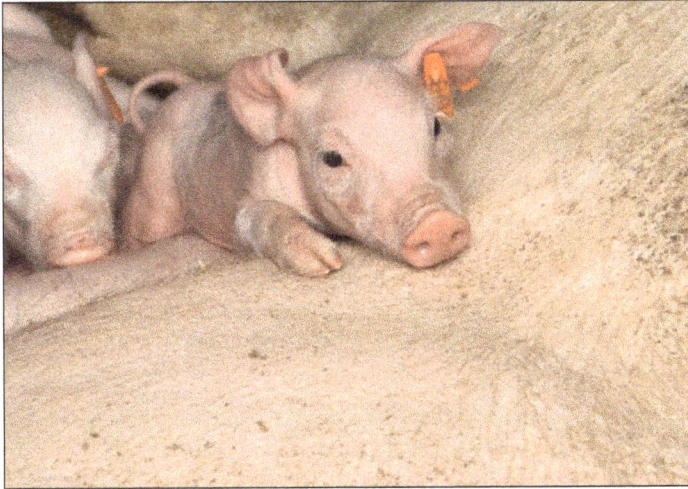

Piglets are castrated within the first week of life.

Many piglets are castrated without any anaesthetic or pain relief (analgesics), which causes them short and long-term pain and stress. It also leaves the piglets more prone to infection from the open wound with limited immunity at such a very young age. The extra time and cost involved in pain relief means that alleviating piglets' distress is rarely considered.

In some countries, such as Denmark and Germany, pain relief is now commonly used, but the timing of the injection is important and it should be given at least half an hour before the procedure, which may not be the case in practice. In the Netherlands CO/O or Isoflurane is used as an anaesthetic. CO/O is known to be aversive to pigs, so while it may make them unconscious, it is a very unpleasant experience.

In a minority of countries, such as Sweden and Lithuania, both anaesthetic and pain relief may be used. The use of both pain relief and a non-aversive anaesthetic is important when surgical castration is performed but this mutilation is causing distress to the pigs and risking their health and welfare. Switzerland has banned castration since 2010.

In some countries pigs are reared to a heavier weight so that certain meat cuts or fat content can be produced. This means there is more risk of boar taint because the pigs reach puberty, as well as the welfare risk of them injuring each other.

Higher Welfare Alternatives for Pigs

There are alternative commercial systems that improve the welfare of pigs by providing a more enriched environment which allows for more natural behavior.

Housing: Higher Welfare Indoor Systems

Pigs are kept in groups on solid floors with straw or other material for bedding and rooting. Although there is no access to the outdoors, there is greater opportunity for natural behavior, free movement within the pen or shed, less crowding, conflict, boredom and tail-biting. Deep bedded systems allow foraging and comfort.

Sows may still give birth in farrowing crates, but in the better systems they give birth in huts or pens.

Outdoor Bred

Sows are kept outside with straw-filled huts for shelter: This is where they will give birth to their piglets. There are no sow stalls or farrowing crates.

Sows have a higher quality of life and are able to act naturally by building nests, rooting, wallowing and foraging. The piglets benefit from the free-range conditions until they are weaned. At weaning, the piglets are taken indoors and reared in extensive or intensive conditions.

Outdoor Reared

Piglets are born outside (without stalls or crates) and spend around half of their lives outside (around 3 months).

Free-range

Whilst there is no legal definition of 'free-range pork', a voluntary industry code in the UK requires that free-range pigs have permanent access to pasture: Born outside (without stalls or crates) and then reared outside throughout their lives.

In the best free-range and organic pig farms, the sows and the growing pigs are kept outside for their entire lives. The piglets stay with their mothers for longer (up to 6 to 8 weeks), mixing of unfamiliar pigs is reduced and tail-docking is not used.

Alternatives to Mutilations

Farming systems should be designed to fulfil the welfare needs of the animals rather than altering the animal, through physical or genetic mutilations to fit a bad system. Mutilations can and should be avoided by better breeding, appropriate enriched environments, management and nutrition.

Alternatives to Tooth Clipping

Breeding sows to produce smaller litters which they can feed properly can reduce injuries caused by fighting for teats. This can also reduce the number of piglets that will starve, provided the sow is properly fed. Some breeds of sow have higher levels of fat and this can help them to maintain high levels of milk.

Keeping the sow in high welfare farrowing systems may also help. Research in Denmark found that sows in free-farrowing systems ate more food than those kept in crates and it was suggested that they were probably producing more milk. Piglets in the free-farrowing systems grew better and were heavier at weaning than those in crates.

There are fewer injuries to the sow's teats and to other piglets, in systems with plenty of space and enrichment such as straw. European Union rules insist that environment and stocking density should be dealt with before resorting to teeth clipping.

Alternatives to Castration

There are alternative options to castrating piglets which can vastly improve their welfare.

In some countries, such as the UK, Ireland and parts of Spain, Portugal and Greece, male piglets are not castrated but are slaughtered at a younger age (with a lower weight), lowering the risk of boar taint developing in the meat that can occur during puberty. In the Netherlands this approach is also being taken, with around 70% of males now reared entire.

Although the pigs are slaughtered at a younger age, as they get close to slaughter weight, some may develop mounting behavior. Gilts (young female pigs) are smaller than males and they can be injured during mounting, sometimes leading to lameness. Both males and females may also suffer from cuts and abrasions leading to skin lesions. It is therefore recommended that the males and females are separated to help reduce this risk.

People's sensitivity to boar taint varies between nationalities and sexes and some argue that even those slaughtered at a younger age may have boar taint. Where this is an issue technology is being developed to detect the scent of boar taint on carcasses at the slaughterhouse. Alternatively a person sensitive to boar taint can be employed to use the human nose to detect the smell after singing a small area of meat while the carcass is on the line. However, countries currently do not agree of what is an acceptable level of 'boar taint' smell and the test is very subjective.

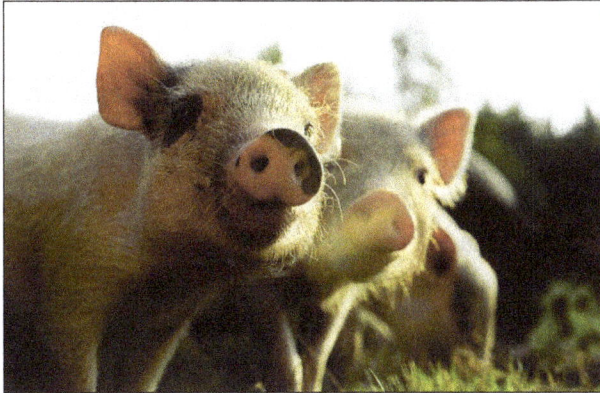

The Welfare of Hens

Designing Housing for Good Bird Welfare

Many of the potential problems that can create stress in alternative systems can be eliminated at the design stage. The following need to be considered when designing new houses:

Siting of Free Range Poultry Houses

The position of a house will influence how well the birds range over the pasture. Soil type and drainage will determine how likely the ground is to become fowl sick through the buildup of soil-borne parasites.

The following points should be taken into account:

- If possible choose free draining, south facing, pasture to minimize the build up of worms and coocidial oocysts. Such pasture should also better retain grass cover.

- Ideally, houses should be positioned in the centre of the land area so that a series of radiating paddocks can be created around the unit. In some cases this is not possible because of local planning constraints or because of the limitations of power or water supplies.

- Siting houses at right angles to the prevailing wind slightly moderates the amount of wind entering the building through the popholes.

- It is important to consider access, not just during good weather, but also during weather conditions when gradients may make lorry access difficult.

- Range areas bordered by dense woodland will be more prone to fox problems. Although the positioning of small, mobile houses may be less critical than that of large fixed buildings, the quality of the pasture is still important, as is the ability to move the houses regularly once they are on site. The maintenance of an adequate supply of electricity and water under all conditions is important. For example, there needs to be some means of preventing overground water pipes from freezing during winter and contingency plans must be drawn up for keeping the birds supplied with water if the pipes do freeze.

Ventilation

The ventilation system needs to be such that the air change rate is adequate for the removal of bird heat from the building during hot weather. This is referred to as the maximum ventilation rate. It also needs to be able to remove stale, smelly air and humidity during periods of low ventilation during cold weather (minimum ventilation rate). Uniform, draught free, distribution of air within the building is important. Ventilation can be achieved either by the use of powered fans or by natural forces. As a guide, maximum ventilation rate may typically be achieved using the equivalent of one 610 mm fan or by allowing 2.6–4.3 m² of inlet and outlet per 1000 layers, depending on the height difference between inlets and outlets. There needs to be some means of providing for minimum ventilation requirements - either using a cycle timer controlling one or more of the fans or by having minimum settings on natural ventilation inlets and outlets. A complement to a ventilation system is the house insulation. Without adequate insulation, the building will tend to overheat in the summer, which will stress the birds. Similarly, the building will be cold and prone to condensation and damp in winter, which will also have an adverse effect on the health, welfare and performance of the birds. As a rule of thumb, a minimum of 100 mm of glass fibre (or equivalent) should be used in the roof and the walls and an adequate vapour barrier (e.g. 1000 gauge polythene) incorporated to prevent deterioration of the material from condensation. This deterioration leads to reduced insulation efficiency.

Ventilation system design can be a fairly complex issue. It may be worth considering professional advice.

Fire Precautions

With the amount of electrical equipment and wiring in most poultry houses, coupled with the combustible nature of many of the structural materials, there is a risk of fire. This risk can be considerably increased where electrical equipment and installations have not been adequately maintained and where they have been subject to rodent damage.

- Make sure electrical equipment and installations are well maintained and inspected regularly.

- Do not allow circuits to be become overloaded by the addition of extra electrical equipment.

- Keep rodents under control at all times to reduce the risk of damage to cables.

- Do not allow smoking in the poultry houses.

Alarms, Failsafes and Generators

There is a statutory requirement for all houses which rely on automated equipment for ventilation to incorporate the following:

- An alarm which will give adequate warning of failure of the system to function properly. The alarm must have some form of back-up power supply (e.g. a battery), so that it will operate in the event of a failure of the mains supply.

- 'Additional equipment' or means of ventilation that will provide adequate ventilation in the event of a failure of the main system. The most appropriate way of meeting this requirement will vary according to individual circumstances and house design. In some situations, for example, having some additional doors or roof openings that can be utilised to ventilate the building by natural forces may be all that is required. In other cases, there may also be a need to incorporate a standby generator.

There is also a requirement to test the alarm system and check any additional emergency equipment at least once a week.

Layout of Equipment and Perches

Inadequate, poorly designed or poorly laid out feeders, drinkers, nestboxes and perches will create stress in the flock and will compromise both bird welfare and performance. There are a number of key issues to consider:

- Numbers of feeders, drinkers and nestboxes must meet the minimum set out in a particular country's legislation.

- Perches should be arranged so that birds can move easily between them and the other equipment, thereby reducing the risk of collisions and subsequent bruising and other damage. Consideration should be given to minimising bird stress and downgrading during catching at the end of the laying period – can the equipment easily be removed from the pens or winched up out of the way?

- Because of the importance of thorough cleaning between flocks, equipment, fixtures and fittings should be selected and installed for ease of cleaning. The ability to remove equipment and fittings in order to achieve a really thorough clean is usually the best option, although this is often not practicable in the case of nestboxes, perches and slatted floors. Where equipment is not removable, it is even more important to give some thought to how less accessible sections or areas of the nestboxes or slatted floors will be cleaned.

Lighting

Lighting should be designed and installed to give an even light distribution and should incorporate some means of adjusting light intensity to control aggressive pecking, should this begin to occur. Light fittings should be installed in a position where they will not be struck by the birds or by the stock keeper working inside the house.

Routine husbandry

Training

No matter how good the design, without a skilled and knowledgeable stock person looking after the chickens, bird welfare and performance are never likely to reach the highest standard. Training can take a variety of forms and should be tailored to the needs and experience of the individual. Many agricultural colleges now offer training to NVQ level 2/3 standard in poultry husbandry and courses can be on a day release basis. Learning stockmanship does not necessarily require attendance on a formal training course, provided that 'on the job' training is adequate and appropriate.

Pullet Rearing

Correctly reared, healthy pullets are essential prerequisites for successful egg production in alternative systems. Underweight, uneven pullets for example will be less able to adapt to life in the laying house and will be more susceptible to stress leading to other welfare problems. It is important therefore that the specification for the pullets is agreed with the rearer at the time the birds are ordered. It is also good practice for the stock keeper to inspect the pullets at least once before delivery to check that all is well. Requirements for pullets destined for free range or barn systems are:

- Floor reared with access to perches and slats from an early age (e.g. from 10 days at the latest).

- Up to breeders target weight.

- (If required) beak trimmed at less than 10 days old.

- Comprehensive vaccination programme as advised by a vet.

- Wormed and resistant to coccidiosis.

- Reared to an agreed lighting programme.

The rearer should match rearing conditions as closely as possible to those that the birds will experience in the laying house. It is good practice, for example, for the drinker system used during rearing to be the same as that in the laying unit. Where this is not possible, the birds may need to be trained to use the unfamiliar drinkers in the laying house. This is particularly important in the case of birds switching from bell drinkers to nipples. Having the same or similar feeding systems in the rearing house as in laying unit also helps to reduce the stress of transition between the two stages.

Inspection and Culling

One of the most important daily tasks for the stock keeper is to thoroughly check the birds for signs of ill health, injury or disease. This is best done first thing in the morning and also last thing in the afternoon/evening prior to lights out. It is important that the whole of the flock is walked and that no birds are missed. It is also important that the lighting is sufficiently bright that all the birds can be clearly seen. This can be achieved by turning the house lights up where there is suitable dimmer fitted or alternatively, by using an additional row of inspection lights or by hand-held torch.

An important skill which comes with practice is the ability to recognise and identify abnormal behavior in the flock. Until the stock keeper has acquired the necessary skills, advice should be sought from more experienced stock keepers or a veterinary surgeon.

Identifying birds with minor injuries or pecking is generally straightforward and birds affected should be removed promptly to a suitable casualty pen where they can be given time to recover. Birds more seriously injured or considered to be unlikely to recover, should be humanely culled as soon as possible.

Where the flock shows signs of ill health or the onset of disease and remedial action undertaken by the stock keeper is not effective, veterinary advice should be sought as soon as possible. It is often helpful in diagnosing disease if dead birds are retained for the vet to examine.

Beak Trimming

Feather pecking can be a problem in alternative systems. Left unchecked, it can lead to more aggressive pecking and ultimately, to cannibalism. The likelihood of feather pecking during lay can be reduced by making strenuous efforts to remove all form of stress. Nevertheless birds destined to be housed in alternative systems may need to have their beaks trimmed during rearing.

Beak trimming must be done by a suitably trained operator and it should be performed when the chicks are less than 10 days old.

Disposal of Dead Birds

There are several reasons why the careful disposal of dead birds is an important part of the health management of alternative systems:

- Reduces the risk of disease spread back to the flock and other species.

- Reduces the likelihood of carcases being removed by scavengers, which can transmit disease.

- Reduces the risk of blow flies (Caliphora sp.), which can also transmit disease. The most effective and reliable way of disposing of dead birds is by burning in a properly constructed incinerator fuelled by gas or oil and incorporating an after-burner. Disposal on an open bonfire tends to be much less reliable and creates dark smoke and odour. This method of disposal is NOT recommended.

Disposal of dead birds in a disposal chamber can be an acceptable alternative to incineration, but must be done in accordance with the guidelines set out in the Code of Good Agricultural Practice for the Protection of Water.

Handling and Moving Birds

Careful handling of the birds during initial stocking and depletion will reduce the risk of stress and will minimize the likelihood of injury or damage. Particular care needs to be taken at depopulation because catching the birds can be difficult and the bone strength and elasticity of older hens is generally poorer than those of point of lay pullets. The following notes should be used as a guide:

- Remove as much of the equipment from the house as possible prior to moving birds in or out of the building. Make sure corridors and gangways are clear.

- Make sure that all staff involved in handling birds are suitably trained and adequately supervised - particularly in the case of inexperienced staff.

- Dim the house lights and work quietly and steadily.

- Catch birds with both legs and do not carry more than three birds in each hand. More detailed advice on bird handling and transport aimed at maintaining high standards of bird welfare is contained in a joint industry code of practice on the 'Handling and Transport of End of Lay Hens', which can be obtained from a number of sources.

Nutrition

Diet can exert a profound influence on bird welfare and performance, so it is essential that the quality and quantity of the rations are adequate. Feeding birds in alternative systems is generally regarded as more difficult than feeding birds in cage systems, because of the additional competition between birds for feeder space and because of greater fluctuations in house temperature. Stock keepers need to be aware of the potential pitfalls that can occur as a result of inadequate nutrition and of the measures that may be required to prevent or rectify them. Some points to bear in mind are:

- Make sure that feeding space is adequate and that the distribution of feeders allows good access by the birds. As a guide, a minimum of 10 cm of linear trough space or 4 cm of circular feeder, per bird is recommended.

- Seasonal changes in temperature can exert a major influence on feed intake - particularly in poorly insulated houses. Food consumption can change by as much as 30–40 g/bird/day from summer to winter, which represents a challenge to the stock keeper and nutritionist in avoiding welfare problems and maintaining performance. Increasing the quantity of feed supplied to the birds during cold weather, coupled with seasonal changes in the concentration of nutrients in the diets, are the key details.

- Birds in alternative systems tend to be more sensitive to marginal dietary deficiencies than birds in cage systems and low levels of intake of some key nutrients can predispose the birds to pecking.

Diet formulation for birds in alternative systems is a specialist subject and advice should be sought when necessary from a poultry nutritionist or suitable consultant.

Pest Control

Mouse and rat infestations are a constant threat to any poultry house because of the warm conditions, the abundance of food available and the very large number of potential harbourages and nesting areas. Uncontrolled populations of rats or mice can create panic and hysteria in flocks and can give rise to sudden, heavy mortality losses due to smothering. Rodents are also prolific carriers of a variety of infections of both poultry and humans.

In recent years, poultry red mite has become a serious problem in alternative systems. The presence of large numbers of red mite will increase stress levels in the birds and predispose them to pecking. Heavy infestations of red mite will cause anaemia and left unchecked will result in deaths.

The key to successful pest control is to adopt a proactive approach, using a range of strategies aimed at prevention. Whilst part of the control programme may involve using the services of a qualified pest controller, excellent on farm control can often be achieved if a thorough and systematic approach is adopted. Some of the elements common to both rodent and red mite control programmes are:

- Houses and equipment should be designed to minimize the number of harbourages and pest-proofing features should be incorporated wherever possible. In the case of red mite, equipment such as feeders, nestboxes, perch frames etc. should be designed to minimize the number of cracks and crevices, since these are the favoured resting areas.

- Repairs to double-skinned walls and roofs should be carried out promptly to reduce the chances of rodents gaining entry to internal voids.

- A regular programme of inspections should be implemented so that infestations can be detected at an early stage. Keeping simple records of the inspections will help to identify increases in pest activity and enable prompt early treatment. Treatments using the appropriate approved products should always be carried out in accordance with the label directions with due regard for the safety of both the birds and the operator.

- As far as possible use products with different active ingredients on a cyclical basis to reduce the risk of resistance developing. This is particularly important in the case of red mite control. It is important not to assume that poor levels of control are due to product resistance – in most cases unsatisfactory performance is due to shortcomings of the operator rather than the product.

- Good housekeeping is essential - particularly in the case of rodent control. Spillages of feed and broken egg etc. should be cleared-up promptly and rubbish and clutter should not be allowed to accumulate either inside or outside the house.

- Thorough cleaning and disinfection of the poultry house at the end of the laying period is also essential. In the case of red mite infestation, this may need to be followed by treatment with an approved residual acaricide once the house is dry, to delay the build-up of mite in the subsequent flock. Records and Record Keeping Record keeping is an important part of any system of livestock production. It is particularly important in the case of free range and barn systems as an aid to the early detection of potential problems. As a minimum records should be kept of mortality and culls, egg numbers, average egg weight (weekly), feed consumption, water usage and house temperature.

As well as these records, it is often a good idea to keep a daily diary. This is particularly useful where more than one person may be responsible for looking after the birds. Diary records might include the incidence of breakdowns or mechanical/electrical failures and the actions taken at the time. Entries might also include records of upsets or disturbances to the flock as a result of adverse weather etc.

Pasture Management

In free range laying systems, good pasture management is essential if the ground is to remain in good condition and the problems of poaching and the build-up of parasitic intestinal worms and coccidial oocysts are to be avoided. Worm infestation and coccidiosis can seriously compromise bird health and welfare. The signs of a worm infestation include a general loss of condition, diarrhoea, loss of egg size and numbers and possibly of yolk colour too. Gapeworm (Syngamous trachea) causes dyspnoea or 'gaping' and head shaking. Left untreated, heavy worm infestations will result in mortality. Many of the external symptoms and effects of coccidiosis are similar to those of worm infestation, although blood may also be present in the droppings. Low level infestations of worms and coccidiosis can increase stress in the flock and precipitate pecking.

Both worm eggs and coccidial oocysts will survive for some time in the soil. This means that the threat of re-infestation is always present and will inevitably carry over to subsequent flocks. Although effective paddock management is the key to avoiding problems during lay, birds should be wormed before delivery and rearing programmes should enable the birds to develop resistance to coccidiosis through the use of coccidiostats in the feed and by vaccination.

Your vet will be able to help you to recognise the symptoms of worm infestation and coccidiosis and provide advice on suitable control strategies and treatment options. Management of Paddocks The land surrounding the laying house should be divided into a series of paddocks which the birds are allowed to use for periods of up to 6 - 8 weeks each. The number of paddocks used will depend on the specific arrangement of the house in relation to the available area, but normally six paddocks is a practical compromise. Similarly, the length of time that the birds are allowed to use individual paddocks will vary depending on soil type, drainage, grass cover and weather conditions. A commonsense approach is required.

Paddocks should be maintained in good condition by the judicious use of chain harrows. This breaks up the soil surface and promotes good drainage and helps reduce the parasite burden by exposing the worm eggs to sunlight. The use of short, resilient grass varieties and clover are generally considered to be most appropriate for free range and the grass should be kept short to reduce the risk of crop impaction.

The area immediately outside the poultry house tends to suffer the greatest amount of damage, so the ground adjacent to the pop holes should be covered with large, rounded stones/pebbles or slats. As well as providing health and welfare benefits the birds' feet will be cleaned as they enter the building, which will help to reduce the number of dirty eggs produced. The incorporation of a covered verandah along the side(s) of the laying house is now common practice. It can be very beneficial as an aid to effective range management and to welfare and production. Providing shelters on the range area, perhaps with some trees, can encourage the birds out to range and spread the wear on the pasture. Shelters also provide protection from the sun in hot weather and from rain and wind during inclement weather. Birds find open space a threat, as it increases the risk of being spotted by predators, so shelters and trees can provide the cover they need to feel safe.

Protection from Predators

Free range layers are attractive to predators. Foxes are the most frequent cause of problems, but mink, dogs and badgers can all cause damage and often kill or maim large numbers of birds – far more than they are able to consume. In addition to direct attacks on the birds, the presence of these predators can cause panic and hysteria in the flock. This can cause losses through smothering and trigger outbreaks of feather pecking.

Siting of the unit can influence the likelihood of such problems. Thick cover, such as conifer plantations, close to the range area will encourage foxes and in some cases hens will be taken in broad daylight. Mink are now found in most areas, but they are most likely to be a problem near rivers and lakes.

Permanent fencing substantial enough to exclude foxes can be extremely expensive and is not normally warranted. Flexible electrified fencing powered by a mains transformer, will generally provide satisfactory levels of protection against most predators and requires less attention than a battery powered unit. The fencing and energiser unit must be well maintained in order to continue to work effectively. Grass underneath the fence must be kept cut to prevent shorting and regular checks should be made on the connections between sections of fence and the transformer. A fencing voltage tester is an essential piece of equipment.

Planning for Problems and Emergencies

Having contingency plans for dealing with problems or emergencies is an essential part of managing a free range or barn unit. The ability to be able to respond quickly to power failure or adverse weather conditions will limit the amount of stress placed on the birds and help to avoid drops in production. Some problems, such as freezing water pipes may be more likely on smaller units where the water supply pipes run above ground. Remote sites may be at greater risk of feed delivery problems during periods of bad weather - particularly when they are at high altitude. Some of the more common problems that can affect free range and barn flocks are:

- Disruption of power supply and fan or feeder failure.

- Adverse weather conditions and disruption to feed/water/electricity supply.

- Heat stress during summer.

The necessary measures will depend on the individual situation. What is important, however, is that contingency plans are drawn up before emergencies occur and that staff are trained to deal with them. Although the risk of fire is probably very low, contingency plans should include a fire drill. A list of emergency numbers next to the telephone, together with written directions to the site for the emergency services, is a sensible practice.

The Welfare of Cows

Generally, animal welfare is considered to be 'good' if the animals are healthy, comfortable, well-nourished and safe and are not suffering from unpleasant states such as pain, fear and distress. Cows also need to be able to express basic behaviors including lying, turning around, scratching and displaying social behaviors to a reasonable degree. In contrast to these positive states are the environments or situations where cows are not functioning well, feeling well or able to have a reasonably natural life.

Morbidity and Mortality

On farms, morbidity (sickness) and mortality (death) are the most fundamental welfare issues. High levels of illness and any subsequent deaths relate to the poor functioning of animals and can also include the other two broad welfare categories, particularly if the illness is chronic and the animal has suffered for an extended period of time or the illness is acute and painful.

Behavioral Abnormalities

When a cow is in a state of poor welfare, her behavior will indicate this. These behavioral changes may include a modified gait, signalling hoof pain and lameness and the duration of lying bouts and the position the cow takes to indicate the comfort of her environment. Social behaviors or a lack thereof, can indicate issues with the ability to express normal behaviors. The existence of stereotypic behaviors, defined as a repeated sequence of behaviors that has no apparent purpose, is the result of frustrations and the inability to perform normal behaviors.

Housing

Housing can have a significant influence on the welfare of cows, affecting all three welfare categories. Whether housed in tie stalls, free stalls or open lounging systems, in order to maximize performance and ensure satisfactory standards of welfare, the accommodation must provide for the animal's basic needs. As an absolute minimum, the housing must provide a comfortable, clean and well-drained dry lying area that provides shelter from adverse weather. The space provided should be enough that the animal can express behaviors that will allow it to be comfortable including standing, turning, scratching and lying. Housing systems should also allow the animal to move without risk of injury. The provision of an environment that fulfils these criteria is a common theme in quantitative measures of dairy cow welfare, highlighting its importance.

Poor housing not only affects the day-to-day comfort of the cow, but also has f low-on effects to their health. Cows at pasture, which is one of the most comfortable environments for them, choose to lie down for 12 to 14 h each day. Reduced lying time is an indication of an uncomfortable lying area or potentially another compromised welfare situation, for example, increased vigilance and fear, with cattle feeling unsafe in their home environment. If cows spend less time lying down, they are likely to spend more time standing in loafing or feeding areas, which can adversely affect hoof health, leading to conditions like lameness. Furthermore, housing and management influence the likelihood of animals experiencing heat stress, which is a significant issue in the tropics.

The provision of pasture has been linked with reduced levels of mastitis, reduced levels of lameness and faster recovery from these issues. When animals are allowed to spend time in an environment they prefer, their affective state is assumed to be more positive because they are provided with a situation they desire. Cows have a preference for lying at pasture rather than indoors, indicating they find it more comfortable. While cows prefer to be indoors, rather than in full sun when it is hot, providing cows with access to both environments will ensure positive welfare. Cows with access to pasture also display abnormal behaviors less frequently and more normal social behaviors than do cows continually kept indoors. Providing cows with pasture access then helps to promote good welfare across the three welfare categories and improves the productivity of the animal by reducing disease and aiding recovery.

'Cow comfort', is dedicated to types of housing systems, the benefits and disadvantages of each for a cow's health and welfare and ways to assess the appropriateness of this housing.

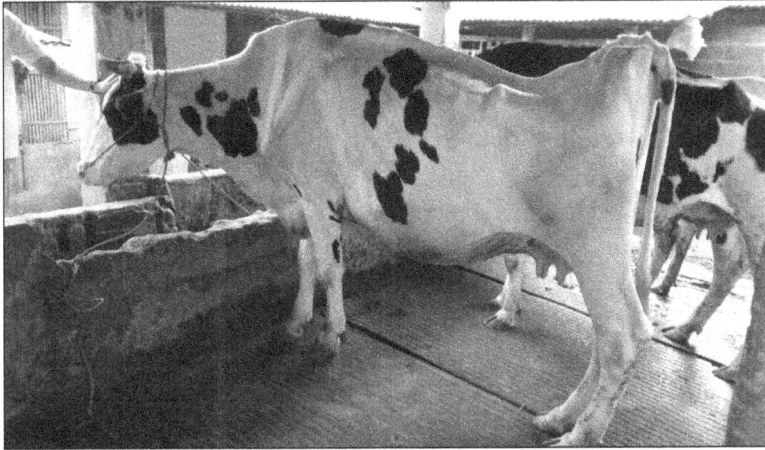

An old cow with permanent skeleton deformities as a result of a lifetime of tethering.

Lameness

Lameness is a major problem on dairy farms, both from the point of animal welfare and farm profits. Lameness can result from infectious diseases or from lesions/injury to the hoof. Management factors have a significant influence on the number and severity of lameness cases. The design of facilities, including uneven concrete floors and uncomfortable stalls with no bedding, are important risk factors for lameness, as is the structural integrity of the cow's hoof. Stockperson ability to identify lameness is also very influential, with farmers/stockpeople only recognising 40 to 50% of lameness problems and only being able to identify these issues when they become severe. These cases of lameness are often well advanced once they are identified for the first time, meaning that the animal is suffering for a long period of time and making the condition difficult to treat. Lameness can be even more difficult to detect in tethered systems and often remains as a shifting lameness condition, misinterpreted or undetected and untreated.

Heat Stress

Heat stress can be common, particularly in high yielding cows in the tropics. Cows experiencing heat stress will show a variety of symptoms including discomfort and distress, that affect their wellbeing. An increased core body temperature, increased respiration rate, drooling and sweating are all signs of their functioning being compromised. General abnormal behaviors include reduced feed intake, agitated and restless behavior and standing for long periods of time, rather than lying down. Weather and climate are the driving factors behind heat stress. However, with the correct management and facility design, heat stress can be dealt with effectively, reducing the physiological stress on the animal.

Tethering

Tethering is a common practice in Asian dairy farms. This type of environment can cause significant welfare issues as it is closely associated with high levels of disease, discomfort and abnormal behaviors in dairy cows. Animals that are continuously tethered are more likely to be dirty than animals that are kept in tie free housing. This is important as dirty cows have a much greater risk of mastitis and lameness and are more likely to pass diseases on to calves as well as zoonotic diseases to humans through their milk. Cows in tie stalls also display both restless behaviors and abnormal behaviors more frequently than cows that are not tethered.

The welfare of tethered cows can be greatly improved by maintaining a clean environment, ensuring that the flooring they have is comfortable, providing water ad libitum and giving them access to pasture and the ability to walk around freely for a few hours each day. These simple changes can significantly improve the milk yields, health and welfare of animals. For example, in a study with shedded cows in Pakistan, the provision of water ad libitum compared to only twice daily, increased milk yields by up to 1.5 L/cow/day.

Painful Husbandry Practices

Some management practices cause pain to animals. These practices should be avoided where possible or if they are necessary, they should be performed by a well-trained technician or veterinarian. It is important to consider ways to limit the pain an animal may experience during these processes. Pain can be significantly alleviated by the provision of pain relief. When pain relief cannot be administered, some methods are considered to be less painful than others. Recommendations on both situations are outlined below.

Tail docking can be a common practice performed on dairy farms that causes significant pain to the animal, but there is no evidence of practical benefit. In the short term, the procedure of tail docking causes significant pain to the cow along with leaving an open wound. In the long term, this can lead to chronic pain, the same way a person with an amputation experiences pain (known as phantom limb pain). Tail docking is practised because it is thought to improve hygiene of the udder, but there is no research to support this. Tail docking, therefore, is an example of a practice that causes unnecessary pain to the animal, without any management benefit and so it should not be performed.

Dehorning and disbudding are common painful husbandry practices performed on dairy farms. Horns on a cow can pose a threat to the farmer and other cows that the horned animal interacts with, therefore dehorning is a necessary management practice. The age at which horn removal is conducted and the method used have an effect on the amount of pain and distress the animal experiences. There are several methods by which horns can be removed. Disbudding is carried out on young calves, before the horn has actually started to grow. Dehorning is the removal of the horn and horn-producing tissue. Cautery disbudding uses a hot iron to remove and burn the horn bud. This technique is suitable for calves 12 weeks or younger and causes the least pain to the animal and the smallest wound area. This is the recommended method and timing of horn removal. While cautery disbudding is the best practice method for disbudding, it can be difficult to perform in SHD situations.

Caustic disbudding uses a paste to remove the horn bud. Along with being painful, this type of disbudding can cause irritation to the surrounding areas of the skin, can damage the eye if the paste runs down the calf's face and can also cause irritation to other animals that the calf comes into contact with. As a result, calves should be housed by themselves in the hours after the paste has been applied and the dehorned area must be kept dry. Pain management for caustic disbudding is difficult to manage and so is not recommended. Amputation dehorning, conducted on animals at a later age, creates a wound that can open the frontal sinus of the animal. This procedure causes extensive pain, long wound healing times and significantly reduced weight gains. It also creates a large risk of infection. Pain relief using both a local anaesthetic and non-steroidal anti-inflammatory are highly recommended in this particular situation and all animals treated with these alleviation methods have shown indicators of a reduced pain response. The wound site will also bleed significantly and clamps or tourniquets should be used to reduce bleeding.

Castration is less common in dairying than it is in beef production, as bull calves are usually sold or slaughtered before they reach sexual maturity. In small holder systems, it is more common to keep bull calves until they reach heavier slaughter weights and so castration can be a usual procedure. There are several different methods for castration and the age of the calf has a significant influence on which method is most effective and least painful.

Calves at a younger age display less pain during castration than older animals. For calves younger than 3 months of age, rubber ring castration has a high success rate and has the best welfare outcome for the animal. As it does not involve a surgical procedure, there is no blood loss or evidence of acute pain, compared to calves castrated with a knife. Calves 3 months or younger are much easier to handle than older animals, making the castration procedure safer for both the handlers and the animal. Rubber ring castration is ineffective on older cattle. For these animals, surgical castration is the best option. It is recommended that older cattle be castrated using an emasculator, as this cuts the blood supply as well as severing the testes and so reduces blood loss. It is strongly recommended that surgical castration be performed on older cattle following the administration of both a local anaesthetic and a non-steroidal anti-inflammatory (ketoprofen), in order to minimize pain.

Calf Management

The provision of the right environment, food and health care to a calf are vitally important to their subsequent productivity and lifespan as an adult. From birth, colostrum needs to be fed and followed by mastitis-free milk in appropriate volumes to ensure the good health and growth of calves. Other factors that need to be managed appropriately to ensure good welfare and growth include care and monitoring of the newborn calf, the appropriate provision of forage for rumen development and a graduated approach to weaning. A detailed manual on the effective rearing of calves on tropical SHD farms is freely available.

Along with appropriate feeding and management to ensure good health, the environment in which calves are kept significantly affects their welfare and development. It is recommended that calves be housed in a way that they can easily stand, lie, turn around, rest comfortably and have visual contact with other calves. Further to this, housing calves in pairs or small groups has been associated with play in calves, which is an indicator of positive welfare and allows them to develop normal social behaviors. Importantly, keeping calves in small groups has not been linked to increased incidences of disease, which is a common argument against group housing.

Equine Management

Owners and persons in charge are required to ensure that they have the skills and personal qualities necessary to be both effective and safe when handling horses. It is necessary that personnel working with horses possess knowledge of their needs and behaviors, an understanding of their husbandry and skill in the practical aspects of equine handling and care. It is important that anyone involved in husbandry procedures such as handling, shoeing, treating, educating, conditioning, breeding, training, riding or driving horses are able to prove competence relevant to the activity being carried out or be under the supervision of a competent person.

It is essential that personnel responsible for horses also have a good knowledge of their normal appearance and behavior and are able to recognise early signs of distress or ill-health so that prompt remedial action can be taken or expert advice sought. A good knowledge of basic equine first aid and access to a veterinarian is essential for anyone caring for horses.

Good equine management skills, appropriate care and timely intervention can lead to positive outcomes for animal behavior and for health and welfare. There are some differences in the types of handling and care required to maintain the welfare of donkeys, mules and horses. Further information on the care of different horses can be obtained by contacting specific equine groups.

Minimum Standard

Horses must be cared for by a sufficient number of personnel, who, collectively, possess the ability, knowledge and competence necessary to maintain the health and welfare of the animals in accordance with this Code.

Example Indicators for Equine Management

- Training/competence in the care of horses can be demonstrated and personnel are aware of how their actions may affect the welfare of the animals.

- Job descriptions or other documentation of expectations of personnel duties include reference to equine health and welfare.

- Owners and people in charge of horses arrange for competent personnel to supervise horses when travelling away.

Recommended Best Practice

- Training and handling procedures should be adapted and modified to suit the individual animal.

- Staff should be trained on the job by supervisors who have competence in handling horses.

- Existing systems and practices for the management of horses should be reviewed regularly to ensure that they continue to be necessary and improved systems incorporated where possible.

- Accurate records should be kept of the history and treatment of the animals.

Food and Water

When considering the amount and type of food, nutrients and water that any equine requires, a number of factors need to be taken into account, including physiological state, the size of the equine, its age, the management system being used, the climate and the amount of work an equine is required to perform.

In their natural state, horses will eat a variety of forages (mainly grasses, which have a high roughage and low energy content) to meet their nutritional needs and, due to the small size of their stomach, they will eat little and often and will normally consume their daily intake over 16-20 hours. When energy requirements are low (such as for horses in good body condition, those in light or no work or dry broodmares), an adequate amount of fresh forage can provide most of the horse's needs. Horses in moderate-to-heavy work generally need supplementary feeding in the form of grains or concentrates, as forages alone will not provide sufficient energy. It is important that they continue to consume some forage, however, to aid digestion and keep healthy. To avoid potentially serious health problems, it is important that if changes are made to the type and quantity of feed, that the changes are made gradually over a period of several days and any contaminated, mouldy or stale leftover food or forage is removed. Feeding levels are best determined by monitoring the body condition of horses. Body condition score (BCS) is a means of taking into account the variability in size and conformation.

The provision of an adequate supply of water is critical for maintaining equine health and welfare. Water needs for different horses vary widely and there will be seasonal variation as water needs will increase when horses are grazing dry summer pastures. Water sources need to be checked to ensure that they are clean, adequate and easily accessible. If water needs are not met, both animal health and welfare will deteriorate.

Most equine pastures contain a large proportion of weeds and rank pasture (areas of paddock under-grazed by horses resulting in the growth of tall grasses and weeds) due to their grazing habits. Horses can be grazed in conjunction with cattle or sheep, which will consume the pasture that horses prefer not to eat, while also reducing the worm contamination on pasture. Where no cattle or other grazers are available, it is important to remove the dung from the paddock as horses will not eat pasture that is contaminated with equine dung. Regular paddock rotation can help to maintain the quality of the pasture.

Donkeys, mules and smaller ponies generally require proportionally more roughage and less protein in their food than larger ponies and horses. Donkeys, mules and smaller ponies usually only need grain and rich feeds such as lucerne or haylage if they are in hard work. Access to high energy pasture needs to be monitored closely to avoid laminitis and obesity, as ponies and donkeys generally tend to be more prone to developing these problems than horses.

In wet weather, higher stocking rates may cause excessive pugging of soil. On small blocks, where the opportunity to spell paddocks and prevent pugging is limited, stocking rate should be reduced and supplementary feeding may be required.

Minimum Standard

- Horses must receive adequate daily quantities of food and nutrients to enable each horse to:
    - Maintain good health.
    - Meet its physiological demands.
    - Minimize metabolic and nutritional disorders.
- If any horse shows signs of being emaciated or if the body condition score of any horse falls below 2 (on a scale of 0-5), urgent remedial action must be taken to improve the condition of the horse.
- If any horse shows signs of being very fat or if the body condition score of any horse is greater than 4 (on a scale of 0-5), urgent remedial action must be taken to reduce the body condition score of the horse.
- All horses must have access to a reliable daily supply of drinking water that is palatable, sufficient for their needs and not harmful to their health.

Example Indicators for Food and Water

- Horses show no signs of problems that are due to poor nutrition.
- Horse body condition score is maintained between 2 and 4.
- Paddock size, pasture cover and feeding frequency and type and amount of supplementary feed is appropriate to the age, physiological state, level of work and breed of the horse.
- Steps are taken to reduce competition for feed between individuals, such as distributing feed in a number of separate piles or feeding individual animals in separate areas.
- If horses become overweight, they are moved to a smaller grazing area or an area providing feed of lower nutritional value.
- Horses have sufficient water to maintain their health and show no signs of dehydration.
- Water quality is monitored and does not contain contaminants at a level harmful to the health of horses.
- Water reticulation systems provide a sufficient amount of water to meet the daily needs of the horses, are monitored and maintained efficiently and any delivery failure is rectified immediately.

Recommended Best Practice

- Any changes to a horse's diet should be introduced gradually over a period of several days and horses monitored closely during this period.

- When feeding baled forage, twine and wrap should be removed to prevent the risk of illness or death from ingestion and to avoid injury from entanglement.

- Horses receiving supplementary concentrated feed should have this fed to them in smaller amounts spread evenly throughout the day, rather than in one large feed.

- When working horses are given a "rest" day (i.e. a day without any work), the concentrate or grain part of the ration should be reduced to decrease the risk of metabolic problems.

- Stallions and pregnant mares should be fed at a level commensurate with their increased energy demands associated with breeding.

- Forage should be fed at floor level and the underlying ground kept reasonably clean, to aid horses' respiratory health.

- Paddocks should be maintained free of plants that are poisonous to horses.

- Watering facilities should be designed to reduce fouling and wastage.

- Troughs should be cleaned often to ensure that water is available and uncontaminated.

Shelter and Housing Facilities

Horses kept outdoors may be exposed to the effects of weather: Heat, cold, rain, snow and wind. In areas lacking natural shelter belts and trees, horses benefit from constructed artificial shelters or covers for protection from the elements.

Horses kept in yards do not have the same freedom of movement as those in open paddocks. They are more susceptible to the chilling effect of cold winds and rain and heat stress from direct summer sun and will require additional shelter to ensure their health and welfare. Lack of adequate shelter and feeding can result in stress, discomfort, loss of body condition and increased susceptibility to disease.

Horses and ponies of different breeds will have differing requirements for shelter. Some breeds of domestic horse, such as the thoroughbred and the Arabian, are recognised as being more susceptible and require additional attention to ensure that their shelter requirements are met. Susceptible horses, ponies or donkeys (i.e. young, old, sick, injured or non-acclimatised animals) will require additional shelter to maintain their health and welfare. The coat of donkeys is less waterproof than that of horses and ponies and so donkeys may be more susceptible to exposure to cold climatic extremes than horses.

Provision of a waterproof, well insulated cover is necessary for non-acclimatised, clipped, sick, injured and old horses for warmth during cold weather. It needs to be ensured that rugs or covers are the correct size and weight to suit each horse and the environmental conditions to which the horses are exposed. Horses will require different rugs or covers for summer and winter. If worn during inclement weather, rugs or covers need to be maintained in a waterproof condition. Unclipped horses and ponies, turned out in paddocks with reasonable shelter, generally adapt well to their environment and when fully acclimatised, may not require covering if feed supplies are adequate.

Minimum Standard

- Horses must have access to shelter to reduce the risk to their health and welfare caused by exposure to cold or wet weather conditions.

- Horses must be provided with the means to minimize the effects of heat stress.

- Covers must be used to protect horses from climatic extremes where other forms of shelter are not sufficient to maintain the horse's health and welfare.

- Where used, covers must be fitted correctly and inspected regularly to ensure that they are providing suitable protection and are not causing the horse discomfort.

- Where horses develop health problems associated with exposure to adverse weather conditions, priority must be given to remedial action that will minimize the consequences of such exposure.

- Additional measures must be taken to enable clipped horses to keep warm in cold weather.

Example Indicators for Shelter

- Horses are not cold (e.g. shivering) or experiencing heat stress (e.g. rapid breathing or panting, excessive sweating).

- Where necessary, horses are covered with rugs or covers to enable them to effectively thermoregulate.

- Horses housed in yards are provided with rugs or covers appropriate to the weather conditions.

- Clipped horses are stabled or provided with additional rugs or covers, shelter and feed appropriate for the weather conditions.

- Horses have access to shelter from sun, rain, wind and adverse weather conditions.

- Natural shade or shelter is available or artificial shelters are provided and are large enough to hold all horses.

- Horses have no skin lesions due to rubbing of the rugs or covers.

- When ambient temperatures are extreme, horses are monitored more frequently than usual, animal behavior is observed and corrective action taken if needed.

Recommended Best Practice

- Horses should not be clipped if the forecast is for cold wet weather unless they are stabled or provided with sufficient rugs or covers, additional roughage and suitable shelter to minimize the effects of exposure.

- Horses should be inspected regularly to ensure that the weight of rug or cover is appropriate for the weather conditions.

- Horse rugs or covers should be inspected daily to ensure they fit correctly and have no loose or broken straps.

- All donkeys should have permanent access to shelter.

Facilities

In the context of this Code, 'facilities' are fixed or portable stalls or yards, which may be used when indoor accommodation is not available or where horses are being held outside for work purposes or to perform husbandry procedures such as shoeing, worming or grooming. These facilities usually provide some shelter from the elements.

Some horses in New Zealand may be kept in a semi-wild state and in this case, special handling facilities may be necessary to enable routine management such as worming and hoof trimming to be performed. When constructing facilities such as these, the design needs to take into account the need to keep stress in these horses to a minimum to reduce danger and avoid injury for both horse and handler.

It is not uncommon for horses or ponies, as a prey and herd animal, to flee as a herd when one horse is panicked. When a large number of horses are being kept within the vicinity of each other, particularly in a novel environment (e.g. at a multiple-day competitive event) and where horses are being contained in temporary yards and pens, this fleeing behavior can result in horses being injured, sometimes fatally. The use of sturdy materials to construct temporary yards, rather than materials such as electric fencing, reduces the chance of horses panicking or joining the fleeing herd, which reduces the risk of injury to horses and persons in the area. As well as being soundly constructed, it is important that yards are also situated in well-drained areas.

Minimum Standard

- All facilities must be designed, constructed, maintained and operated in a manner that minimizes the likelihood of distress or injury to the horses.

- All fittings and internal surfaces must be constructed and maintained to ensure that there are no hazards likely to cause injury to horses.

- Faeces and urine must not be permitted to accumulate to such an extent that they pose a threat to the health and welfare of the horses.

Example Indicators for Facilities

- Handlers are trained and familiar with the operation of facilities and understand how incorrect operation may affect the horses in their care.

- Floor surfaces are not slippery.

- Potential hazards such as windows, ventilators, light bulbs, power cables and associated fittings are covered or placed out of reach of horses.

- Grain based feeds, health remedies, toxic materials and associated equipment are securely stored and unable to be accessed by horses.

- Sharp objects, protrusions, edges, gaps and damaged flooring likely to cause injury have been removed, repaired or covered.

- All stable and barn doorways are wide enough for a horse and handler to move through easily.

- No toxic paint or timber preservatives are used.

- Personnel take action to rectify any problems or potential problems, with facilities that are apparent upon inspection of horses within the facilities.

Recommended Best Practice

- Yards and pens used to contain horses for unsupervised periods should not be constructed with electrified tape or electrified wire as the only barrier.

- Horses should be yarded within visual contact of familiar horses to reduce stress.

- Horses should be inspected regularly in facilities to ensure that they are in good health and have sustained no injuries.

Housing

Horses may be held in indoor housing in stables, loose boxes or stalls. When horses are housed, they are totally dependent on their handlers for all daily requirements, welfare and safety and handlers must be aware that there are additional responsibilities of care to those horses being managed extensively outdoors.

Loose boxes are commonly used for overnight or long-term individual accommodation of horses. Housing horses in loose boxes that are too small may increase the risk of injury to both horse and handler. If horses are to be housed in loose boxes for an extended period of time, the provision of bedding is necessary to give them the opportunity to rest.

It is important that priority is given to the health and safety of both horses and handlers when planning the layout of stables, loose boxes and stalls. Housing should be dry, well-ventilated and draught-free. Non-slip floor surfaces designed to direct liquid effluent away from the animal accommodation will help reduce effluent build up. Regular checking and filling of holes which may develop in the floor will help to maintain an even surface. Good hygiene is important in order to maintain the health and welfare of horses and to minimize disease and distress. Fire is a significant threat in a stable environment but the risk can be minimized by taking precautions.

Minimum Standard

- All housing for horses must be designed, constructed, maintained and operated in a manner that minimizes the likelihood of distress or injury to the horses.

- When housed, horses must be confined in a manner which prevents them causing injury to themselves or adjacent animals and have sufficient room to lie down, readily rise and turn around in comfort.

- Horses may be tied in a stall, but for no more than 6 hours in a 24 hour period, unless under veterinary recommendation and while untied must receive daily exercise.

- Horses must be able to lie down and rest comfortably for a sufficient time each day to meet their behavioral needs.

- Ventilation must ensure that housed horses do not become heat or cold stressed and prevent a buildup of harmful concentrations of noxious gases.

- Immediate and appropriate action must be taken to reduce ammonia levels if they exceed 15 ppm at horse level.

- Bedding must be of good quality, friable and with minimal risk of toxic agent contamination.

- Horses housed in buildings must be monitored at a frequency that ensures their health and welfare.

- Natural or comparable artificial lighting must be provided during daylight hours.

- Floors must be constructed of a non-slip surface or material and must be designed to drain liquid effluent away.

- Water containers and feed bins should be constructed and sited in a manner that minimizes the risk of injury to horses.

- Persons in charge of horses housed in buildings must have contingency plans to address any event which could result in a potentially significant welfare impact on the horses.

Example Indicators for Housing

- Horses are able to exhibit signs of relaxation when housed (lying down or neck low, drooping lower lip, nostrils narrowed).

- When the horse is standing with all four feet on the floor there is sufficient space above it to enable the full range of head and neck motion without touching the ceiling.

- All stable and barn doorways are wide enough for a horse and handler to move through easily.

- Adequate lighting is provided to allow inspection of all horses •Levels of ammonia are no more than 15ppm at any time.

- Bedding is clean and dry, provides warmth and protects against abrasion.

- Where a large number of horses are housed together, a roster system is used to ensure all animals have regular supervision by competent personnel.

- Contingency plans are in place for dealing with any hazards or emergencies and include the ability to rapidly release horses into a safe and secure environment.

Restraint and Containment

The construction of suitable fencing is vital to ensure that horses do not become entangled in the fencing material or escape and become injured roaming away from the property. The suitability of fencing varies according to the breed, sex and disposition of the horses, as well as stocking density and paddock size. It is important that fences are readily visible to horses and are well maintained, with no sharp protrusions from the fence on the inner side.

In the context of this Code, 'tethering' refers to securing a horse for the purpose of grazing. This is different from 'tying up' a horse for management purposes such as grooming or attention by a farrier. Tethering is sometimes used to contain horses within a specified area without the necessity to erect boundary fences. Tethering has the potential to cause injury and is recommended to be used only for short time periods and when other forms of grazing or containment are unavailable. Only horses adequately trained to accept the practice can be tethered in relative safety and, even then, will require close supervision.

Equipment such as the twitch or hobbles may be used in situations where horses need to be restrained for short periods of time for management purposes.

Post-and-rail type fences painted with non-toxic preparations provide an ideal visual barrier for premises designed mainly for horses. A popular alternative to post and rail fencing, which also provides a good visual barrier, is a single top rail attached to a conventional post-and-wire fence.

If electric fencing is used to contain horses, it needs to be designed, installed and maintained so that the fence does not cause more than a momentary discomfort to the animal. It is important that power units are earthed correctly and fences checked daily to ensure that they are taut and not posing a risk to the horses. If wire with a potential to cause injury to horses, such as barbed wire, is used to contain horses in paddocks, an inner fence (e.g. electric fencing) can be used to reduce the risk of a horse making direct contact with the barbed wire.

Tethering is not suitable for long-term management of horses as it restricts the animal's freedom to exercise itself, find its own food and water, escape attacks from predators and take its own measures to reduce the effects of extremes of temperature. Tethering also risks the animal becoming entangled or injuring itself on the tethering equipment. The longer the tether used, the less chance that it will become dangerously twisted and cause injury. It is recommended that the tether is 9m or longer, is fixed as low as possible to the anchor post and includes a swivelling device on the tether. It is important that the area chosen to tether the horse is free of obstructions that may entangle the tether. When tethering horses in close proximity to other tethered animals, they need to be sufficient distance away from each other to avoid becoming entangled.

Hobbles can be used to temporarily limit the locomotion of a horse by inhibiting the action of one or more legs. They are used in situations where effective restraint is required including medical treatment or surgery, to restrain mares being served at stud or to shoe difficult horses. A number of types of hobbles are available and they are generally made of rope, leather or synthetic materials. Horses need to be gradually introduced to hobbles using recognised techniques until they become accustomed to the new equipment.

Exerting pressure on the upper lip of a horse using a nose twitch can be used to restrain the animal in certain situations. Placing pressure on the upper lip calms the horse by causing endorphins to be released from the brain. As such, a nose twitch is only to be used on the upper lip.

Minimum Standard

- Any method to restrain or contain horses must be used in a way that minimizes the possibility of injury, harm or distress to the horses.

- Fences must be designed, constructed and maintained to minimize risk of injury to horses.

- When restraining horses, the mildest effective method of restraint available must be used and be applied for the minimum period required.

- Horses that are restrained by tethering must be:

  - Trained to the conditions.

  - Provided with food, water, shade and protection from extremes of heat and cold.

  - Able to walk and move around without undue hindrance.

  - Kept under general surveillance.

- Horses must not be tethered for longer than 15 hours without being released for exercise.

- Horses must not be tethered if they are physiologically compromised in such a way that tethering may affect their health or welfare.

- A tether must be sited so as to prevent the horse reaching any public access-way or becoming entangled with objects or other animals.

Example Indicators for Restraint and Containment

- Hobbles used to restrain a horse are used for short periods of time only.

- The horse has been trained to accept the use of hobbles and remains calm during their use.

- The nose twitch is only used on the upper lip of the horse.

- Wire and electric fencing is kept at a sufficient tension so horses cannot become entangled in it.

- Horses are only introduced to a new paddock in the dark if the paddock is known to be safe, secure and free from hazards.

- The height, strength and quality of fences and gates being used to contain horses are sufficient to prevent them escaping and are clearly visible.

- Gateways are wide enough to allow for the easy and safe passage of horses.

- Non-toxic preparations are used if painting or treating wooden fencing rails.

- Electric fencing used for fencing horses is highly visible.

- Horses that are tethered are calm, have been trained to accept tethering and to accept human approach.

- Horses are not tethered if they are very young, pregnant, nursing, sick or injured.

- Horses that have been tethered during the day are placed in a paddock or loose box overnight.

- Food and water requirements for tethered horses are met according to food and water minimum standards and indicators.

- Sites that are to be used for tethering horses are examined beforehand for potentially harmful objects that a horse could eat such as toxic plants or litter and for objects or vegetation that might snag on the tether or head collar and prevent the horse's movement.

- Tethered horses have the ability to walk and move around within the constraints of the tethered range.

Recommended Best Practice

- Wire with the potential to cause serious injury, such as high-tensile steel or barbed wire, should not be used when constructing fences for horses.

- When using electric fencing, horses should be supervised until they have become accustomed to the boundaries of the new paddock.

- Measures should be taken to ensure that boundary fences are visible to horses.

- Items of machinery, equipment or rubbish (especially wire) should be removed from paddocks used to accommodate horses.

- Horses should not be tethered.

- If horses are tethered, wide ropes made of hemp or other soft material should be used instead of nylon rope, which can cause serious burns if the horse becomes entangled.

Behavior

Horses are kept under a variety of conditions, from extensive grazing to intensive housing in yards, pens and stables. Horses are highly social and hierarchical in nature and thrive best in herds, where they can establish hierarchies. Whenever animals are introduced into a herd, they will be challenged as newcomers and will have to establish their place in the group. These challenges can be aggressive and lead to injury and distress. Such behavior needs to be managed and this is particularly important when introducing young horses into a herd for the first time. The risk of injury increases where horses are overcrowded and competition for food, water and space may lead to fighting. Subordinate animals need to have sufficient space to escape bullying by dominant animals.

Signs of injury, aggression or stress include continual harassment, hair loss, fighting, excessive fence pacing and isolation. A large paddock can be used to minimize confrontation and, where possible, paddocks with broken contours and natural cover will assist in reducing stress. Colts, stallions, mares close to foaling and sick animals generally require segregation from other groups to reduce the risk of injury and transfer of disease.

When mixing horses, consideration needs to be given to differences in the individuals, such as the temperament of the animals to be mixed, physiological status of the horses and differences in breed, age and body size, as well as the availability of food and water, ground conditions and size of the paddock.

Exercise is extremely important for a horse's physical and mental health, particularly where they are stabled for many hours of the day. Insufficient exercise can lead to behavioral problems and the development of stereotypical behaviors. Horses are usually exercised by being ridden or turned loose into a paddock to exercise themselves, but they can also be exercised in other ways such as lunging them or walking them in hand or on a walker.

Horses, donkeys and mules are all social animals and need to be provided with companions to maintain their welfare. While interaction with humans may provide a substitute for some of their social and behavioral needs, the provision of social companions of their own species is preferable. Horses can, however, live with companions such as sheep, cattle or goats. If it is not possible to keep a horse in a herd with others, providing them with the opportunity to see or hear other horses (or other animals) can provide some welfare benefits.

Donkeys bond strongly to their companions. Care needs to be taken not to separate bonded partnerships in order to minimize the risk of stress and illness that this may cause, particularly if the donkey only has one other companion.

Horses are not always kept as riding or working animals. They can be kept for a number of other reasons including as pets or as companions for other horses. In cases such as these, even though the horse is not being worked, it still needs to be provided with a standard of care that will maintain its health and welfare.

Minimum Standard

- When horses are mixed into new groups, they must be managed to minimize the effects of aggression and injury.

- Horses must receive daily exercise sufficient to maintain their health and welfare.

Example Indicators for Behavior

- Horses are active and alert and do not exhibit signs of discomfort, injury or distress.

- Stallions are kept in a separate paddock if they are likely to cause injury to other individuals in a herd.

- Personnel observe the temperament and the social structure of the horses under their care and are aware which horses can and cannot be mixed.

- Horses are provided with sufficient space to enable subordinate horses to move away from those individuals exhibiting threatening behavior.

- When horses are first mixed, management practices are used that aim to reduce the chances of competition and aggression between individuals occurring, for example, spreading additional feed (hay) over a large surface area, feeding individuals in separate areas, providing additional space etc.

- Horses are observed closely when unfamiliar horses are first placed together and then daily until settled, to monitor for signs of injury or continued aggression.

- Horses subjected to persistent bullying are removed from the herd.

- The level of exercise is appropriate for the age and level of fitness of the horse.

Recommended Best Practice

- The introduction of new horses to the herd should not occur more frequently than necessary because of the social distress involved while the introduced and resident horses re-establish a hierarchy.

- If any horses are subjected to persistent bullying, they should be removed from the paddock, checked for illness and injury and, if returned to the group, be monitored closely thereafter to ensure that confrontation is minimized.

- Horses should be kept with at least with one other social companion. If this is not possible, horses should be kept where they can see or hear other horses (or other animals).

- Horses should be provided with an area in which they are able to move freely and obtain daily exercise sufficient to meet their health and welfare.

- Horses should be given the opportunity to graze daily.

Handling, Training and Equipment

Equine Handling and Training

Horses naturally exist as prey animals and so are likely to flee in response to situations or objects that they are unsure of. The risk of injury to both handlers and horses is reduced when good handling skills are used and the horse is held in appropriate facilities. Knowledge of appropriate handling and management skills can lead to positive welfare outcomes for the horse. Young horses (under two years old), benefit from being introduced to basic training and positive handling techniques that will instil confidence in them and positively influence their relationship with their handlers. Horses pushed beyond their level of capability at a young age are more likely to sustain injuries or develop undesirable behavioral traits that can continue to be present as an adult. A competent person will ensure that horses are trained in a way that is not physically or psychologically damaging. For this reason, it is important that persons training horses are experienced, confident and competent in this role.

Reinforcing and rewarding positive behavior is crucial when training horses to perform to their full potential. Horses exhibiting abnormal or undesirable physiological and behavioral responses to handling, training and confinement can do so for a number of reasons, including negative prior experience, frustration or pain. Responses may include aggressive threats, biting and kicking. Behaviors such as pacing, weaving and crib biting are more likely to be associated with restricted housing conditions and the feeding of concentrated low fibre foods. Factors such as early weaning and the horse's temperament may also contribute to the development of these behaviors. Pacing, weaving and crib biting behaviors need to be addressed through changes in the management of the horse as these behaviors will not be resolved by disciplinary intervention.

Appropriate techniques for correcting undesirable behaviors will vary depending on the underlying reason for the behavior. Undesirable behaviors are likely to become increasingly problematic if not corrected promptly and, if they occur, it is necessary to seek advice from a person experienced in equine handling.

The age that horses begin their training can vary considerably depending on their breed and the discipline for which they are to be used. The weight of rider and amount of work they are asked to perform needs to be commensurate with their size and development. Thoroughbred racehorses often have small, light riders on their backs as early as 15 months of age, in order to race as two or three year olds. Horses used in other disciplines often begin their training at a later age and may be three or four years old before they are first backed and ridden.

Horses respond best when aids and instructions are humane, clear and consistent. Ill-timed or inappropriate reprimands are counterproductive and may result in the development of unwanted behaviors. The whip needs to be used only as an additional aid for a horse, not as a punishment. Often, the use of positive reinforcement behavioral techniques can bring changes in behavior, creating the same results as restrictive or harsher methods, without reducing the horse's welfare.

Some horses, such as stallions or those that are young or unbroken, may be unpredictable and require more advanced handling skills to ensure the safety of both horse and handler. Geldings (castrated males) are in general, calmer and easier to handle than stallions and will not seek to mate with mares. It is recommended that colts are gelded within their first year and preferably before they reach sexual maturity.

Some equine facilities, such as riding schools, offer advice and training days to enable those who are responsible for horses to learn how to handle or improve their handling skills. Equine related organisations or clubs can also offer advice on horse husbandry and care.

Minimum Standard

- Horses must be handled and trained at all times in such a way as to minimize the risk of pain, injury or distress.

- Horses must not be worked at such an intensity that is likely to cause exhaustion, heat stress, injury or distress.

- Electric prodders must not be used on horses.

- Horses must not be struck or prodded with a goad in the udder, anus, genitals or eyes.

    ○ Horses must not be prodded in sensitive areas.

    ○ Horses must not be struck around their heads.

- The whip, lead or any other similar object must only be used for safety, correction and encouragement and not used in an unnecessary, excessive or improper manner.

Example Indicators for Equine Handling and Training

- Handlers' behavior towards horses is patient.

- Horses are handled in such a manner that they remain relaxed and do not exhibit signs of discomfort or anxiety (such as hind leg kicking, flared nostrils, contracted lips, visible white of the eyes or tail swishes).

- Handlers are able to recognise the different behavior patterns of horses and react appropriately.

- Handlers appreciate how individual horses may react to and interact with other horses, animals, humans, strange noises, sights and smells.

- Handlers are trained in the use of equipment used to move and restrain horses.

- Horses are introduced to basic training and are backed or started in harness, at a suitable level of maturity.

- Horses are not expected to accept practices and perform procedures prior to the level of maturity where they are able to physically and psychologically cope with what is being expected of them.

- Horses are trained by competent persons using accepted techniques.

- The mildest form of discipline that will achieve the required behavioral change is used.

Recommended Best Practice

- Appropriate advice (for example, from a person knowledgeable in equine behavior) should be sought at the first signs of unwanted behavior occurring. This may prevent more persistent behavioral problems developing which are likely to be more difficult to cure.

- Riders should not be heavier than is appropriate for the equine in question, taking into account the size of the animal, its breed, physiological status and workload that it is being asked to perform.

Saddlery and Equipment

The equipment used with horses can have a large influence on their health and welfare. It is important that all equipment used to handle, ride or drive horses is of a suitable size and is correctly fitted to reduce rubbing or slipping and minimize discomfort. For reasons of comfort, hygiene and safety it is necessary that all equipment is maintained in a clean, supple condition, free from cracks and other features likely to cause injury.

Much of the equipment used on horses is to help guide or control a horse and influence its movement and behavior and so the incorrect use and handling of this type of equipment has the potential to cause pain and distress. For this reason, it is important that handlers and riders are aware of the potential effects that incorrect and harsh use of equipment can have on the health and welfare of a horse. It is important that techniques, methods and equipment that have a mild effect on horses are used in place of severe equipment wherever possible. However, how the equipment is used by the handler or rider will largely determine the effect that any piece of equipment has on a horse. Ropes that are used for educating and restraining horses can cause significant injury to both horse and handler if they are of the wrong type.

Halters or headcollars are sometimes left on horses that have a history of being difficult to catch when turning them out into paddocks. However, this practice can be potentially hazardous as the headcollar may catch on items in the paddock and cause injury. If halters or headcollars are left on horses when turning them out, it is necessary to check frequently to ensure that the headcollar is not damaged and is not chaffing or causing injury. Young horses outgrow their halters rapidly, which can result in pressure injury if they are not adjusted and changed as necessary.

The use of restrictive equipment (e.g. harsh bits and over tightened nosebands) used for controlling a horse needs to be reduced to a minimum through the application of appropriate, effective and safe training and handling techniques so as to maintain the horse's welfare. It is important that all equipment is assessed for its suitability and fit before use, with consideration given to the horse's natural movement, behavior, temperament and physical capabilities. If in doubt or where expertise is required (e.g. when fitting saddles) this needs to be sought to ensure that the equipment is not causing the horse pain or discomfort. If boots or leg bandages are used, they need to be suitable for the purpose and correctly fitted to avoid discomfort or injury and left on only for the minimum length of time necessary.

Minimum Standard

- Equipment used on horses must be maintained in good condition and be fitted so as not to cause injury.

- Equipment must be used in such a way as to avoid pain, injury or distress to the horse.

- Example indicators for Saddlery and Equipment.

- Equipment is regularly cleaned and inspected to ensure that leather/synthetic fibre etc. is supple and all parts of the equipment are in good order.

- Bits are clean and have no rough or sharp edges.

- Equipment does not pinch, rub or cut horses on which it is used.

- Every effort is made to ensure that equipment is fitted correctly for the individual horse on which it is being used.

- Equipment that is placed next to the horse's skin is kept clean, soft and free from debris.

- Equipment that is restrictive for the horse is used by knowledgeable and competent persons only.

Recommended Best Practice

- Ropes used for educating and restraining horses should be pliable, at least 15 mm thick and not made of nylon.

- Ropes should not be attached directly to a horse's legs.

- Where leg restraint is essential, felt-lined leather straps should be used for this purpose.

- Covers should be removed from horses on a weekly basis and aired and loose hair and cakedon dirt removed from the cover.

- All horses, especially young and inexperienced ones, should be handled gently with equipment that exerts a mild effect only.

- Horses should be monitored when being brought back into work to ensure that the equipment does not cause injury or discomfort while the skin hardens with consistent use of the equipment.

- Halters or headcollars should not be left on horses when they are turned out into the paddock.

Husbandry Practices

Breeding and Foaling

The majority of mares are sexually mature at two years of age and will begin to regularly come into season after this age. Jenny donkeys mature later than mares and are not bred until three years of age. As day length increases they will start cycling and come into season every 21 days until day length decreases in autumn and cycling ceases. When a mare is in season, she is more willing to accept a stallion and at this stage, a mare and stallion can be mated for breeding purposes.

Breeding management techniques and programmes that optimise genetic potential are used in all sectors of the equine industry in New Zealand. In addition to selecting animals with desirable genotypes for breeding, there are a number of established and developing technologies being used to facilitate genetic gains and better manage animals.

Precautions can be taken to reduce the chances of either the mare or stallion becoming injured, acquiring or spreading infection during the breeding process.

Inexperienced mares or those who have experienced foaling difficulties previously are more likely to experience problems and care needs to be taken that these horses have experienced persons on hand to assist if required. Difficulties during foaling are a veterinary emergency and help needs to be sought as soon as possible.

Horses usually give birth to one foal only. Twin births do happen, but it is rare that both foals survive and usually one or both of the foals die during the pregnancy. Pregnancy can be confirmed by ultrasound, blood test, urine test or manual palpation.

Minimum Standard

- Owners or persons in charge of mating horses must ensure that they possess the appropriate experience and level of competency in the technique used so that the health and welfare of the horses is not compromised.

- Horses that are foaling or are due to foal, must be provided with a suitable area in a safe, sheltered and quiet environment.

- Horses that are due to foal must be observed discreetly and as frequently as required to ensure that they are not experiencing difficulties.

- If a horse is exhibiting signs to indicate that she is experiencing difficulties at any point during or following foaling, expert assistance must be provided immediately.

- Laparoscopic artificial insemination must only be carried out by veterinarians or trained and competent operators under veterinary supervision.

- Cervical artificial insemination and pregnancy diagnosis must only be carried out by persons trained and competent in the techniques.

- Rectal pregnancy diagnosis must only be carried out by persons trained and competent in the techniques.

Example Indicators for Breeding and Foaling

- The person supervising a mare that is due to foal knows the indicators that the mare may be experiencing problems foaling.

- Contact details for a veterinarian are accessible to all personnel.

- Horses that are foaling are given a suitable safe and quiet place to enable them to foal, for the foal to suckle and for the mare to bond with her foal.

- Persons in charge of breeding horses have received training in the relevant techniques (natural insemination, artificial insemination or embryo transfer).

Recommended Best Practice

- When selecting animals for breeding, attention should be given to selecting animals of appropriate size, breed and foaling experience.

- If foaling is to take place in a paddock, the area should be free from hazards such as ponds and ditches in which the foal can become injured or drown and free from large livestock such as other horses or cattle, which are likely to be curious of the new foal and may accidently injure it.

- If foaling is to take place in a foaling box, the box should be thoroughly disinfected and sufficient straw provided to create a warm but well ventilated environment. Potential hazards such as hay nets or bucket holders should be removed before foaling.

- Boxes provided for foaling should be substantially larger (preferably twice as big) as those used for housing a single horse so as to minimize the risk of the mare injuring the foal.

- Mares in late pregnancy should be observed at least twice daily for signs of impending foaling.

Rearing and Weaning

Foals rely on the dam's milk to obtain nutrients for the first few weeks of life. Colostrum is the first milk produced by the dam after foaling and contains nutrients and antibodies that are essential to protect the foal from disease. The newborn foal absorbs antibodies from colostrum, but begins to lose that ability about six hours after birth. It is important that foals receive sufficient colostrum as soon as possible after birth to ensure their health and welfare.

Weaning foals from their dam combines a number of factors with the potential to compromise animal welfare – the physical separation of dam and foal, changes to the foal's feeding regime and cessation of milk being taken from the dam. In some cases, weaning may also mean a change in the environment for the foal and mixing with other new social groups.

Weaning is stressful for mare and foal, but if the process is properly managed, foals generally appear to adapt within a few days without any long lasting consequences to their health and welfare.

Colostrum, either fresh or stored, can provide local immunity in the gut and is a highly digestible, high quality food. Antibodies cannot be absorbed by the foal beyond 24-36 hours after birth, so colostrum needs to be fed as soon as possible after birth.

Weaning can be undertaken abruptly (with dam and foal kept out of visual and auditory contact from each other) or progressively (gradually removed from each other but kept in adjacent paddocks). The latter method may be less stressful for horses, but requires good fences and greater resources. There is some evidence that weaning foals in pairs or groups, in an environment which is as familiar as possible and providing them with access to clean water and a high fibre diet, is beneficial for their health and welfare.

Minimum Standard

- Newborn foals must receive sufficient colostrum or a good quality commercial colostrum substitute to ensure their health and welfare.

- Weaning must be managed in a way that avoids undue stress on the dam and foal and minimizes negative impacts on their health and welfare.

Example Indicators for Rearing and Weaning

- Handlers are able to recognise if a foal is not receiving adequate feed and will remedy the situation.

- Foals are not weaned until they are receiving at least 75% of their daily feed requirements from solid feed.

Recommended Best Practice

- Foals should receive colostrum as soon as possible after birth, preferably within the first six hours.

- Horses should not be weaned from their dams until they are at a level of maturity where minimal negative consequences are likely to result.

- Prior to weaning, foals should be introduced to the feed that they will be expected to consume following weaning, to help reduce weight loss and growth problems in the foal after being weaned.

- Where foals are unable to be reared with their natural mother, alternative equine company should be provided.

Identification

Identification of horses using specified systems is a compulsory requirement in some areas of horse sport such as thoroughbred and standardbred racing. However, identification can also be used as a temporary method of tracking a horse when it is sold or being transported and can also be a way of proving ownership in the case of horse theft. There are a number of different methods of identification, which vary in their permanency and the amount of pain that they cause the horse when applied. Methods of identification include hot and cold branding, microchipping and DNA analysis.

Minimum Standard

- All identification procedures must be applied by a competent operator.

- Pain relief must be used with hot branding.

Example Indicators for Identification

- No injuries or infections are apparent at the site of identification.

- One application to the skin, for the minimum time, is required to produce a brand.

- Horses show minimal reaction to hot branding.

Recommended Best Practice

- Freeze branding, if undertaken, should only be used with pain relief and carried out by a competent equine handler trained in the procedure. The brand site should be closely shaved before branding.

- Freeze branding should be performed using liquid nitrogen, rather than dry ice, as the brand is applied to the skin for a shorter period, with a similar result.

- Microchipping should be administered by a veterinarian or trained equine handler who ensures good aseptic technique.

- Hot branding should not be used.

Pre-transport Selection

Where specific guidelines for the selection and transport of horses exist, they should be consulted. Otherwise, transport should generally be in accordance with the Animal Welfare. All persons in charge of horses, including staff and contract transport operators, should be aware of the requirements for pre-transport selection and transport of horses.

In cases of doubt about the condition of an animal, a veterinarian needs to be consulted. A veterinarian can certify an animal as fit for transport, in which case the appropriate documentation needs to accompany the animal on its journey.

Transport can be a stressful experience for horses, particularly for those animals that have not been transported previously, that have had a negative past experience while being transported or that are not accustomed to human contact. Good handling techniques will help to reduce anxiety during the process.

All precautions should be taken to ensure the safety and security of horses during transportation. Horses are transported on land, sea or in the air in a variety of trailers and containers, from small boxes that carry one horse alone to large trucks or containers that are capable of carrying a large number of horses simultaneously.

Minimum Standard

- All horses selected for transport must be examined by the person in charge prior to loading to ensure that they are fit for transport and are able to withstand the journey without suffering unreasonable or unnecessary pain or distress.

- Any horse likely to give birth during transport or be affected by metabolic complications of late pregnancy as a result of the journey, must not be selected for transport.

- Proper care must be taken when deciding if it is appropriate to transport young, old, pregnant or otherwise physiologically or behaviorally compromised horses.

Example Indicators for Pre-transport Selection

- Transported horses do not display symptoms of unreasonable pain or distress.

- No horse gives birth during transport.

- Foals under four months of age are transported with their dam.

Recommended Best Practice

- Every effort should be made to ensure that horses are transported for the shortest possible time.

- When undertaking long journeys, horses should be familiarised with the feed and provided with the same type of feed that they are used to eating at home, both at rest stops during the journey and upon arrival.

- When undertaking long journeys, horses should be provided with water with which they have been familiarised.

Health, Injury and Disease

Health and welfare are closely associated and owners and people in charge of horses have a responsibility to, as far as possible, prevent ill-health in their horses and treat it where it occurs. Every person responsible for the care of horses needs to be able to recognise signs of ill-health, have knowledge of basic equine first aid and have access to a veterinarian to diagnose and treat any serious illness or injury. Potential problems need to be noted as early as possible and steps taken to rectify the problem. Animal health programmes need to include disease prevention strategies. The ability to detect ill-health early in horses is crucial for successful diagnosis and treatment.

Regular examination of the hooves of horses can ensure that signs of injury, other abnormalities, loose shoes and impacted foreign material are detected before they cause further problems to the health of the horse.

The dental health of horses can have a large influence on their health and welfare. Horses with worn, sharp or otherwise abnormal teeth often experience discomfort or pain and are unable to chew their food properly, which can result in poor digestion or malnutrition.

Parasite infestation can cause disease and death. It is important that a parasite management programme is in place, as large parasite burdens can cause disease, loss of weight and a gradual deterioration in the health of horses. Management strategies such as pasture rotation, faecal egg count monitoring, cross grazing the pasture with other animal species, harrowing or regular removal of faeces can be used to control parasites. A holistic approach encompassing a number of management strategies is optimal for minimising parasitic burdens.

Products such as worming pastes are available when quick and effective measures are needed to reduce worm burdens. There are a range of alternative therapies available for the treatment of various conditions in horses. When using alternative therapies, the person in charge needs to ensure that the use of these therapies do not cause harm to horses.

The optimal frequency for trimming a horse's hooves to maintain its health and welfare will depend on factors such as age, time of year, nutrition, management, the present condition of the hoof and the presence of injury. Unless running on dry abrasive surfaces, hooves need regular trimming to avoid cracking and disease. Horses standing in excess moisture, such as that which occurs in stabled horses under conditions of poor stable management or pastured horses standing in excess moisture for extended periods of time can suffer skin problems or hoof problems such as thrush (an infection of the frog of the hoof which may cause tenderness of the foot and lameness).

Where abnormal heat or painful pressure points are found in the hoof, a veterinarian or competent farrier can provide advice on the cause and appropriate action to prevent further problems developing.

Following trimming of the hoof, horses can have shoes fitted, be left unshod or the hooves can be trimmed leaving the hoof shaped as a 'barefoot trim'. The most appropriate method for a particular horse will depend on a number of factors such as the individual horse's hooves, the management schedule that the horse is kept under and its workload. Shoes, if used, need to be removed and adjusted or replaced regularly in response to hoof wall growth or when shoes have moved off the wall.

Hoof trimming and shoe fitting needs to be carried out by persons trained and competent in equine anatomy and hoof care. Trimming of hooves and fitting shoes by persons who have not received adequate training in equine anatomy and hoof care can cause lameness, muscular problems and impaired movement which can possibly result in irreparable damage to the horse.

Sharp and uneven points can develop on a horse's teeth. Regular attention is required to file these edges so that the horse can chew more effectively. Older horses (i.e. those over 16 years of age) may require extra dental care and attention than younger horses.

As a result of being ridden, horses and ponies can develop muscular pain, including back pain. If horses are experiencing pain, they may change their behavior in an attempt to escape the discomfort. This can be interpreted as 'disobedience' or 'misbehavior' by the novice rider. Both gradual or sudden changes in equine behavior need to be investigated and, if necessary, a veterinarian called to perform an assessment of the horse to determine if the horse is experiencing pain, before other methods of correction are considered. All those responsible for managing horses, even if the horses are in different ownership, need to devise and implement a parasite control programme to apply to all horses in the same establishment.

Minimum Standard

- Those responsible for the welfare of horses must be competent at recognising the signs of ill-health or injury and take prompt remedial action, as appropriate.

- Medication must only be used in accordance with registration conditions and manufacturer's instructions or professional advice.

- Hooves must be trimmed as required to permit normal mobility and to maintain hoof health, shape and function.

- Teeth must be maintained as required to permit normal grazing and chewing.

Example Indicators for Health, Injury and Disease

- Horses are active, bright, alert, move freely and actively graze.

- Persons working with horses demonstrate a good knowledge of equine first aid, are able to recognise key physical and behavioral signs that an horse is unwell, in pain or distressed and will undertake prompt action and treatment as necessary.

- Hygiene standards and management procedures protect against ill-health and spread of disease.

- When the early signs of a disease outbreak are recognised or suspected, expert advice is sought promptly and any intervention is documented.

- A regular health programme is implemented.

- Expert advice and treatment is sought for any irregularities in the hoof which are causing lameness or may cause problems if not remedied.

- Horses are not losing condition, resisting bridling, feed-packing in cheeks or dropping hard feed while eating as a result of dental abnormalities.

- When using a roster system, full documentation is maintained and is available to all personnel outlining any health problems or potential health problems, that have been apparent upon inspection of horses.

Recommended Best Practice

- Following illness or injury, the owner or person in charge should follow veterinary instructions regarding the resumption of work for the horse.

- Horses should have an annual health check conducted by a veterinarian.

- Horses should receive regular expert care from a qualified and competent hoof care professional to maintain the health of the hoof.

- Equine teeth should be examined and treated as necessary, but at least annually for dental conditions that may cause pain or interfere with normal feeding, digestion or work.

- A record should be maintained of any medicinal treatment given to horses.

- Horses should be vaccinated according to veterinary recommendations, to protect them from infectious diseases.

Animal Health and Disease Management

Animal health focuses primarily on ensuring that the animals are healthy, disease-free and well looked after. Diseases like anthrax, black-leg, blue tongue, rinderpest, footrot, calf scour, etc. are common in animals and their treatment practices fall under the domain of disease management. This chapter delves into the concept of animal health and disease management to provide an in-depth understanding of the subject.

Animal Health

Animal health is a state of complete physical, mental and social well-being and not merely the absence of disease or infirmity'. More recently, the concept of 'mental health' has quite sensibly been defined as 'more than the absence of mental disorders or disabilities, a state of well-being in which the individual realizes his or her own abilities, can cope with the normal stresses of life, can work productively and fruitfully and is able to make a contribution to his or her community'.

It should be noted that this concept is only gradually gaining ground in veterinary circles. Since its creation in 1924, the key activities of the OIE have been to monitor and control animal diseases. It was not until the OIE's Third Strategic Plan for 2001–2005 that the organization included the improvement of animal health, veterinary public health and animal welfare worldwide in its mandate. This mandate was reaffirmed in subsequent Strategic Plans, the latest of which extends into 2015. Nonetheless, an examination of the OIE's specific missions reflects the importance of diseases and the broadening of the definition of 'animal health' seems to have more to do with adding 'animal welfare' than with changing the definition of animal health as such, which would bring it more into line with the WHO definition.

That said, scientific advances in the fields of ethology and neurosciences are forcing us to revise our perception of the mental complexity of animals. Animals as 'sentient beings', as they are described in the Treaty of Lisbon, must be considered as capable of feeling emotions, having needs and a degree of consciousness. The concept of mental health should therefore apply equally to animals. An animal can, for example, suffer from 'anxiety', 'depression' or even 'compulsive disorders', which are some of the new challenges facing 'veterinary behavioral medicine'. In addition to the absence of these pathologies, an animal in good mental health would be one with 'a life worth living', as demonstrated by recent advances in certain aspects of animal ethics.

Appearance of the Healthy Animal

- The healthy animal is alert and aware of its surroundings. It is active and holds its head up watching what is happening around it.

- It should stand on all of its feet. The separation of an animal from the others in its group is often a sign of a health problem.

- An animal which is not interested in its surroundings and does not want to move has health problems.

Movement (GAIT)

- The healthy animal will walk easily and steadily with all of its feet taking its weight.

- Steps should be regular. Irregular movement results from pain in the feet or limbs.

- Horses normally stand during the day.

- If you go near an animal that is lying down it should stand up quickly otherwise it has health problems.

Eyes

The eyes should be bright and alert with no discharge at the corners.

Ears

- Most animals have erect ears which move in the direction of any sound.

- Ear movements will also be quick to get rid of flies, he body temperature of the pig can be checked by touching the ear when an unusually high temperature will be noticed.

Nose and Muzzle

- The nose should be clean with no discharge.

- In cattle and buffalo the muzzle should be moist not dry.

- In sheep and goats, the nose should be cool and dry.

- Healthy animals frequently lick their noses with their tongues.

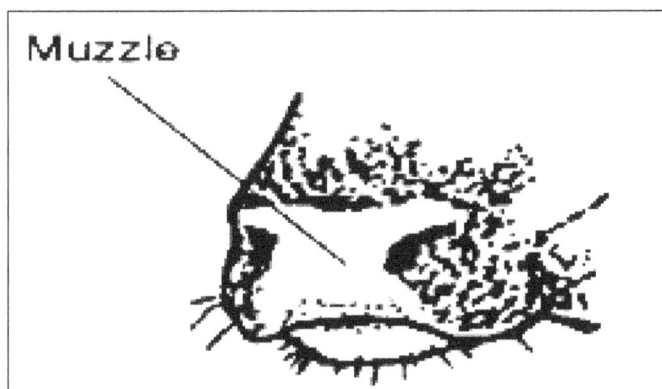

Nose and muzzle.

Mouth

There should be no saliva dripping from the mouth. If chewing is slow or incomplete there must be a problem with the teeth.

The coat

- In short-haired animals, e.g. goat and cattle, the hair or coat of the healthy animal will be smooth and shiny.

- Healthy cattle, buffalo and their calves lick their coat and the lick marks will show.

- Horses should not sweat when resting.

- In poultry, the feathers should be smooth and glossy and not ruffled.

- In pigs a curly tail is a sign of good health while a scaly skin points to health problems.

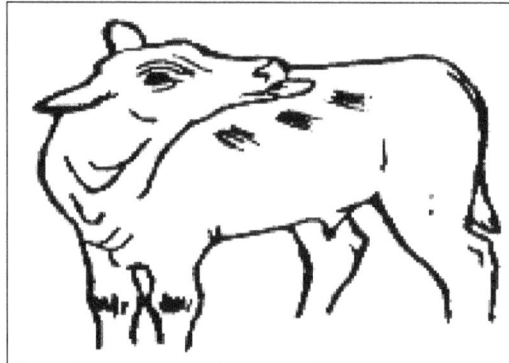

The coat.

Behavior

If a horse, cow or buffalo keeps looking at its flanks or kicks at its belly it has a pain in the stomach.

Breathing

- Breathing should be smooth and regular at rest. Remember that movement and hot weather will increase the rate of breathing.

- If the animal is resting in the shade it should be difficult to notice the chest moving as it breathes.

Pulse

Taking the pulse is important when examining an animal. In man the pulse can be easily taken but in animals it is more difficult and requires practice.

- In sheep and goats, you can feel the pulse on the inside of the top of the back leg. The rate of the pulse is 70 - 130 per minute in the adult.

- The pulse of cattle is taken at a point on the underside of the base of the tail, the normal rate is 40 - 80 per minute in the adult. In buffalo the pulse rate is 40 - 60 per minute.

- The pulse of the horse is taken on the inside of the cheek. The normal rate is 35 - 40 per minute.

- The pulse of the camel is taken at a point on the underside of the root of the tail. The normal rate is 35 - 45 beats per minute.

Remember that the pulse will be higher in the young animal. To take the pulse you should feel for it with the first two fingers of the hand.

In the llama, alpaca and the pig there is no point at which the pulse can be taken. In these animals, the beat of the heart itself must be felt for.

Droppings or Dung

- The droppings of the healthy animal will be firm. Very soft droppings (diarrhea) is a sign of ill health.

- If the animal has difficulty in defecating (constipation) this is also a bad health sign.

Urine

- The urine should be clear and the animal shows no signs of pain or difficulty in urinating.

- Horses, mules and donkeys can have thick yellow urine which is normal.

Appetite and Rumination

- If feed is available, the healthy animal will have a full belly.

- Pigs will naturally rush at their feed, if they do not something is wrong.

- Sheep, goats, cattle, buffalo and camels chew the cud (ruminate) for 6 to 8 hours each day. It is a sign of ill health when these animals stop ruminating.

Milk

- In the milking animal, a sudden change in the amount of milk produced can mean a health problem.

- Any sign of blood or other matter in the milk points to infection in the udder.

- There should be no swelling of the udder and no sign of pain when it is touched. There should be no injury to the teat.

Body Temperature

If you suspect that an animal is sick you should take its temperature. Taking the temperature may show a higher than normal body temperature which is sign of an infection.

Keeping the Livestock Healthy

The most important things a farmer can provide animals are lots of clean water, feed and a healthy environment. These simple, yet crucial, items allow the animals to behave naturally and go through natural processes such as eating, resting, growing and, for some animals, making milk.

There are many different ways that farmers help to prevent sickness and injury on their farms. One way is for farmers to vaccinate their animals against diseases, very similar to the way humans are vaccinated. Farmers work with veterinarians to develop vaccination programs that outline which vaccinations to give and at what age each is to be given.

Animals need their "toe nails" clipped just like we do. But instead of using a clipper, animals like cattle, horses, pigs, goats and sheep need something a bit different. They get their hooves trimmed. It is important that livestock get their feet trimmed because it can prevent lameness. Trimming feet also gives the producer a chance to inspect his animals' hooves and catch infections.

The cow enters the chute, which holds her comfortably in place while her feet are trimmed. The hoof trimmer lifts the cow so that he can work on her feet. He begins by scrapping her feet free of manure and then the excess growth is removed with a clipper. The foot is then examined for any indication of infection. The cow is then lowered to the ground and let loose. Cows typically have their hooves trimmed twice a year.

Horse shoes aren't just for luck. They serve a very important purpose for horses. Horse shoes help to maintain hoof health. Special types of horse shoes have been developed for different types of work, just like an athlete wears special shoes for his or her sport.

Farmers can protect their animals' feet through grooving the barn floor and installing rubber mats at feed alleys, where animals stand to eat their food. The grooved floors will prevent the animals from falling or slipping. The rubber mats act as a cushion when the animal is eating and causes less wear on feet.

Deworming is a method of protection that helps to prevent animals, especially those on pasture, from getting parasites. Farmers can give dewormers by mouth, injection or pour them onto the animal's back.

Some farmers may choose to dehorn their cattle, sheep or goats. Dehorning is a process where the horn bud of the animal is removed. This means that the horn is not able to grow back. Dehorning can protect other animals from being injured and farmers from being harmed.

Tail docking is when part or all of the tail is removed from the animal. This practice most commonly occurs in sheep and pigs. Sheep may have their tails docked because it prevents flies from infesting the hind wool. Sheep may get manure on their hind wool and it can become matted. Flies may lay their eggs here and the maggots could infest the animal. Pigs have their tails docked because some pigs may bite other pigs' tails. This is a health concern because open wounds on the pigs could become infected.

Farmers might use a ventilation system and fans to keep air moving through barns, not only to provide fresh air for livestock but to keep them cool. Sprinklers in barns also come in handy when it is very hot and animals need to cool off.

Farms also work with a nutritionist and veterinarian, who come out to the farm to make decisions on how best to care for the animals. A nutritionist is someone who formulates the diets for the animals to ensure proper growth and development. A veterinarian is an animal doctor who checks for illnesses and treats sick animals. Veterinarians also help to set vaccination schedules and administer shots.

When animals do have a health problem, farmers use antibiotics and other medications to treat illnesses. In the U.S., many livestock producers also give their animals low doses of certain antibiotics in their feed to improve overall health and help animals gain weight. This is called "subtherapeutic" use because instead of curing a specific disease, the antibiotics are used to improve overall growth and health.

It is important that farmers monitor people coming and going on the farm. Biosecurity is a preventative measure to keep out diseases that may be tracked onto the farm by other animals, people or farm equipment. Farmers may restrict certain people from coming on their farm if they know that person has been in contact with diseased animals. The farmer may also ask that people clean their shoes or vehicle tires before entering the farm area. Proper biosecurity helps the farm keep disease out and away from healthy animals.

Farmers often buy new animals and bring them on to the farm, but they can take preventative measures to avoid unwanted diseases that the new animal may have from entering the herd by placing the animal in quarantine. Quarantine is the separation of newly received animals from those already in the facility until the health of the new animals has been checked by a veterinarian and found to be disease-free.

Keeping the Wildlife Safe in Cities

There are certain ways to keep the wildlife in cities and parks safe. Some of them are as follows:

- Always keep dogs on a leash: Unleashed dogs kill animals — they are, after all, carnivores by nature. They can destroy nests or harass ground dwelling birds and small animals to the point that the parents abandon their young.

- Keep your cats indoors: Domestic cats are the single largest cause of bird deaths. Every year, cats kill approximately 2.4 billion birds and 12.3 billion mammals in the United States.

- Put decals on your windows during migratory season: To prevent birds hitting glass, apply translucent contact paper or bird tape to the outside of your windows. For maximum effectiveness, the tape or stickers should be installed no more than 4″ if vertical and 2″ if horizontal.

- Do not litter: Many types of litter can be harmful to animals: Discarded gum, for example, has been known to kill birds and animals can become entangled in six-pack rings. Discarded food may be eaten by wild animals, but they do best on a natural diet of food grown wild in the park. Moreover, frequent feeding can make wildlife dependent on human food.

- Stick to the official trails when walking in Parks: Short-cuts, "social trails" and informal paths not only disturb animals, especially those who are breeding, they also cause habitat fragmentation. When a habitat becomes fragmented by a new path, it is opened for predators, invasive plants and animals and parasites. These, in turn, can make the habitat less useful for native animals.

- Enjoy wildlife from a distance: It is generally not safe for you to get too close to wild animals and they need their distance from you. By keeping about 50 feet between you and any small mammal or birds you observe, you can let them continue their feeding, resting or breeding activities while being smart and safe yourself.

- Do not catch and remove animals from their homes: It is illegal and wrong to remove animals from parks. They are not domestic and they do not make good pets. Many are extremely difficult to care for, even by experts. If you find an animal that may need help, contact park staff for advice. Don't take matters into your own hands.

- Consider volunteering to help improve park habitat: Many parks host special clean-up events and have volunteer corps that maintain trails and remove trash and invasive plant species.

Keeping Wildlife Out of your Home

Even those of us who love wild animals are not pleased when the animals move into our homes. A few relatively simple measures can help prevent or resolve conflicts between you and your wildlife neighbors.

- Make sure all your garbage cans have secure lids. If they do not, use bungee cords to keep the lids on tight.

- Keep dumpsters away from fences and trim branches that overhang them to keep animals out. If an animal is stuck in a dumpster, place a large limb in the container so it can climb out. Be patient; animals do not always leave immediately.

- Don't feed your pets outside: Leaving pet food out attracts animals both large and small. Even if your pet eats most of its food soon after you put it out, small particles left behind can still attract wild animals.

- Hang bird feeders out of reach of other animals: Given the chance, squirrels, rodents and other animals will eat the seed you leave out for birds. Be sure to hang your feeder in a way so that other animals cannot get to it.

- Fence your vegetable gardens: Some gardens attract animals. If you discover that your garden is attracting wild animals, put up fences and other barriers.

- Close-off entry points to your house: Put caps on chimneys and vents. Make sure window screens and screen doors are secure. Enclose crawl spaces under porches and homes with hardware cloth. Bury the hardware cloth several inches into the ground and make sure that you are not sealing in animals who may be in these spaces. Caulk or otherwise seal openings in eaves, corners and foundations.

- Cut back branches that overhang your roof: Cutting back branches helps keep animals off the roof and out of dormers and attics.

- Be mindful of small animals when mowing your lawn: Before you mow, do a walk-through of your lawn to look for rabbits, turtles, toads, fledgling birds and other animals. Leave the animals in place and work around them. When the animals are gone, you can return to complete the mowing.

- If you need to remove an animal from your home, do it humanely. Animals can often be humanely evicted from attics, garages, sheds and crawl spaces using a bright light, a loud radio or a safe repellent such as ammonia-soaked rags. It may take several days for a mother to move all her babies. To see if the animal has left and not returned, sprinkle baby powder around the entrance hole and look for tracks. Trapping animals and releasing them elsewhere is generally not effective in the long run and it's not humane. Relocated animals often can't survive in unfamiliar locations.

Animal Disease

Animal disease is an impairment of the normal state of an animal that interrupts or modifies its vital functions.

Diseases of animals remain a concern principally because of the economic losses they cause and the possible transmission of the causative agents to humans. The branch of medicine called veterinary medicine deals with the study, prevention and treatment of diseases not only in domesticated animals but also in wild animals and in animals used in scientific research. The prevention, control and eradication of diseases of economically important animals are agricultural concerns. Programs for the control of diseases communicable from animals to man, called zoonoses.

Importance

Economic Importance

About 50 percent of the world's population suffers from chronic malnutrition and hunger. Inadequate diet claims many thousands of lives each day. When the lack of adequate food to meet present needs for an estimated world population of more than 4,600,000,000 in the 1980s is coupled with the prediction that the population may increase to 7,000,000,000 by the year 2000, it becomes obvious that animal-food supplies must be increased. One way in which this might be accomplished is by learning to control the diseases that afflict animals throughout the world, especially in the developing nations of Asia and Africa, where the population is expanding most rapidly. Most of the information concerning animal diseases, however, applies to domesticated animals such as pigs, cattle and sheep, which are relatively unimportant as food sources in these nations. Remarkably little is known of the diseases of the goat, the water buffalo, the camel, the elephant, the yak, the llama or the alpaca; all are domesticated animals upon which the economies of many developing countries depend. It is in these countries that increased animal production resulting from the development of methods for the control and eradication of diseases affecting these animals is most urgently needed.

Despite the development of various effective methods of disease control, substantial quantities of meat and milk are lost each year throughout the world. In countries in which animal-disease control is not yet adequately developed, the loss of animal protein from disease is about 30 to 40 percent of the quantity available in certain underdeveloped areas. In addition, such countries also suffer losses resulting from poor husbandry practices.

Animals in Research: The Biomedical Model

Although in modern times the practice of veterinary medicine has been separated from that of human medicine, the observations of the physician and the veterinarian continue to add to the common body of medical knowledge. Of the more than 1,200,000 species of animals thus far identified, only a few have been utilized in research. Veterinary medicine plays an ever-increasing role in the health of man through the use of animals as biomedical models with similar disease counterparts in man. This use of animals as models is important because research on many genetic and chronic diseases of man cannot be carried out using humans.

Hundreds of thousands of mice and monkeys are utilized each year in research laboratories in the U.S. alone. Animal studies are used in the development of new surgical techniques (e.g. organ transplantations), in the testing of new drugs for safety and in nutritional research. Animals are especially valuable in research involving chronic degenerative diseases, because such diseases can be induced in animals experimentally with relative ease. The importance of chronic degenerative diseases, such as cancer and cardiovascular diseases, has increased in parallel with the growing number of communicable diseases that have been brought under control.

Examples of animal diseases that are quite similar to commonly occurring human diseases include chronic emphysema in the horse; leukemia in cats and cattle; muscular dystrophies in chickens and mice; atherosclerosis in pigs and pigeons; blood-coagulation disorders and nephritis in dogs; gastric ulcers in swine; vascular aneurysms (permanent and abnormal blood-filled area of a blood vessel) in turkeys; diabetes mellitus in Chinese hamsters; milk allergy and gallstones in rabbits; hepatitis in dogs and horses; hydrocephalus (fluid in the head) and skin allergies in many species; epilepsy in dogs and gerbils; hereditary deafness in many small animals; cataracts in the eyes of dogs and mice; and urinary stones in dogs and cattle.

The study of animals with diseases similar to those that affect man has increased knowledge of the diseases in man; knowledge of nutrition, for example, based largely on the results of animal studies, has improved the health of animals, including man. Animal investigations have been used extensively in the treatment of shock, in open-heart surgery, in organ transplantations and in the testing of new drugs. Other important contributions to human health undoubtedly will result from new research discoveries involving the study of animal diseases.

Role of Ecology

Epidemiology, the study of epidemics, is sometimes defined as the medical aspect of ecology, for it is the study of diseases in animal populations. Hence the epidemiologist is concerned with the interactions of organisms and their environments as related to the presence of disease. The multiple-causality concept of disease embraced by epidemiology involves combinations of environmental factors and host factors, in addition to the determination of the specific causative agent of a given disease. Environmental factors include geographical features, climate and concentration of certain elements in soil and water. Host factors include age, breed, sex and the physiological state of an animal as well as the general immunity of a herd resulting from previous contact with a disease. Epidemiology, therefore, is concerned with the determination of the individual animals that are affected by a disease, the environmental circumstances under which it may occur, the causative agents and the ways in which transmission occurs in nature. The epidemiologist, who utilizes many scientific disciplines (e.g., medicine, zoology, mathematics, anthropology), attempts to determine the types of diseases that exist in a specific geographical area and to control them by modifying the environment.

Diseases in animal populations are characterized by certain features. Some outbreaks are termed sporadic diseases because they appear only occasionally in individuals within an animal population. Diseases normally present in an area are referred to as endemic or enzootic, diseases and they usually reflect a relatively stable relationship between the causative agent and the animals affected by it. Diseases that occasionally occur at higher than normal rates in animal populations are referred to as epidemic or epizootic, diseases and they generally represent an unstable relationship between the causative agent and affected animals.

The effect of diseases on a stable ecological system, which is the result of the dominance of some plants and animals and the subordination or extinction of others, depends on the degree to which the causative agents of diseases and their hosts are part of the system. Epidemic diseases result from an ecological imbalance; endemic diseases often represent a balanced state. Ecological imbalance and, hence, epidemic disease may be either naturally caused or induced by man. A breakdown in sanitation in a city, for example, offers conditions favourable for an increase in the rodent population, with the possibility that diseases such as plague may be introduced into and spread among the human population. In this case, an epidemic would result as much from an alteration in the environment as from the presence of the causative agent Pasteurella pestis, since, in relatively balanced ecological systems, the causative agent exists enzootically in the rodents (i.e., they serve as reservoirs for the disease) and seldom involves man. In a similar manner, an increase in the number of epidemics of viral encephalitis, a brain disease, in man has resulted from the ecological imbalance of mosquitoes and wild birds caused by man's exploitation of lowland for farming. Driven from their natural habitat of reeds and rushes, the wild birds, important natural hosts for the virus that causes the disease, are forced to feed near farms; mosquitoes transmit the virus from birds to cattle and man.

Causes of Diseases in Animals

In order to understand what causes disease in animals, we first need to know what disease is. Disease (also known as sickness) is any process that interferes with the normal functioning of the body. We do not normally consider injuries such as broken legs and cuts as diseases.

There are many causes of disease in animals. Knowledge of what causes disease and how animals can get a disease will help us knows how to prevent disease and treat sick animals.

- Parasites: Parasites are organisms that have to live on or in other organisms, such as animals, in order to survive. Most parasites are easy to see, although some mites and the early stages of worms can only be seen under a microscope. Parasites can result in irritation and skin damage in animals. Some parasites can also pass diseases such as Redwater in cattle.

  Types of Parasites:

  - External parasites: Flies, lice, fleas, ticks and mites can cause serious diseases in animals. Some live on the animals for their entire lives, others only spend part of their lives there, while others only visit to feed.

  - Internal parasites: Internal parasites (including roundworms, flukes and tapeworms) can cause serious diseases and loss of production in animals. They usually live in the stomach and intestines but also in other parts of the body such as the lungs and liver.

- Microbes (germs): Microbes (germs) are usually too small to be seen with the naked eye and only a microscope will enable you to see what a microbe looks like. Just because you do not see microbes with your naked eye, does not mean they cannot cause disease in animals.

Some microbes are harmless. For example, bacteria surround animals and people and they even live on our skin and inside our nose, mouth and stomach, but these bacteria do not normally cause problems. Also, some microbes are even helpful, such as the ones in our gut which help us to digest food. However, many different microbes can cause disease in animals, but there are four main types.

- Viruses: Viruses are the smallest of all microbes. They must live inside cells in order to survive and breed. Viruses cause about 60% of disease outbreaks in animals and humans. Examples of diseases in animals caused by viruses are rabies, Newcastle disease and Bovine ephemeral fever, also known as three-day stiff-sickness (TDS).

  It is usually difficult to treat diseases caused by viruses because the viruses live inside animal cells. Therefore, any medicine that can kill the viruses will also harm the animals in which the viruses are present.

- Bacteria: Bacteria can live in animals and in the environment. Not all bacteria cause disease. People and animals have bacteria living on and in them that do not cause disease. Examples of diseases in animals caused by bacteria are Anthrax, Black Quarter and Tuberculosis. Bacteria can infect wounds and that is why wounds should be treated.

- Fungi: Fungi include mould on stale food and mushrooms. Fungi need to grow on organic material in order to feed and this can include animals and humans. An example of a fungal disease in animals is ringworm. Some fungi are normally harmless, but can cause disease in some situations, especially after prolonged use of antibiotics. Some fungi can also produce toxins or poisons which can be a problem when food becomes stale or wet.

- Protozoa: Some protozoa can live outside the cells, especially the types that cause Trichomonosis, a venereal disease in cattle. Others need to live inside cells and include those causing Coccidiosis, Redwater, Heartwater and Gallsickness.

- Poisoning: Animals can be poisoned by chemicals (such as insecticides and dips), poisonous plants and fungal toxins. Animals can also be poisoned when bitten by snakes, scorpions and spiders.

- Dietary problems: Lack of enough food or lack of adequate the components (such as phosphorus) can diseases in animals. Malnourishment in animals may lead to other serious diseases.

- Metabolic diseases: Metabolic diseases are an upset in the normal functioning of the animal (that is not caused by infection, poisoning or feed deficiencies) and usually result from intensive animal production. An example is milk fever in highly-productive dairy cows.

- Congenital diseases: In some cases, animals can be born with a disease. Some of these may be inherited (passed on from the parents). This is rare and inherited diseases are usually seen at birth. An example of congenital disease include hydrocephalus, which is a swelling of the brain caused by fluid and can be clearly seen as a swelling of the head.

- Environmental Condition: Environmental problems, such as littering, contribute to some diseases in animals, for example, animals may eat plastic bags or wires and this can harm the animal's health.

- Cancer: Cancer occurs when some of the cells in the body grow abnormally. In some instances viruses can cause cancer.

- Allergies: Allergy is a damaging immune response by the body to a substance some diseases are caused by allergies, which is when the body's own immune system attacks part of the body.

- Degenerative disease: Just like in humans, some diseases are associated with old age in animals.

How to Prevent Diseases in Animals

- Be sure not to bring infection onto your farm or spread it around your farm.

- Where possible, limit and control farm visitors – people and vehicles.

- Have pressure washers, brushes, water and disinfectant available and make sure visitors use them.

- Don't share injecting and dosing equipment – if it can't be avoided, cleanse and disinfect thoroughly.

- Clean and then disinfect any farm machinery/equipment if you are sharing these with a neighbouring farm.

- Introduce a pest control programme.

- Fence off streams and rivers – supply clean fresh drinking water.

- Keep livestock away from freshly spread slurry.

- Ensure your livestock identification and record keeping is accurate and up-to-date.

- Dispose of fallen stock (dead animals) properly.

- Make a herd/flock health plan with your vet including isolation for new or returning stock.

- Know the health status of any animals or birds you are buying or moving.

- Be vigilant to spot any signs of disease among your animals or birds and report suspicions of noticeable disease to your vet.

- Train staff on the principles of hygiene and disease security.

- Include signs directing visitors to the farmhouse/office and urging visitors not to feed animals or get in close contact.

- Keep your farmyard and surroundings clean and tidy to discourage vermin.

- Provide cleaning and disinfectant materials for all visitors and workers.

- Wash your hands with soap and water after handling livestock.

- Avoid wearing dirty clothes and footwear off the farm - this is important when visiting markets, shows, farms and other premises where there are livestock.

- Clean and disinfect all shared and hired equipment before and after use.

- Make sure that animals kept indoors have fresh clean dry bedding.

- Dispose of used bedding away from livestock, humans and watercourses as it can cause contamination.

- Clean and disinfect buildings and equipment after use by livestock.

- Keep incoming and returning stock separate from the rest of the herd/flock.

- Use separate equipment and staff or handle isolated stock last.

- Have water bowls or drinkers above the level for faecal contamination.

- Avoid contamination of watercourses.

- Clean feed and water troughs regularly.

- Discourage dogs and cats from walking in feed troughs.

- Keep feed in a clean, dry store.

- Keep feed stores covered and shut to ensure no access by dogs, cats, vermin and wildlife.

Detection and Diagnosis

Reactions of Tissue to Disease

Disease may be defined as an injurious deviation from a normal physiological state of an organism sufficient to produce overt signs or symptoms. The deviation may be either an obvious organic change in the tissue composing an organ or a functional disturbance whose organic changes are not obvious. The severity of the changes that occur in cells and tissues subjected to injurious agents is dependent upon both the sensitivity of the tissue concerned and the nature and time course of the agent. A mildly injurious agent that is present for short periods of time may either have little effect or stimulate cells to increased activity. Strongly injurious agents in prolonged contact with cells cause characteristic changes in them by interfering with normal cell processes. Most causative agents of disease fall into the latter category.

Characteristics of Cell and Tissue Changes

Changes in cells and tissues as a result of disease include degenerative and infiltrative changes. Degenerative changes are characterized by the deterioration of cells or a tissue from a higher to a lower form, especially to a less functionally active form. When chemical changes occur in the tissue, the process is one of degeneration. When the changes involve the accumulation of materials within the cells comprising tissues, the process is called infiltration. Diseases such as pneumonia, metal poisoning or septicemia (the persistence of disease-causing bacteria in the bloodstream) may cause the mildest type of degeneration—parenchymatous changes or cloudy swelling of the cells; the cells first affected are the specialized cells of the liver and the kidney.

Serious cellular damage may cause the uptake of water by cells (hydropic degeneration), which lose their structural features as they fill with water. The causes for the accumulation in cells of abnormal amounts of fats (fatty infiltration and degeneration) have not yet been established with certainty but probably involve fat metabolism. Poisons such as phosphorus may cause sudden increases in the accumulation of fats in the liver. An abnormal protein material may accumulate in connective-tissue components of small arteries as a result of chronic pneumonia, chronic bacterial infections and prolonged antitoxin production (in horses); the condition is known as amyloid degeneration and infiltration. Hyaline degeneration, characterized by tissues that become clear and appear glasslike, usually occurs in connective-tissue components of small blood vessels as a result of conditions that may occur in kidney structures (glomeruli) of animals with nephritis or in lymph glands of animals with tuberculosis. Certain structures (glomeruli) of animals with nephritis result in degeneration.

The condition in which mucus, a secretion of mucous membranes lining the inside surfaces of organs, is produced in excess and accumulates in greater than normal amounts is referred to as mucoid degeneration. Major causes of this condition include chronic irritation of mucous membranes and certain mucus-producing tumours. Abnormal amounts of glycogen, which is the principal storage carbohydrate of animals, may occur in the liver as a result of certain inherited diseases of animals; the condition is known as glycogen infiltration. The abnormal deposition of calcium salts, which is known as hypercalcification, may occur as a result of several diseases involving the blood vessels and the heart, the urinary system, the gallbladder and the bonelike tissue called cartilage. Pigments (coloured molecules) from coal dust or asbestos dust may infiltrate the lungs of certain dogs in two types of lung disease: Anthracosis and asbestosis. Abnormal amounts of iron-containing coloured molecules (hemosiderin) resulting from the breakdown of hemoglobin, the oxygen-carrying protein of red blood cells, are often deposited in the liver and the spleen after diseases that involve excessive breakdown of red blood cells. A dark-coloured molecule (melanin) occurs abnormally in the livers of certain sheep suffering from Dubin–Johnson syndrome and in certain tumours called melanomas. Uric acid infiltration, which occurs in poultry, is characterized by the deposition of uric acid salts.

Necrosis, the death of cells or tissues, takes place if the blood supply to tissues is restricted; poisons produced by microbes, chemical poisons and extreme heat or electricity also may cause necrosis. The rotting of the dead tissue is known as gangrene.

Atrophy of animal tissue involves a process of tissue wasting, in which a decrease occurs in the size or number of functional cells—e.g., in inherited muscular dystrophy of chickens. Hypertrophy—an increase in the size of the cells in a tissue or an organ—occurs in heart muscle during diseases involving the heart valves, in certain pneumonias and in some diseases of the endocrine glands. Aplasia is the term used when an entire organ is missing from an animal; hypoplasia indicates arrested or incomplete development of an organ and hyperplasia an increase in the production of the number of cells—e.g., the persistent callus that forms on the elbows of some dogs. Metaplasia is used to describe the change of one cell type into another; it may occur in chronic irritation of tissues and in certain cancerous tumours.

Characteristics of Inflammatory Reactions

When tissues are injured, they become inflamed. The inflammation may be acute, in which case the inflammatory processes are active or chronic, in which case the processes occur slowly and new connective tissue is formed. The reaction of inflamed tissues is a combination of defensive and repair mechanisms. Acute inflammation is characterized by redness, heat, swelling, sensitivity and impaired function. Several types of acute inflammation are known. Mild acute inflammations of mucous membranes resulting in the production of thin watery material (exudate) are called catarrhal inflammations; parenchymatous inflammations occur in organs undergoing degeneration. If the exudate formed in response to an injury is of a serious nature—that is, resembling blood plasma—the process is called serous inflammation. In fibrinous inflammation, a protein (fibrin) forms on membranes, including those in the lungs. In suppurative inflammation, dead tissue is replaced with pus composed of colourless blood cells (leucocytes) and tissue juices.

During the inflammatory reaction, the injured tissue is surrounded by an area of rapidly dividing cells. Specialized cells called macrophages enter the tissue and remove blood and tissue debris. Other cells, called neutrophils, ingest disease-causing bacteria and other foreign material. In chronic inflammations, the connective tissue contains fibroblasts, cells that divide and form new connective or scar, tissue.

Characteristics of Circulatory Disturbances

An increase in the rate of blood flow to a body part, which is referred to by the term congestion or hyperemia, occurs during inflammation; a diminished blood flow to tissues is referred to by the term ischemia or a local anemia. Examples of hemorrhage, the escape of blood from vessels, include epistaxis or nosebleeds, in racehorses; hematemesis or regurgitation of blood, in dogs with uremia; hemoptysis or blood loss from lungs; hematuria or blood in urine, of cattle with inflammation of the urinary bladder. Edema, a condition that is characterized by abnormal accumulations of fluid in tissues, occurs not only in a tissue during inflammation but also over the entire body if the concentration of blood-serum proteins, especially albumin, is low. A thrombosis, which is a blood clot in a blood vessel, may block or slow circulation of blood to tissues; if blood vessels become blocked, the condition is known as an embolism. The term infarction describes the necrosis that occurs in tissues whose blood supply is blocked by an embolism.

Methods of Examination

Before an unhealthy animal receives treatment, an attempt is made to diagnose the disease. Both clinical findings, which include symptoms that are obvious to a no specialist and clinical signs that can be appreciated only by a veterinarian and laboratory test results may be necessary to establish the cause of a disease. A clinical examination should indicate if the animal is in good physical condition, is eating adequately, is bright and alert and is functioning in an apparently normal manner. Many disease processes are either inflammatory or result from tumours. Malignant tumours (e.g., melanomas in horses, squamous cell carcinomas in small animals) tend to spread rapidly and usually cause death. Other diseases cause the circulatory disturbances or the degenerative and infiltrative changes that are summarized in the preceding section. If a specific diagnosis is not possible, the symptoms of the animal are treated.

The veterinarian must diagnose a disease on the basis of a variety of examinations and tests, since he obviously cannot interrogate the animal. Methods used in the preparation of a diagnosis include inspection—a visual examination of the animal; palpation—the application of firm pressure with the fingers to tissues to determine characteristics such as abnormal shapes and possible tumours, the presence of pain and tissue consistency; percussion—the application of a short, sharp blow to a tissue to provoke an audible response from body parts directly beneath; auscultation—the act of listening to sounds that are produced by the body during the performance of functions (e.g., breathing, intestinal movements); smells—the recognition of characteristic odours associated with certain diseases; and miscellaneous diagnostic procedures, such as eye examinations, the collection of urine and heart, esophageal and stomach studies.

General Inspection

Deviation of various characteristics from the normal, observation of which constitutes the general inspection of an animal, is a useful aid in diagnosing disease. The general inspection includes examination of appearance; behaviour; body condition; respiratory movements; state of skin, coat and abdomen; and various common actions.

The appearance of an animal may be of diagnostic significance; small size in a pig may result from retardation of growth, which is caused by hog-cholera virus. Observation of the behaviour of an animal is of value in diagnosing neurological diseases; e.g., muscle spasms occur in lockjaw (tetanus) in dogs, nervousness and convulsions in dogs with distemper, dullness in horses with equine viral encephalitis and excitement in animals suffering from lead poisoning. Subtle behavioral changes may not be noticeable. The general condition of the body is of value in diagnosing diseases that cause excessive leanness (emaciation), including certain cancers or other chronic diseases, such as a deficiency in the output of the adrenal glands or tuberculosis. Defective teeth also may point to malnutrition and result in emaciation.

The respiratory movements of an animal are important diagnostic criteria; breathing is rapid in young animals, in small animals and in animals whose body temperature is higher than normal. Specific respiratory movements are characteristic of certain diseases—e.g., certain movements in horses with heaves (emphysema) or the abdominal breathing of animals suffering from painful lung diseases. The appearance of the skin and hair may indicate dehydration by lack of pliability and lustre; or the presence of parasites such as lice, mites or fleas; or the presence of ringworm infections and allergic reactions by the skin changes they cause. The poisoning of sheep by molybdenum in their hay may be diagnosed by the loss of colour in the wool of black sheep. Distension of the abdomen may indicate bloat in cattle or colic in horses.

Abnormal activities may have special diagnostic meaning to the veterinarian. Straining during urination is associated with bladder stones; increased frequency of urination is associated with kidney disease (nephritis), bladder infections and a disease of the pituitary gland (diabetes insipidus). Excessive salivation and grinding of teeth may be caused by an abnormality in the mouth. Coughing is associated with pneumonia. Some diseases cause postural changes, for example, a horse with tetanus may stand in a stiff manner. An abnormal gait in an animal made to move may furnish evidence as to the cause of a disease, as louping ill in sheep.

Clinical Examination

Following the general inspection of an animal thought to have contracted a disease, a more thorough clinical examination is necessary, during which various features of the animal are studied. These include the visible mucous membranes (conjunctiva of the eye, nasal mucosa, inside surface of the mouth and tongue); the eye itself; and such body surfaces as the ears, horns (if present) and limbs. In addition, the pulse rate and the temperature are measured.

The veterinarian examines the visible mucous membranes of the eye, nose and mouth to determine if jaundice, hemorrhages or anemia are present. The conjunctiva or lining of the eye, may exhibit pus in pinkeye infections, have a yellow appearance in jaundice or exhibit small hemorrhages in certain systemic diseases. Examination of the nose may reveal ulcers and vesicles (small sacs containing liquid), as in foot-and-mouth disease, a viral disease of cattle or vesicular exanthema, a viral disease of swine. Ulceration of the tongue may be apparent in animals suffering from actinobacillosis, a disease of bacterial origin.

A detailed examination of the eye may show abnormalities of the cornea resulting from such diseases as infectious hepatitis in dogs, bovine catarrhal fever and equine influenza. Cataract, a condition in which the passage of light through the lens of the eye is obstructed, may result from a disorder of carbohydrate metabolism (diabetes mellitus), infections or a hereditary defect.

An elevated temperature or fever, resulting from the multiplication of disease-causing organisms may be the earliest sign of disease. The increase in temperature activates the body mechanisms that are necessary to fight off foreign substances. Measuring the pulse rate is useful in determining the character of the heartbeat and of the circulatory system.

Tests as Diagnostic Aids

In many cases, the final diagnosis of an animal disease is dependent upon a laboratory test. Some involve measuring the amount of certain chemical constituents of the blood or body fluids, determining the presence of toxins (poisons) or examining the urine and feces. Other tests are designed to identify the causative agents of the disease. The removal and examination of tissue or other material from the body (biopsy) is used to diagnose the nature of abnormalities such as tumours. Specific skin tests are used to confirm the diagnoses of various diseases—e.g., tuberculosis and Johne's disease in cattle and glanders in horses.

Confirmation of the presence in the blood of abnormal quantities of certain constituents aids in diagnosing certain diseases. Abnormal levels of protein in the blood are associated with some cancers of the bone, such as multiple myeloma in horses and dogs. Animals with diabetes mellitus have a high level of the carbohydrate glucose and the steroid cholesterol in the blood. The combination of an increase in the blood level of cholesterol and a decrease in the level of iodine bound to protein indicates hypothyroidism (underactive thyroid gland). A low level of calcium in the serum component of blood confirms milk fever in lactating dairy cattle. An increase in the activities of certain enzymes (biological catalysts) in the blood indicates liver damage. An increase in the blood level of the bile constituent bilirubin is used as a diagnostic test for hemolytic crisis, a disease in which red blood cells are rapidly destroyed by organisms such as Babesia species in dogs and in cattle and Anaplasma species in cattle.

The examination of the formed elements of blood, including the oxygen-carrying red blood cells (erythrocytes), the white blood cells (neutrophils, eosinophils, basophils, lymphocytes and monocytes) and the platelets, which function in blood coagulation, is helpful in diagnosing certain diseases. Examination of the blood cells of cattle may reveal abnormal lymphocytic cells characteristic of leukemia. Low numbers of leucocytes indicate the presence of viral diseases, such as hog cholera and infectious hepatitis in dogs. Neutrophil levels increase in chronic bacterial diseases, such as canine pneumonia and uterine infections in female animals. Elevated monocyte levels occur in chronic granulomatous diseases; e.g., histoplasmosis and tuberculosis. Canine parasitism and allergic skin disorders are characterized by elevated eosinophil levels. Prolonged clotting time may be associated with a deficiency of platelets.

Anemia has many causes. They include hemorrhages from blood loss after injuries; the destruction of red blood cells by the rickettsia Haemobartonella felis in cats; incompatible blood transfusions in dogs; the inadequate production of normal red blood cells, which occurs in iron or cobalt deficiency after exposure to radioactive substances; general malnutrition; and contact with substances that depress the activity of bone marrow.

Poisonings occur commonly in animals. Some species are more sensitive to certain poisons than others. Swine develop mercury poisoning if they eat too much grain that has been treated with mercury compounds to retard spoilage. Dogs may be poisoned by the arsenic found in pesticides or by strychnine, which is found in rat poison. Many plants are poisonous if eaten, such as bracken fern, which poisons cattle and horses and ragwort, which contains a substance poisonous to the liver of cattle.

Examination of an animal's urine may reveal evidence of kidney diseases or diseases of the entire urinary system or a generalized systemic disease. The presence of protein in the urine of dogs indicates acute kidney disease (nephritis). Although constituents of bile normally are found in the urine of dogs, the quantity increases in dogs with the presence of infectious hepatitis, a disease of the liver. The presence of abnormal amounts of the simple carbohydrate glucose and of ketone bodies (organic compounds involved in metabolism) in an animal's urine is used to diagnose diabetes mellitus, a disease in which the pancreas cannot form adequate quantities of a substance (insulin) important in regulating carbohydrate metabolism. The urine of horses with azoturia (excessive quantities of nitrogen-containing compounds in the urine) or muscle breakdown may contain a dark-coloured molecule called myoglobin.

The presence of eggs or parts of worms in the excrement of animals suspected of suffering from intestinal parasites, such as roundworms, tapeworms or flatworms, aids in diagnosis. Feces that are light in colour, have a rancid odour, contain fat and are poorly formed may indicate the existence of a chronic disease of the pancreas. Clay-coloured fatty feces suggest obstruction of the bile duct, which conveys bile to the intestine during digestion.

The identification of a disease-causing microorganism within an animal enables the veterinarian to choose the best drug for therapy. Agglutination tests, which utilize serum samples of animals and microorganisms suspected of causing a disease, many times confirm the presence of the following bacterial diseases: Brucellosis in cattle and swine, salmonellosis in swine, leptospirosis in cattle and actinobacillosis in swine and cattle. Other tests measure the antibodies (specific proteins formed in response to a foreign substance in the body) formed against a disease-causing agent, such as those that cause brucellosis, foot-and-mouth disease, infectious hepatitis in dogs and fowl pest.

The modern veterinary diagnostic laboratory performs, in addition to the tests, tests of cells in the bone marrow; specific-organ-function tests (liver, kidney, pancreas, thyroid, adrenal and pituitary glands); radioisotope tests, tissue biopsies and histochemical analyses; and tests concerning blood coagulation and body fluids.

Common Animal Diseases and their Management

Anthrax

Anhrax, a highly infectious and fatal disease of cattle, is caused by a relatively large spore-forming rectangular shaped bacterium called Bacillus anthracis. Anthrax causes acute mortality in ruminants. The bacteria produce extremely potent toxins which are responsible for the ill effects, causing a high mortality rate. Signs of the illness usually appear 3 to 7 days after the spores are swallowed or inhaled. Once signs begin in animals, they usually die within two days.

Hoofed animals, such as deer, cattle, goats and sheep, are the main animals affected by this disease. They usually get the disease by swallowing anthrax spores while grazing on pasture contaminated (made impure) with anthrax spores. Inhaling (breathing in) the spores, which are odorless, colorless and tasteless, may also cause infection in animals and people.

Symptoms

- Sudden death (often within 2 or 3 hours of being apparently normal) is by far the most common sign.

- Very occasionally some animals may show trembling, a high temperature.

- Difficulty breathing, collapse and convulsions before death. This usually occurs over a period of 24 hours.

- After death blood, may not clot, resulting in a small amount of bloody discharge from the nose, mouth and other openings.

Treatment and Control

- Due to the acute nature of the disease resulting in sudden death, treatment is usually not possible in animals even though Anthrax bacilli are clines. Treatment is of use in cases showing sub-acute form of the disease.

- In most cases, early treatment can cure anthrax. The cutaneous (skin) form of anthrax can be treated with common antibiotics.

Preventive Measures

- Regular annual vaccination of animals in endemic areas will prevent the disease from occurring.

- Vaccination may be carried out at least a month prior to expected disease occurrence in endemic areas.

- Never open a carcass of an animal suspected to have died from anthrax.

Contact a veterinarian immediately if the following symptoms are seen and seek advice on control measures to be adopted:

- Fever (106-108 °F), loss of appetite, depression and dullness.

- Suspended rumination. Rapid pulse and heart rates.

- Difficult breathing (dyspnoea).

- Lameness in affected leg.

- Crepitation swelling over hip, back & shoulder.

- Swelling is hot & painful in early stages whereas cold and painless inter.

- Recumbency (prostration) followed by death within 12-48 hrs.

Black Quarter (Black-leg)

It is an acute infectious and highly fatal, bacterial disease of cattle. Buffaloes, sheep and goats are also affected. Young cattle between 6-24 months of age, in good body condition are mostly affected. It is soil-borne infection which generally occurs during rainy season.

Causal Organism

It is a bacterial disease caused by Clostridium chauvoei.

Symptoms

- Fever (106-108 °F), Loss of appetite, Depression and dullness.

- Suspended rumination.

- Rapid pulse and heart rates.

- Difficult breathing (dyspnoea).

- Lameness in affected leg.

- Crepitation swelling over hip, back & shoulder.

- Swelling is hot & painful in early stages whereas cold and painless inter.

- Recumbency (prostration) followed by death within 12-48 hrs.

Treatment

- Early treatment can be possible to complete cure of the animal.

- Consult with veterinarian immediately.

Ethnovet Practice

The following measure is to be taken up in the month of May/June every year.

Exudates of thirugukalli (Euphorbia tirucalli), kodikalli (Sareostemma brevistigma), aththi (Ficus racemosa), banyan tree (Ficus bengalensis), madara (Calotropis gigantea) are taken at the rate of 1 to 15 drops each in a stainless-steel vessel and mixed with 50 ml of sesame oil and ragi flour are added and made into a paste. This paste is applied as dot (coin size) in each animal in the groin region. (the above material may be used for about 50 animals).

Rabies (Mad Dog Disease)

Rabies is a disease of dogs, foxes, wolves, hyaenas and in some places; it is a disease of bats which feed on blood.

The disease is passed to other animals or to people if they are bitten by an animal with rabies. The germs which cause rabies live in the saliva of the sick (rabid) animal. This is a killer disease but not every dog which bites is infected with rabies.

When the rabid animal bites another animal or human, the germs which live in its saliva pass into the body through the wound caused by the bite. The germs travel along the nerves to the brain. The time between the bite and the first appearance of signs that the bitten animal or human has been infected can take from 2 to 10 weeks or more. The time taken depends on the distance of the bite from the brain. If the bite is on the face or head, the bitten animal or human will quickly show signs, but if the bite is on the leg it will take much longer for signs to develop.

General Signs of Rabies

You should first look for the marks of the bite and discover where and when the animal was bitten. All rabid animals show similar signs in the beginning.

- They change their normal behaviour and behave very strangely.

- They stop eating or drinking.

- Male animal will try to mate (mount) other animals.

- There is no change in the body temperature.

- These signs will continue for 3 to 5 days. Then, before it dies, the animal will develop one or the other of two types of the disease:

  - The furious (mad) type of the disease makes the animal aggressive and it will bite anything.

  - The quiet (dumb) type when the animal is quiet and does not move.

Rabies in the Dog

Dogs show either of the two types of rabies:

- A dog with the dumb or quiet type of the disease cannot move. It looks as if it has a bone stuck in the mouth and saliva drips from the mouth.

- Rabies in the dog lasts about 10 days before the animal dies. If the animal does not die after this length of time then it may not be suffering from rabies.

Rabies in Sheep, Goats and Cattle

Rabies is characterised by the animals becoming restless and excited. They may bite themselves and saliva drips from the mouth. The most important sign in cattle is that the animal bellows (calls) very frequently and with strange sound. The animals will become paralysed and die.

Rabies in the Horse and Camel

The horse will show the furious (mad) type of the disease. It will kick and bite and show signs similar to colic. The animal will die after paralysis of the back legs.

In the camel the signs of rabies are similar to those shown by an animal in the rut.

What to do with a Biting Dog

Remember that not every dog which bites has rabies. If the dog belongs to somebody ask the owner about its normal behaviour. If the dog is showing signs of rabies you must inform your veterinary officer immediately. The dog must be shot and if it has bitten anybody, they must be taken to a hospital immediately for vaccination.

Control of Rabies

Dogs in your community can be vaccinated against rabies. You should ask your veterinary service about vaccination against rabies. If there is an outbreak of rabies, the livestock in your community can be vaccinated too.

Treatment (ethnovet practices): Leaves of chirchra (Achyranthes aspera) 100gm and onion 50 gm are ground well and smeared over the bitten place. The extract of these ingredients is administered orally twice in a day.

Blue Tongue

Bluetongue, a disease which is transmitted by midges, infects domestic and wild ruminants and also camelids, however sheep are particularly badly affected. Cattle, although infected more frequently than sheep, do not always show signs of disease. Virus spreads between animals occurs via the midges of Cullicoides species.

The likelihood of mechanical transmission between herds and flocks or indeed within a herd or flock, by unhygienic practices (the use of contaminated surgical equipment or hypodermic needles) may be a possibility.

Clinical Signs Include

- Sheep: Eye and nasal discharges, drooling, high body temperature, swelling in mouth, head and neck, lameness and wasting of muscles in hind legs, haemorrages into or under skin, inflammation of the coronary band, respiratory problems, fever, lethargy.

- In cattle: Nasal discharge, swelling of head and neck, conjunctivitis, swelling inside and ulceration of the mouth, swollen teats, tiredness, saliva drooling, fever. A blue tongue is rarely a clinical sign of infection.

Control

Inspect stock closely, particularly focusing on the lining of the mouth and nose and the coronary band (where the hoof stops and the skin starts). If an animal is suspected as having bluetongue, it must be reported as quickly as possible. Telephone your local animal health office immediately.

Preventive Measures and Treatment (Ethovet)

Since the animal is not taking any feed the starvation may lead to death. So the animal has to be administered orally the following food. Banana fruits (one) smeared with sesame oil (50 ml) for 2 to 3 times. By this animal will recover little. However, this will not control the disease fully. Next the leaf pulp of "sothukathalai"(Aloe vera) has to be administered daily. Administering of Aloe vera has to be continued for more days till the animal fully recovers from this disease. By this treatment the infected animal will recover from the disease. The disease will not spread to other animals if all animals are administered with Aloe vera as a preventive treatment. Administering aloe vera also increases the body weight of animals as it is against all intestinal parasite.

Pox

- Epidemiology: Sheep-pox is a highly contagious disease. It causes a mortality of 20 to 50 percent in animals below the age of 6 months and causes damage to the wool and skin in adults. Of the pock diseases, sheep-pox ranks only second to human small-pox in virulence. The disease is transmissible to in-contact goats but not to other species of animals. It, however, spreads slowly.

- Symptoms: The disease in characterized by high fever and symptoms of pneumonia and acute enteritis. Skin lesions appear particularly in parts free from wool, notably around the eyes, inner side of the thigh, udder and under surface of the tail. The internal organs such as trachea, lungs, kidneys and intestines are also affected. The disease results in emaciation and, as already mentioned, frequent deaths of affected animals.

- Treatment, prevention and control: The diseased animal should be treated with palliatives. In the young ones nursing is more important than medication. The infected litter should be burnt and the bedding changed every day. Affected animals should be kept on soft diet. The ulcers on the skin should be washed with potassium permanganate lotion and dusted with boric acid; strict hygienic measures should be adopted.

- Preventive measures and treatment (ethnovet): External application of paste prepared by grinding neem leaves, tulsi leaves each 100 gm and turmeric powder- 50gm sprinkled with sufficient water. Continue for 3 to 5 days. Administer orally the same mixture by diluting with water.

Brucellosis of Sheep

- Transmission: The mode of entry is by ingestion or via conjunctiva. The aborted foetus, vaginal discharge and milk from infected goats contain a large number or organisms.

- Symptoms in infected goats and sheep state of abortion may occur followed by a quiescent period during which a few abortions occur. The aborted animals do not breed. After 2 years or more another abortion storm is likely to occur.

- Diagnosis, treatment and control: It is not possible to diagnose brucellosis on the basis of symptoms alone. The suspicion is aroused when humans in contact suffer from undulant fever and there is poor breeding record in goat herd and evidence of mastitis. The diagnosis can be done by the isolation of organisms and by serological tests.

- There is no adequate treatment: This is based on hygiene, vaccination, testing and disposal. Good management practice is essential. Separate quarters should be provided for kidding. Immunization can be done with attenuated as well as killed vaccines. The test and disposal procedure is highly desirable.

Tetanus

This is an infectious, non-febrile disease of animals and man and is characterized by spasmodic tetany and hyperaesthesia. This disease is prevalent all over the world.

- Transmission: Infection takes place by contamination of wounds. Deep punctured wounds provide favourable conditions for the spores to germinate multiply and produce toxin which is subsequently absorbed in the animal body. The micro-organism is present in soil and in animal faeces and is carried into the wound by a penetrating object. The organism is present in the intestine of normal animals and under some undetermined conditions multiplies rapidly and produces toxin in sufficient quantities to be absorbed and cause the disease.

- Symptoms: The incubation period is generally 1-2 weeks but it may be as short as 3 days. Tetanus affects many species of domesticated animals but occurs particularly in horses and lambs; less frequently in adult sheep, goats, cattle, pigs, dog and cats; and rarely in poultry. The initial symptoms are mild stiffness and an unwillingness to move all the animals. More severe symptoms develop after 12-24 hours which are stiffness of limbs, neck, head, tail and twitching of muscles. The spasms develop in response to noise. In terminal stages ears are erect, nostrils dilated, nictitating membrane protruded. Mastication becomes very difficult because mouth cannot be opened, hence the name lockjaw.

- Treatment: The treatment is carried out by first injecting antitoxin then treating the wound. Penicillin parenterally is beneficial. Muscular relaxation is achieved by injection of relaxants. The animal should be kept in a dark room and fed with the help of stomach tube.

- Control: Proper hygiene and cleanliness at castration and other surgical procedures should be observed. Sheep should be given 2 injections based 3 weeks apart to develop a solid immunity.

Listeriosis

- Transmission: The organisms are excreted in the faeces, urine, aborted foetuses, uterine discharge and milk of infected animals. The organisms are sufficiently resistant to remain viable in animal and human faeces, sewage, soil, silage and dust foe several weeks and months. The blood sucking arthropods may spread infection since organisms have been isolated from cattle ticks and tabanid flies. Under natural conditions certain predisposing factors are related to clinical infection.

- Symptoms: In farm animals the disease occurs towards the end of winter or early spring. The first signs of meningo- encephalitis are stiffness of neck, incoordinated movement of limbs and tendency to move in circles or to lean against a fence or wall. There may be paralysis of muscles of jaw and pharynx. Incoordination becomes progressively more severe until the animal can no longer stand. The cattle which are not severely affected may survive. Abortions in cattle usually occur after 4-8 months of pregnancy and at a comparatively later stage in sheep. In pigs and horses, clinical signs are not common but may develop as encephalitis and septicaemia. In poultry, the disease usually causes sudden death, occasionally there are signs of torticollis, weakness and inco-ordination of the legs.

- Treatment: Tetracyclines are very effective in meningo-encephalities of cattle less so in sheep. The recovery rate depends on the speed with which the treatment is commenced.

- Control: When outbreaks occur all affected animals should be slaughtered and buried along with litter and bedding. The vaccines, living or killed, have little effect on the pathogenesis of infection under natural conditions; tetracycline's are very effective for treatment of listeriosis.

Campylobactor Abortion (Vibriosis)

- Transmission: Transmission occurs by coitus. The affected bulls carry the organisms in preputial cavity indefinitely. Mature cows and heifers also carry the infection for long periods. Infected semen from an infected bull is the important means of the disease. The organism survives low temperature used in semen storage.

- Symptoms: Infertility may cause become apparent only when the percentage of pregnancies in a dairy herd is low. The infertility rate in heifers is more than in cows. Abortions usually occur between fifth and sixth month of pregnancy. Infected bulls show no symptoms and their semen is normal. Healthy bulls become infected during coitus with diseased cow. Among sheep the disease is characterized by abortion occurring towards the end of gestation. Usually abortion is preceded by vaginal discharge for several days. The aborted foetus is edematous with petechial hemorrhages on serous surfaces and necrotic foci in the liver.

- Control: Abortion rate can be reduced by antibiotic therapy and particularly by using chlortetracycline and concurrently with the development of specific immunity. The use of killed vaccines may reduce the incidence of disease in a herd but does not eradicate the infection. The bulls can be treated by injecting antibiotic cream in the prepuce. There is no direct treatment of females.

Johne`s Disease

Johne`s disease is a specific chronic contagious enteritis of cattle, sheep, goat, buffaloes and occasionally of pigs. The disease is characterized by progressive emaciation and in cattle and buffaloes by chronic diarrhea and thickening of the intestine.

Transmission under natural conditions the disease spread by ingestion of feed and water contaminated by the faeces of infected animals. The infection occurs mostly in the early month of life. The incubation period extends from 12 months to several years. The animal aged 3 to 6 years mostly suffer from the disease. Affected animals may not show clinical symptoms continue to discharge organisms in faeces. The organisms persist in pastures for about 1 year. The organisms are susceptible to sunlight, drying and high ph of soil; continuous contact of urine with faeces reduces the life of bacteria. In cattle clinical signs appear mainly during 2-6 years of age. The infected animals which are apparently healthy, often show clinical signs after parturition.

Treatment the organisms is more resistant to chemotherapeutic agents invitro than mycotuberculosis. Because of this the practical utility of treatment in clinical cases is poor.

Control the affected animal should be segregated and their faeces properly disposed of. Alive vaccine has been developed. It reduces the incidence of clinical disease. It consists of a non-pathogenic strain of jhone`s bacillus with an adjuvant. The calves soon after birth are inoculated with vaccine subcontaneously. The vaccinated animals become reactors of jhonin. Vaccination is generally done in heavily infected herds.

Bovine Ephemeral Fever

Bovine ephemeral fever is an insect-transmitted, noncontagious, viral disease of cattle and water buffalo that is seen in Africa, the middle-east, Australia and Asia.

Etiology and Epidemiology

Bovine ephemeral fever virus (befv) is classified as a member of the genus Ephemerovirus in the family Rhabdoviridae (single-stranded, negative sense rna).

The prevalence, geographic range and severity of the disease vary from year to year and epidemics occur periodically. During epidemics, onset is rapid; many animals are affected within days or 2–3 wk. Bovine ephemeral fever is most prevalent in the wet season in the tropics and in summer to early autumn in the subtropics or temperate regions (when conditions favor multiplication of biting insects); it disappears abruptly in winter. Virus spread appears to be limited by latitude rather than topography or availability of susceptible hosts. Morbidity may be as high as 80%; overall mortality is usually 1%–2%, although it can be higher in lactating cows, bulls in good condition and fat steers (10%–30%).

Clinical Findings

Signs, which occur suddenly and vary in severity, can include biphasic to polyphasic fever (40°–42 °C [104°–107.6 °F]), shivering, inappetence, lacrimation, serous nasal discharge, drooling, increased heart rate, tachypnea or dyspnea, atony of forestomachs, depression, stiffness and lameness and a sudden decrease in milk yield.

Affected cattle may become recumbent and paralyzed for 8 hr to >1 wk. After recovery, milk production often fails to return to normal levels until the next lactation. Abortion, with total loss of the season's lactation, occurs in about 5% of cows pregnant for 8–9 months. The virus does not appear to cross the placenta or affect the fertility of the cow. Bulls, heavy cattle and high-lactating dairy cows are the most severely affected, but spontaneous recovery usually occurs within a few days. More insidious losses may result from decreased muscle mass and lowered fertility in bulls.

Lesions

The most common lesions include polyserositis affecting pleural, pericardial and peritoneal surfaces; serofibrinous polysynovitis, polyarthritis, polytendinitis and cellulitis; and focal necrosis of skeletal muscles. Generalized edema of lymph nodes and lungs, as well as atelectasis, also may be present.

Treatment and Control

Complete rest is the most effective treatment and recovering animals should not be stressed or worked because relapse is likely. Anti-inflammatory drugs given early and in repeated doses for 2–3 days are effective. Oral dosing should be avoided unless the swallowing reflex is functional. Signs of hypocalcemia are treated as for milk fever. Antibiotic treatment to control secondary infection and rehydration with isotonic fluids may be warranted.

Rinderpest

Rinderpest is the most destructive of the virus diseases of cloven-footed animals, such as cattle, buffaloes, sheep, goats, pigs and wild ruminants. The virus is found notable in the saliva, discharge from eyes and nostrils and in the urine and faeces. It is present in the circulating blood during the febrile stage and is later concentrated in different organs, especially in the spleen, lymph nodes and liver. Outside the animal body, the virus is rapidly destroyed by direct sunlight and disinfectants. Cold preserves the virus. The virus is usually spread by contaminated feed and water. Rise in temperature up to 104 – 107 °F. Lacrimation and redness of eye. Foul odour from mouth. Discrete necrotic foci develop in the buccal mucosa, inside lip and on the tongue. Bloody mucoid diarrhea is noticed.

Treatment

Symptomatic treatment can be help early cure of the animals. Consult with veterinary doctor.

Mastitis

Mastitis or inflammation of the mammary gland, is the most common and the most expensive disease of dairy cattle throughout most of the world. Although stress and physical injuries may cause inflammation of the gland, infection by invading bacteria or other microorganisms (fungi, yeasts and possibly viruses) is the primary cause of mastitis. Infections begin when microorganisms penetrate the teat canal and multiply in the mammary gland.

Treatment

- Success depends on the nature of the aetiological agent involved, the severity of the disease and the extent of fibrosis.

- Complete recovery with freedom from bacterial infection can be obtained in cases of recent infection and in those where fibrosis has taken place only to a small extent.

- Such drugs as acriflavine, gramicidin and tyrothricin have now ceased to be in use and have given place to the more effective drugs, such as sulphonamides, penicillin and streptomycin.

Foot Rot

Foot rot is a common cause of lameness in cattle and occurs most frequently when cattle on pasture are forced to walk through mud to obtain water and feed. However, it may occur among cattle in paddocks as well, under apparently excellent conditions. Foot rot is caused when a cut or scratch in the skin allows infection to penetrate between the claws or around the top of the hoof. Individual cases should be kept in a dry place and treated promptly with medication as directed by a veterinarian. If the disease becomes a herd problem a foot bath containing a 5% solution of copper sulphate placed where cattle are forced to walk though it once or twice a day will help to reduce the number of new infections. In addition, drain mud holes and cement areas around the water troughs where cattle are likely to pick up the infection. Keep pens and areas where cattle gather as clean as possible. Proper nutrition regarding protein, minerals and vitamins will maximize hoof health.

Bovine Rhinotracheitis

Infectious bovine rhinotracheitis (ibr) is a highly contagious, infectious respiratory disease that is caused by bovine herpesvirus-1 (bhv-1). It can affect young and older cattle. In addition to causing respiratory disease, this virus can cause conjunctivitis, abortions, encephalitis and generalised systemic infections. Ibr is characterized by acute inflammation of the upper respiratory tract.

Treatment

There is no direct treatment for viral diseases. Infected animals should be isolated from the rest of the herd and treated with anti-inflammatory drugs and antibiotics for secondary infections if necessary. Carrier cattle should be identified and removed from the herd.

Prevention

Control of the disease is based on the use of vaccines.

Piglet Diarrhea or Scour

Of all the diseases in the sucking piglet, diarrhea is the most common and probably the most important. In some outbreaks, it is responsible for high morbidity and mortality. The main bacterial causes are E. Coli and Clostridia and the main parasite is Coccidia.

Clinical Signs

Scour in the piglet can occur at any age during sucking but there are often two peak periods, before 5 days and between 7 and 14 days.

Acute Disease

The only sign may be a perfectly good pig found dead. Post-mortem examinations show severe acute enteritis, so sudden that there may be no evidence of scour externally. Clinically affected piglets huddle together shivering or lie in a corner. The skin around the rectum and tail will be wet. Look around the pen for evidence of a watery to salad cream consistency scour. In many cases, there is a distinctive smell. As the diarrhea progresses the piglet becomes dehydrated, with sunken eyes and a thick leathery skin. The scour often sticks to the skin of other piglets giving them an orange to white color.

Prior to death piglets may be found on their sides paddling and frothing at the mouth.

Sub-acute Disease

The symptoms are similar but the effects on the piglet are less dramatic, more prolonged and mortality tends to be lower. This type of scour is often seen between 7 to 14 days of age manifest by a watery to thin salad cream consistency diarrhea, often white to yellow in color.

Treatment

- In severe outbreaks of E. Coli disease the sows feed can be top dressed with the appropriate antibiotic daily, from entry into the farrowing house and for up to 14 days post-farrowing. This can be effective in reducing bacterial output in the sows faeces.

- Observe litters for the presence of diarrhea both night and morning.

- Study the history of the disease on your farm. Is it sporadic, in one piglet in a litter or total litters?

- In the light of the history either treat the individual pig or on the first signs of disease treat the whole litter.

- If a litter is badly scoured dose night and morning for a minimum of two days.

- Assess the response to treatment. If there is no change within 12 hours, then change to another medicine as advised by your veterinarian.

- Always treat piglets less than 7 days of age by mouth.

- For older pigs where the disease is less acute injections are equally effective and easier to administer.

- Provide electrolytes in drinkers. These prevent dehydration and maintain body electrolyte balances.

- Cover the pen, the creep area and where the pigs defecate with straw, shredded paper, shavings or sawdust.

- Provide an additional lamp to provide an extra source of heat.

- Use binding agents such as chalk, kaolin or activated attapulgite to absorb toxins from the gut.

Management Control and Prevention

- Adopt procedures to prevent the spread of the scour - disinfect boots between pens, use a disposable plastic apron when dosing piglets to prevent heavy contamination of clothing, wash hands after handling a scoured litter, disinfect brushes and shovels between pen.

- Ensure that farrowing houses are only used on an all-in all-out basis with a pressure wash and disinfection between each batch.

- Farrowing pens must be dry before the house is repopulated. Remember that moisture, warmth, waste food and faeces are ideal for bacterial multiplication.

- Pen floors should be well maintained. Poor pen hygiene associated with bad drainage predisposes to scour.

- Look carefully at the part of the pen floor where there are piglet faeces. Is this poorly drained? Do large wet patches develop? If so cover them with extra bedding daily and remove. This is a most important aspect of control.

- Check nipple drinkers and feeding troughs for leakages.

- Ensure that faeces are removed daily from behind the sow from the day she enters the farrowing crates until at least 7 days post-farrowing if the floors are slatted. Also remove faeces daily throughout lactation if they are solid concrete.

- Maintain creep environments that are always warm and comfortable. Fluctuating temperatures are a major trigger factor to scour particularly from 7 to 14 days of age.

- Consider vaccinating against E. coli (make sure first that this is the cause of the problem however). E. Coli vaccines only protect the piglet for the first 5 to 7 days of age.

- Assess the environment of the entire farrowing house. Poor environments allow heavy bacterial multiplication and a much higher bacterial challenge is likely to break down the colostral immunity.

- Check the sow's health. Animals affected with enteric or respiratory disease, lameness or mastitis predisposes the litter to scour.

- Where farrowing house floors are very poor, pitted and difficult to clean, brush them over with lime wash containing a phenolic disinfectant.

- Colostrum management: It is vital that the piglet receives the maximum amount of colostrum within the first 12 hours of birth. High levels of antibody are only absorbed during this period. Factors such as poor teat access, poor crate design and particularly the development of agalactia in the sow, associated with udder oedema, reduce intake.

PPR (Goat Plague)

PPR (Peste des petits ruminants) is a most important viral disease of goat capable of heavy mortality and commonly called as goat plague.

Etiology

The causative virus was first thought to be an aberrant strain of rinderpest virus that had lost its ability to infect cattle. Later molecular studies showed that it was distinct from, but closely related to, rinderpest virus.

Clinical Signs

The clinical sign of PPR in goats is often fulminating and fatal although apparent infection occurs in endemic areas. Incubation period may range from 2-6 days in field conditions. In acute form, there is sudden onset of fever with rectal temperature of at least 40°- 41 °C. The affected goats show dullness, sneezing, serous discharge from the eyes and nostrils. During this stage farmers often think that the animal has developed cold exposure and may attempt to provide protection for cold. In the process goats, may be congregated and accentuate the process of transmission. After 2-3 days, discrete lesions develop in the mouth and extend over the entire oral mucosa, forming diphtheric plaques.

During this stage profound halitosis (foul smell) is easily appreciable and the animal is unable to eat due to sore mouth and swollen lips. Latter ocular discharge becomes mucopurulent and the exudate dries up, matting the eyelids and partially occluding the nostrils. Diarrhea develops 3-4 days after the fever and is profuse and faeces may be mucoid or bloody depending upon the damage. Dyspnea and coughing occur later due to secondary pneumonia. Death occurs within one week of the onset of the illness.

Treatment and Control

No specific treatment is recommended for ppr being viral disease. However, mortality rates can be reduced by the use of drugs that control the bacterial and parasitic complications. Specifically, oxytetracycline and chlortetracycline are recommended to prevent secondary pulmonary infections. Lesions around the eyes, nostrils and mouth should be cleaned twice daily with sterile cotton swab. Our experience indicates that fluid therapy and anti-microbial such as enrofloxacin or ceftiofur on recommended doses along with mouth wash with 5% boro-glycerine can be of benefit in reducing the mortality during outbreak of ppr in goats. Health workers should inspect first the unaffected goats followed by treatment of affected goats. Immediate isolation of affected goats from clinically healthy goats is most importance measure in controlling the spread of infection. Nutritious soft, moist, palatable diet should be given to the affected goats. Provide parenteral energy infusion in anorectic goats along with appetizers.

Immediately measures should be taken for notification of disease to nearest government veterinary hospital. Carcasses of affected goats should be burned or buried. Proper disposal of contact fomites, decontamination is must. Vaccination is the most effective way to control ppr.

Bovine Babesiosis (Tick Fever)

Cause

Bovine babesiosis (bb) is a tick-borne disease of cattle. Transmission of b bovis takes place when engorging adult female ticks pick up the infection. They pass it on to their progeny via their eggs. Larvae (or seed ticks) then pass it on in turn when feeding on another animal. B bigemina is also passed from one generation of ticks to the next. Engorging adult ticks pick up the infection and nymphal and adult stages (not larval stages) of the next generation pass it on to other cattle. Morbidity and mortality vary greatly and are influenced by prevailing treatments employed in an area, previous exposure to a species/strain of parasite and vaccination status. In endemic areas, cattle become infected at a young age and develop a long-term immunity. However, outbreaks can occur in these endemic areas if exposure to ticks by young animals is interrupted or immuno-naïve cattle are introduced. The introduction of babesia infected ticks into previously tick-free areas may also lead to outbreaks of disease.

Symptoms

- High fever.

- Neurologic signs such as incoordination, teeth grinding and mania. Some cattle may be found on the ground with the involuntary movements of the legs. When the nervous symptoms of cerebral babesiosis develop, the outcome is almost always fatal.

- Dark colored urine.

- Anorexia.

- Animals likely to separate from herd, be weak, depressed and reluctant to move.

- N b. Bigemina parasitaemia often exceeds 10 percent and may be as high as 30 percent.

Clinical symptoms for babesia divergens are similar to b. Bigemina infections. The survivors may be weak and in reduced condition, although they usually recover fully. Subacute infections, with less apparent clinical signs, are also seen.

Treatment

Mild cases may recover without treatment. Sick animals can be treated with an antiparasitic drug. Treatment is most likely to be successful if the disease is diagnosed early; it may fail if the animal has been weakened by anemia. Imidocarb has been reported to protect animals from disease but immunity can develop. There are also concerns with regard to residues in milk and meat. In some cases blood transfusions and other supportive therapy should be considered.

Prevention

Effective control of tick fevers has been achieved by a combination of measures directed at both the disease and the tick vector. Tick control by acaracide dipping is widely used in endemic areas. Dipping may be done as frequently as every 4-6 weeks in heavily infested areas. The occurrence of resistance of ticks, chemical residues in cattle and environmental concerns over the continued use of insecticides has led to use of integrated strategies for tick control. Babesiosis vaccines are readily available and are highly effective. Anti-tick vaccines are also available in some countries and can be used as part of an integrated program for the control of ticks. Babesiosis can be eradicated by eliminating the host tick(s). In the us, this was accomplished by treating all cattle every two to three weeks with acaricides. In countries where eradication is not feasible, tick control can reduce the incidence of disease.

Treatment for Control of Tick (Ethnovet)

Mix common salt and little camphor in castor oil or neem oil and apply over the affected area. Whole plant extract of ghaner (lantana camara) should be diluted with the urine of cattle and apply externally. Boil 250 gm of tobacco in 2 litres of water and add 5 litres of water and sprayed over the body of 10-20 animals.

Theileriosis

Theileriases are a group of tickborne diseases caused by theileria spp. Both theileria and babesia are members of the suborder piroplasmorina. Although babesia are primarily parasites of rbcs, theileria use, successively, wbcs and rbcs for completion of their life cycle in mammalian hosts. The infective sporozoite stage of the parasite is transmitted in the saliva of infected ticks as they feed. Sporozoites invade leukocytes and, within a few days, develop to schizonts. In the most pathogenic species of theileria (eg, t parva and t annulata), parasite multiplication occurs predominantly within the host wbcs, whereas less pathogenic species multiply mainly in rbcs. Development of the schizont stage of pathogenic theileria causes the host wbc to divide; at each cell division, the parasite also divides. Mortality in such stock is relatively low, but introduced cattle are particularly vulnerable. Unlike in babesiosis, in theileriasis there is no evidence of increased resistance in calves <6 mo old.

East Coast Fever

East coast fever, an acute disease of cattle, is usually characterized by high fever, swelling of the lymph nodes, dyspnea and high mortality. Caused by theileria parva and transmitted by the tick vector rhipicephalus appendiculatus, it is a serious problem in east and southern africa.

Etiology and Transmission

The african buffalo (syncerus caffer) is an important wildlife reservoir of t parva, but infection is asymptomatic in buffalo. T parva transmitted by ticks from either cattle or buffalo cause severe disease in cattle, but buffalo-derived parasites differentiate poorly to merozoites in cattle and generally are not transmitted by ticks. Hence, buffalo t parva are maintained as a separate population. Buffalo t parvawere previously considered a separate subspecies (t parva lawrencei), but dna typing indicate that the cattle and buffalo parasites are a single species. T parva is usually highly pathogenic, causing high levels of mortality, although some less pathogenic isolates have been identified.

Pathogenesis, Clinical Findings and Diagnosis

T parva sporozoites are injected into cattle by infected vector ticks. An occult phase of 5–10 days follows before infected lymphocytes can be detected in giemsa-stained smears of cells aspirated from the local draining lymph node. Subsequently, the number of parasitized cells increases rapidly throughout the lymphoid system and from about day 14 onward, cells undergoing merogony are observed. This is associated with widespread lymphocytolysis, marked lymphoid depletion and leukopenia. Piroplasms in rbcs infected by the resultant merozoites assume various forms, but typically they are small and rod-shaped or oval.

Clinical signs vary according to the level of challenge and they range from in apparent or mild to severe and fatal. Typically, fever occurs 7–10 days after parasites are introduced by feeding ticks, continues throughout the course of infection and may be >106 °F (41 °C). Lymph node swelling becomes pronounced and generalized. Lymphoblasts in giemsa-stained smears of needle aspirates from lymph nodes contain multinuclear schizonts. Anorexia develops and the animal rapidly loses condition; lacrimation and nasal discharge may occur. Terminally, dyspnea is common. Just before death, a sharp decrease in body temperature is usual and pulmonary exudate pours from the nostrils. Death usually occurs 18–24 days after infection. The most striking postmortem lesions are lymph node enlargement and massive pulmonary edema and hyperemia. Hemorrhages are common on the serosal and mucosal surfaces of many organs, sometimes together with obvious areas of necrosis in the lymph nodes and thymus. Anemia is not a major diagnostic sign (as it is in babesiosis) because there is minimal division of the parasites in rbcs and thus no massive destruction of them.

Animals that recover are immune to subsequent challenge with the same strains but may be susceptible to some heterologous strains. Most recovered or immunized animals remain carriers of the infection.

Treatment and Control

Treatment with parvaquone and its derivative buparvaquone is highly effective when administered in the early stages of clinical disease but is less effective in the advanced stages, in which there is extensive destruction of lymphoid and hematopoietic tissues. Immunization of cattle against t parva using an infection-and-treatment procedure is practical and continues to gain acceptance in some regions. The components for this procedure are a cryopreserved sporozoite stabilate of the appropriate strain(s) oftheileria derived from infected ticks and a single dose of long-acting oxytetracycline given simultaneously; although oxytetracycline has little therapeutic effect when administered after development of disease, it inhibits development of the parasite when given at the outset of infection. Cattle should be immunized 3–4 wk before being allowed on infected pasture. Parasitized bovine cells containing the schizont stage of t parva and t annulata can be cultivated in vitro as continuously growing cell lines. In the case of t annulata, cattle can be infected with a few thousand cultured cells. Attenuated strains produced by serial passage of such cultures form the basis of live vaccines used in several countries, including israel, iran, india and the former ussr.

Incidence of east coast fever can be reduced by rigid tick control, but this is not feasible in many areas because of cost and the high frequency of acaricidal treatment required.

Ringworm

This is the most common infectious skin disease affecting beef cattle. It is caused by a fungus and is transmissible to man. Typically, the disease appears as crusty grey patches usually in the region of the head and neck and particularly around the eyes.

As a first step in controlling the disease, it is recommended that, whenever possible, affected animals should be segregated and their pens or stalls cleaned and disinfected. Clean cattle which have been in contact with the disease should be watched closely for the appearance of lesions and treated promptly. Proper nutrition, particularly high levels of vitamin a, copper and zinc while not a cure, will help to raise the resistance of the animal and in so doing offer some measure of control. Contact your vet and or feed store for products to treat this disease. Using a wormer like ivomec will kill lice and help prevent cattle from scratching causing skin damage and a place for the fungus to enter.

Milk Fever

Milk fever, also known as Parturient hypocalcaemia and parturient paresis, is a disease which has assumed considerable importance with the development of heavy milking cows. Decrease in the levels of ionized calcium in tissue fluids is basically the cause of the disease. In all adult cows, there is a fall in serum-calcium level with the onset of lactation at calving. The disease usually occurs in 5 to 10-year-old cows and is chiefly caused by a sudden decrease in blood-calcium level, generally within 48 hours after calving.

Symptoms

- In classical cases, hypocalcaemia is the cause of clinical symptoms. Hypophosphataemia and variations in the concentration of serum-magnesium may play some subsidiary role.

- The clinical symptoms develop usually in one to three days after calving. They are characterized by loss of appetite, constipation and restlessness, but there is no rise in temperature.

Calf Scour

Calves may develop scours due to bacterial or virus infections. Scours is known as "calf scours" or neonatal calf diarrhea. The primary causes of scours include: Rota virus, Corona virus, Cryptosporidium parvum, Salmonella and Escherichia coli.

- Determine if treatment is required: Calves that are moving around in the pasture, with their tails up, probably do not need treatment. Check to see if the diarrhea is yellow or white. If this is the case, treatment is probably not needed.

- Determine if the calf is looking listless: Calves that are lethargic or not participating much in the playful activities with other calves are a red flag to pay attention to. Calves that are also losing condition are also cause for alarm.

- Check to see if the calf is dehydrated: You can check for dehydration by pulling on the calf's neck skin. If the skin "tents" this is a sign of dehydration.

- Determine the calf's body temperature. A normal body temperature ranges from 100.5 °F (38.1 °C) to 102.5 °F (39.2 °C). Anything outside of this range is a sign for treatment.

- Separate the sick calf or calves from the healthy herd. You'll want to do this to avoid spreading the disease further.

- Administer fluids using your veterinarian-approved electrolyte solution. You may need to inject the fluids via iv or orally.

- Follow appropriate nursing care protocol using your vet's guidelines. This may include providing shelter, feed and a warm place to sleep.

- A drawback from providing shelter is maintaining infectious control. You will have to work extra to get rid of soiled bedding and disinfect everything that a calf will touch, from the floor to the fence panels and even the feed bucket.

- Enthnovet practice: Ingredients needed: Vasambu (Acorus calamus) leaves 2 numbers, dried ginger (Zingiber officinale) 50 gm, guava (Psidium guajava) tender leaves 200 gm. The above materials are ground and made into a bolus and administered orally one or two times.

Scrapie

Scrapie is a neurodegenerative disease, caused by a prion that affects sheep and less frequently, goats. Infected animals do not usually become ill for years; however, the clinical signs are progressive and invariably fatal once they develop. Scrapie can be transmitted between animals, either directly or via the environment and infected premises are difficult to decontaminate. The presence of classical scrapie can result in trade sanctions and many countries are conducting control or eradication programs. Breeding sheep for genetic resistance is an important tool in many of these programs; however, the understanding of resistance genes is still incomplete in goats.

As a result of increased surveillance, atypical scrapie prions have been detected in both sheep and goats. Atypical scrapie often occurs in sheep that are genetically resistant to classical scrapie. It has been reported in countries that do not have classical scrapie. Atypical/Nor98 prions do not seem to be transmitted readily between animals in nature and are rarely detected in more than one animal in a herd or flock. It is possible that they arise spontaneously in sheep, similarly to some genetic prion diseases in humans.

Scrapie is a member of the transmissible spongiform encephalopathies (TSEs), a group of neurodegenerative disorders caused by prions, infectious proteins that seem to replicate by converting a normal cellular protein into copies of the prion. The cellular protein, which is called PrPc, is found on the surface of neurons. The pathogenic isoforms of PrPc found in animals with scrapie are designated PrPres ('res' refers to the proteinase K-resistant nature of prions, compared to normal PrPc). Other names used for this protein are PrPSc ('Sc' for scrapie), PrPTSE or PrPd ('d' for disease-associated).

Classical scrapie is an infectious disease that can be caused by multiple strains of the classical scrapie prion. Atypical (or Nor98) scrapie prions were first detected in Norway in 1998, although they have also been found in older archived samples from Europe. Several lines of evidence, including the apparently sporadic nature of atypical/Nor98 cases and their relatively homogeneous distribution across small ruminant populations, have led to the suggestion that these prions may arise spontaneously, similarly to some diseases in other species. However, this agent can be difficult to detect. At one time, it was uncertain whether atypical scrapie was caused by one agent or by different prions in different animals. Recent experiments suggest that most of these infections are caused by the same prion. One group reported that, in one experimentally infected animal, atypical/Nor98 changed into a phenotype indistinguishable from CH1641, an unusual classical scrapie strain that has some similarities to bovine spongiform encephalopathy (BSE) in immunoblots, while some other animals developed atypical/Nor98 scrapie.

Species Affected

Classical Scrapie

Classical scrapie can affect domesticated sheep and goats, mouflon (Ovis musimon) and possibly other animals closely related to sheep and goats. An in vitro prion conversion test has suggested that bighorn sheep (Ovis canadensis) might be susceptible; however, this still needs to be confirmed by direct evidence of infection in these animals. Cattle and pigs were not susceptible to oral inoculation, although cattle have been infected by intracerebral inoculation, a route that bypasses normal species barriers to prions.

Squirrel monkeys (Saimiri sciureus) became infected when they were fed tissues that contained hamster-adapted scrapie prions; however, chimpanzees (Pan troglodytes), capuchin monkeys (subfamily Cebinae), cynomolgus macaques (Macaca fascicularis) and woolly monkeys (Lagothrix sp.) did not appear susceptible to oral inoculation. Mink (Mustela vison), rats, mice, hamsters, rabbits, various species of voles and several primate species - chimpanzees, capuchin and woolly monkeys and marmosets (Callithrix jacchus) – have infected experimentally by intracerebral inoculation. Some of these studies (e.g., those in rabbits) used rodent-adapted scrapie prions rather than those from sheep or goats. Ferrets did not develop clinical signs after inoculation by an unspecified route and cats were resistant to intracerebral inoculation. One study reported that sea bream (Sparus aurata) appeared to be susceptible to oral inoculation.

Atypical Scrapie

Atypical (Nor98) scrapie has been reported in sheep and goats. Attempts to infect laboratory mice (nontransgenic) and bank voles by intracerebral inoculation were unsuccessful.

Geographic Distribution

Classical scrapie has been reported on all major continents and on many islands. Recent surveillance suggests that this disease is either absent or minimally present in some countries. However, small numbers of infected animals can be difficult to detect and the World Organization for Animal Health (OIE) requires that a country conduct active surveillance, with a high probability of detecting low levels of scrapie, for at least 7 years before it can be considered scrapie-free. Australia and New Zealand, where scrapie was last reported in the 1950s, are widely recognized to be scrapie-free. Some countries perform little or no active surveillance for scrapie and the presence or absence of this disease is uncertain.

Atypical/Nor98 scrapie has been detected in most European countries, North America, New Zealand, Australia and some other nations. If it is a spontaneous genetic disease, it is likely to occur in all areas where small ruminants are found. The presence of atypical/Nor98 scrapie does not affect a country's scrapie status for international trade.

Transmission

Infected animals carry the scrapie prion for life and can transmit the agent even if they remain asymptomatic. Infections are thought to occur primarily by ingestion, but sheep can also be infected experimentally via the conjunctiva or nasal cavity, by injection into various body sites and probably through abraded skin. Most sheep are thought to become infected from their dam, either at or soon after birth. Older animals can be infected, but are more resistant. The placenta can contain high levels of scrapie prions in some sheep and licking or ingesting fetal membranes and fluids is thought to be an important route of infection in this species. Goats also have scrapie prions in the placenta, though in much smaller amounts. Milk from both sheep and goats is known to be infectious. One study demonstrated that, in sheep, both colostrum and milk from infected ewes can transmit scrapie One recent experiment suggested that prenatal transmission can occur in lambs derived by caesarian section and immediately separated from their dams and highly sensitive techniques have detected small amounts of scrapie prions in fetal tissues of offspring from both subclinically infected and symptomatic sheep.

Highly sensitive techniques have found low levels of scrapie prions in the urine and saliva of symptomatic sheep; in the oral cavity of some subclinically infected sheep; and in feces from subclinical and symptomatic sheep. How much these sources contribute to transmission is still uncertain. Iatrogenic transmission is also possible. Prions have been detected intermittently in the blood of some animals, up to a year before the onset of clinical signs. Transmission via blood becomes increasingly efficient as the animal nears the clinical stage. Some animals were infected by two vaccines that had inadvertently been prepared with central nervous system (CNS) and lymphoid tissues from infected sheep. Most studies indicate that there is little or no risk of transmission in semen; however, one group detected scrapie prions and infectivity in the semen of sheep inoculated with one laboratory strain.

Epidemiological evidence suggests that sheep can be infected from contaminated environments, including pastures. One study recovered scrapie prions from various environmental sources, such as feed and water troughs, 20 days after infected sheep were removed. Prions were found both indoors and outside, although they seemed more likely to be recovered from metal objects (e.g., water troughs, metal gates) indoors. In another study, scrapie prions were detected on various surfaces, in ambient dust samples and on pastures up to 30 m from the open ends of infected barns that had housed sheep a year earlier. In Iceland, scrapie recurred on some premises restocked 2-3 years after decontamination and in one barn where small ruminants had been absent for 16 years. Prions can bind to soil and persist for varying periods depending on the type of soil. They remain infectious for animals when bound to soil. Rodent-adapted scrapie prions were isolated from an experimentally contaminated soil sample after 3 years and prions from sheep were still present for at least 18 months in some types of soils in the laboratory. Repeated cycles of wetting and drying are reported to decrease, though not necessarily eliminate, infectivity in soil. Prions can also remain infectious after passage through the digestive tracts of scavengers or predators; this has been demonstrated experimentally for coyotes and crows.

Scrapie Prions in the Tissues of Sheep and Goats

Scrapie prions occur in the CNS of sheep, but they have also been found in many tissues outside the CNS, including the peripheral nervous system, many lymphoid tissues, salivary glands, adrenal gland and kidney; in the nerves or sensory structures (muscle spindles) of skeletal muscle; occasionally in various other tissues and organs; and in association with chronic inflammatory lesions caused by other pathogens. Whether an animal has prions outside the CNS may depend on factors such as its resistance to scrapie (e.g., its genotype), the stage of the disease and possibly the prion dose. In some animals, there may be little or no accumulation outside the CNS.

A limited number of studies in goats have found scrapie prions in the CNS, retina, peripheral nervous system, adrenal gland, salivary gland, kidney, muscle, pancreas, liver and various lymphoid tissues including the spleen, lymph nodes, gut-associated lymphoid tissues (GALT), tonsil and lymphoid tissues in the nictitating membrane and tongue. Lymphoid tissues can contain prions in both symptomatic and asymptomatic goats. Very small amounts of prions were also found in the nasal mucosa, associated with nerves.

Atypical Scrapie

Epidemiological evidence suggests that atypical scrapie is either not a contagious disease in the field or transmission occurs inefficiently and at a very low rate. Except in very large flocks, infections have only been identified in a single animal per flock or herd. However, laboratory experiments have demonstrated that atypical scrapie prions can be transmitted orally in newborn lambs. Highly sensitive tests found infectivity in the CNS and ileum of some of these lambs by 12 months and some animals later developed neurological signs. In an ongoing experiment, there was no evidence of infection in lambs inoculated when they were 3-months old.

Atypical scrapie prions have mainly been found in the CNS. Highly sensitive bioassays have detected infectivity in lymphoid tissues, muscles and the peripheral nervous system of experimentally infected sheep, although prions were not found in these tissues with the standard techniques used to detect scrapie.

Disinfection

Complete decontamination of prion-contaminated tissues, surfaces and environments can be difficult. These agents are very resistant to most disinfectants, including formalin and alcohol. They are also resistant to heat or ultraviolet, microwave and ionizing radiation, particularly when they are protected in organic material or preserved with aldehyde fixatives or when the prion titer is high. Prions can bind tightly to some surfaces, including stainless steel and plastic, without losing infectivity. Prions bound to metal seem to be highly resistant to decontamination.

Relatively few prion decontamination techniques have been published and confirmed to be effective for routine use. Some laboratories pre-treat tissues with formic acid to decrease infectivity before sectioning tissue blocks. A 1-2 N sodium hydroxide solution or a sodium hypochlorite solution containing at least 2% (20,000 ppm) available chlorine, has traditionally been recommended for equipment and surfaces. Surfaces should be treated for more than 1 hour at 20 °C (68 °F). Overnight disinfection is recommended for equipment. Cleaning before disinfection removes organic material that may protect prions.

Experimentally, some milder treatments have also been effective against certain prions, under some conditions. They include a specific phenolic disinfectant, various alkaline and enzymatic detergents (although the efficacy of specific agents within these classes varies), hydrogen peroxide gas plasma, radiofrequency gas plasma and sodium dodecyl sulfate plus acetic acid. These agents might be useful for items that cannot withstand harsher decontamination procedures.

Physical inactivation of prions can be carried out by porous load autoclaving at 134 °C (273 °F) for 18 minutes at 30 lb/in². Resistance to heat may vary with the specific prion, the degree of contamination and type of sample. Tissue films containing prions are more difficult to decontaminate by steam after they have dried, after use, they be kept moist or wet until decontamination is performed. The cleaning agent used before autoclaving should also be chosen with care, as certain agents (e.g., some enzymatic treatments) can increase the resistance of prions to steam sterilization. Dry heat is less effective than moist heat; some prions can survive dry heat at temperatures as high as 360 °C (680 °F) for an hour and one group even reported that infectivity survived incineration at 600 °C (1112 °F). A combination of chemical and physical decontamination can be more effective than either procedure alone and effective combinations of chemical agents (e.g., NaOH) and autoclaving have been published.

It should be noted that even the harshest combination of chemical and physical disinfection is not guaranteed to destroy all prions in all types of samples. Decontaminating contaminated facilities, especially sites such as animal pens, may be very difficult. In one study, genetically susceptible sheep became infected with scrapie prions after being placed in pens that had been pressure washed and decontaminated with high concentrations of sodium hypochlorite (20,000 ppm free chorine solution) for one hour, followed by painting and full re-galvanization or replacement of metalwork. Reports from an eradication program in Iceland indicated that scrapie recurred on some farms despite decontamination (500 ppm chlorine), power washing and no restocking for 2 years or more. Decontaminating soil contaminated with prions is currently impractical, although some agents, including an aqueous subtilisin-based enzymatic treatment (effective at ambient temperatures), appear promising in the laboratory. Incineration is commonly used for carcasses, but two studies found that composting may reduce or eliminate scrapie and other prions in tissues, while another suggested that soil microorganisms might degrade prions in buried carcasses.

Incubation Period

The incubation period for classical scrapie is estimated to be 2-7 years in most animals, with peak prevalence occurring at 2-5 years of age in sheep. Signs of illness are rare in animals less than a year old.

The incubation period for atypical scrapie is uncertain, but it is usually seen in older animals than classical scrapie. In the laboratory, however, some orally inoculated newborn lambs had neurological signs by 2 years of age.

Clinical Signs

Classical Scrapie

The signs of classical scrapie can be variable in sheep and may be influenced by factors such as the animal's susceptibility and the strain of the prion. The first clinical signs are usually behavioral. Affected sheep tend to stand apart from the flock and may either trail or lead when the flock is driven. Other common signs include hypersensitivity to stimuli, a fixed stare, ataxia and a high-stepping or unusual hopping gait. Animals may also develop tremors (especially of the head and neck), grind their teeth, have an impaired menace response or carry their heads low. Some animals may unexpectedly collapse when they are handled. Blindfolding may reveal incoordination, loss of balance or circling in an animal that is able to compensate for neurological deficits when it is able to see. Visual impairment is also possible, though uncommon. Many sheep become intensely pruritic and may rub, scrape or chew at these areas. In a pruritic animal, scratching the dorsum or pressure over the base of the tail may cause a characteristic nibbling response or rhythmic head and body movements (the scratch reflex test). Loss of condition is common in the early stages and significant weight loss or emaciation may be seen late. The fleece may be dry and brittle. Drinking behavior and urination can also change, with some sheep drinking small quantities of water often. Most animals die within a few weeks to several months after the onset of clinical signs.

Some goats have neurological and behavioral signs similar to those in sheep. However, pruritus seems to be less common; if it occurs, it is typically less intense and often localized over the tailhead or withers. Pruritic goats may nibble at affected body sites rather than rub and the scratch reflex test is often negative. Many goats are reported to be difficult to milk. There are also reports of cases where the animal had only nonspecific signs (e.g., listlessness, weight loss and premature cessation of lactation). As in sheep, the disease is progressive and fatal, with death usually occurring within a few months.

Atypical Scrapie

Incoordination and ataxia seem to be the most prominent clinical signs in sheep with atypical/Nor98 scrapie. Pruritus appears to be minimal or uncommon, although it has been seen in some animals. Loss of body condition, anxiety, tremors, abnormal menace responses or a subdued mental status have been reported in some cases, but not others. Some cases of atypical scrapie have been found by routine surveillance in apparently healthy flocks or herds at slaughter.

Post Mortem Lesions

There are no characteristic gross lesions in classical or atypical scrapie, although there may be nonspecific changes such as wasting or emaciation and skin or wool lesions resulting from pruritus. The histopathological lesions of scrapie are usually (though not always) bilaterally symmetrical. The characteristic lesions of classical scrapie are noninflammatory spongiform changes, with neuronal vacuolation, in the CNS. Astrocytosis may be seen to a greater or lesser extent and amyloid plaques may occur in some animals. Lesions are usually present in the brainstem of animals with classical scrapie, although they are not limited to this location. In contrast, animals with atypical/Nor98 scrapie tend to have minimal or no spongiform lesions in the brainstem, although some animals may have lesions in more rostral parts of the CNS, such as the cerebellar cortex, cerebral cortex and basal ganglion.

Diagnostic Tests

Both classical and atypical scrapie can be diagnosed after death by detecting prions in the CNS. Prions can usually be found in the brainstem of animals with classical scrapie and these animals are typically diagnosed by sampling the medulla oblongata at the level of the obex. Prions are much less likely to accumulate in this area in animals with atypical/Nor98 scrapie and may be absent. Some animals with atypical/Nor98 scrapie have had significant prion deposits in the cerebellar cortex, cerebral cortex, substantia nigra, thalamus and basal nuclei; however, the specific prion staining pattern differs between animals. Sampling both the cerebellum and medulla is more likely to detect both classical and atypical cases than sampling the medulla alone.

Classical scrapie can be diagnosed in live sheep by detecting prions in biopsies from the nictitating membrane (third eyelid test), palatine tonsil or rectoanal mucosaassociated lymphoid tissue. They have also been found sometimes in superficial lymph nodes. Third eyelid and rectal mucosa biopsies can be taken without sedation, using only topical anesthesia and restraint. Palatine tonsil biopsies require anesthesia and are less practical for field use. In sheep and goats with classical scrapie, prions can sometimes be found in peripheral lymphoid tissues before they appear in the brain. The usual diagnostic tests have not, to date, found prions outside the CNS of animals with atypical scrapie.

Immunoblotting (Western blotting) and immunohistochemistry are the most specific assays for detecting prions. Immunoblotting can also distinguish atypical/Nor98 scrapie from classical scrapie. Various rapid tests for classical scrapie, based on enzyme-linked immunosorbent assays (ELISAs), automated immunoblotting or other techniques, are available in some countries. Rapid tests allow large numbers of samples to be screened and are often used in surveillance and slaughter testing. Some rapid tests can also detect atypical scrapie; however, their sensitivity varies. In autolyzed brains, scrapie may occasionally be diagnosed by finding characteristic prion fibrils, called scrapie-associated fibrils, with electron microscopy; however, this test has low sensitivity and is no longer commonly used. Histological examination of the brain can be helpful in diagnosis (although it is not generally used as the sole confirmatory test), but some animals in the early stages of infection have few or no spongiform changes. A combination of tests may be used to certify flocks as scrapie-negative.

Highly sensitive assays, including protein misfolding cyclic amplification (PMCA) and quaking-induced conversion (QuIC) or real-time quaking-induced conversion (RT-QuIC), may be able to identify infected animals earlier than immunoblotting or immunohistochemistry. These techniques detect tiny amounts of prions by their ability to convert PrPc (the normal cellular protein) into prions in vitro. They are mainly used in research at present, but are being investigated for possible diagnostic use in sheep and goats. Scrapie can also be detected by inoculation into mice (rodent bioassays); however, an incubation period of several months makes this technique impractical for routine diagnosis. Serology is not useful for diagnosis, as antibodies are not made against prions.

Scrapie may need to be distinguished from BSE, which can infect sheep in the laboratory and has been detected in rarely in naturally infected goats. In most cases, this can be accomplished with conventional prion tests. BSE is more difficult to distinguish from certain rare classical scrapie prions, such as CH1641. A limited number of assays such as PMCA, certain special types of immunoblots, PrPSc profiling or epitope mapping can differentiate the latter two agents.

Treatment

There is no treatment for scrapie or any other prion disease.

Control

Disease Reporting

Veterinarians who encounter or suspect scrapie should follow their national and local guidelines for disease reporting. Scrapie is a reportable disease in many countries where it is endemic, especially when control programs are in place. Scrapie is reportable in the United States.

Prevention

Classical scrapie mainly seems to be introduced via animal movements, although other possibilities, such as exposure in contaminated feed (e.g., hay) have also been suggested. The risk of introducing scrapie can be reduced by maintaining a closed flock/herd or minimizing outside purchases of stock. If replacement animals must be added, they should be from herds that test negative for this disease and are managed in a way that makes them unlikely to become infected. Milk and colostrum from potentially infected sheep or goats should not be fed to scrapie-free flocks. Selecting genetically resistant sheep as replacements and breeding rams may also be helpful in reducing the flock's risk of infection. Certification programs can help identify classical scrapie-free flocks.

In sheep flocks that have become infected, control measures can include removing animals that test positive in live animal tests, are at an elevated risk of infection and are genetically susceptible to scrapie. Lambs seem to become infected mainly from their dams and removing the offspring of infected ewes may contribute to control. In addition, some countries cull members of the infected animal's birth cohort that were raised with it during the first year of life. Reducing exposure to high concentrations of prions (e.g., in the placenta) may reduce transmission within the flock. Breeding genetically susceptible, infected ewes to a resistant ram can decrease or eliminate prions in the fetal membranes and fluids. If a ewe of unknown scrapie status was not bred to a resistant ram, separating her from the rest of the flock before lambing and until there is no vaginal discharge, may help protect other animals. Control is more difficult in herds of goats, where genetic resistance to scrapie is incompletely understood. Complete depopulation, followed by cleaning and disinfection, is sometimes used on infected farms, particularly in goat herds; however, decontamination of the farm is difficult and the disease may recur. Two studies suggest that it might be possible to derive a classical scrapie-free sheep flock from an infected flock by embryo transfer.

The components of official scrapie control/eradication programs often include surveillance (e.g., at slaughter, on farms and in diagnostic samples sent to laboratories), flock/herd certification programs, quarantines or depopulation of infected herds, tracing of infected animals and programs to increase genetic resistance in sheep. A few countries have successfully excluded classical scrapie with import controls, although their sheep populations are genetically susceptible. There are no control methods for atypical scrapie, which seems to occur sporadically and at low levels and does not appear to spread readily between animals in the field.

Genotype and Classical Scrapie Susceptibility in Sheep

Sheep with that are genetically resistant to scrapie may either have no evidence of infection after exposure or develop clinical signs after longer incubation periods than susceptible animals. The genotype also influences transmission. A genetically resistant fetus suppresses the appearance of prions in the placenta of an infected, scrapiesusceptible dam (except when a resistant fetus develops in the same uterine horn as a susceptible fetus). Breeding these ewes to a resistant ram can decrease the amount of prion contamination in the environment at lambing. Ewes with resistant genotypes do not produce scrapie-positive placentas, regardless of the genotype of the fetus.

Polymorphisms in the PrP gene at codons 136, 154 and 171 play a major role in resistance to classical scrapie, although other PrP codons and other genes also seem to have some influence. At codon 136, alanine (A) is linked to resistance and valine (V) associated with susceptibility to some scrapie strains. Sheep with histidine (H) at codon 154 are relatively resistant to classical scrapie, with prolonged survival and a longer incubation period, while sheep with arginine (R) are more susceptible. Arginine (R) at codon 171 is linked to resistance, while glutamine (Q) and histidine (H) have been associated with susceptibility. The effects of some uncommon amino acids at codons 136, 154 or 171 are unknown. However, lysine (K) at codon 171 appeared to prolong the incubation time in the Barbado breed of sheep. The relative frequency of resistant genotypes can differ between sheep breeds and this is thought to be a major influence on overall breed susceptibility to classical scrapie.

The five most common PrP alleles in sheep are A136R154R171 (abbreviated ARR), ARQ, AHQ, ARH and VRQ. Sheep with the ARR/ARR genotype are highly resistant to classical scrapie (cases are very rare); homozygous or heterozygous AHQ and heterozygous ARR animals usually have marginal susceptibility; and VRQ/VRQ, ARQ/VRQ and ARQ/ARQ sheep are expected to be most susceptible. Some countries use all three codons to classify sheep as susceptible or resistant, while the U.S. eradication program employs codons 136 and 171.

Genotype and Classical Scrapie Susceptibility in Goats

Scrapie resistance is still incompletely understood in goats; however, a number of polymorphisms that seem to influence resistance have been identified. Some alleles apparently linked to resistance include serine (S) or aspartic acid (D), rather than asparagine (N), at codon 146; histidine (H) rather than arginine (R) at codon 154; glutamine (Q) rather than arginine (R) at codon 211; and glutamine (Q) rather than lysine (K) at codon 222. K222, which seems to confer strong (but not absolute) resistance to classical scrapie and has also been linked to resistance to BSE, has been proposed as a possible target for breeding goats. Some studies have also suggested that polymorphisms at codons 127, 142, 143 and 145 may influence susceptibility, although other studies found little or no effect for some of these codons. The influence of the animal's genotype might differ between goat populations and scrapie strains and the effects of combined genotypes are still uncertain.

Genotype and Atypical Scrapie Susceptibility in Sheep and Goats

Atypical/Nor98 scrapie often occurs in sheep that are genetically resistant to classical scrapie. Genotypes reported to be common in infected sheep include AHQ, ARR, ARH and ARQ. Animals with the VRQ genotype, which are very susceptible to classical scrapie, seem to be relatively resistant to atypical scrapie. Histidine (H) at the PrP gene codon 154 has been linked to increased susceptibility to atypical scrapie in both sheep and goats. Sheep with the ARQ genotype that have a phenylalanine (F) residue at codon 141 (AF141RQ) are reported to be more susceptible to atypical scrapie than ARQ sheep with leucine (L) at this position. Atypical scrapie has also been reported more often in ARR and ARQ genotypes with a leucine at position 141 (AL141RQ).

Morbidity and Mortality

Classical Scrapie

Scrapie is always fatal once the clinical signs appear. Classical scrapie is most common in 2 to 5 year-old sheep and signs of illness are rare in animals less than a year of age. The percentage of a flock or herd affected by scrapie varies, depending on the genotypes of the animals, flock management and other factors. If there are no control measures, the number of infected animals tends to increase over time and clinical signs start to occur at a younger age. The annual mortality rate may be as high as 10-20% in some severely affected flocks with a high percentage of genetically susceptible sheep, but it is often lower. In some flocks or herds, many infected animals may be slaughtered for meat or culled before they show clinical signs.

Classical scrapie can be a significant problem in some areas, while other regions report few or no cases. The U.S. and E.U. both conduct control/eradication programs. In the E.U., 17 countries reported classical scrapie in sheep between 2002 and 2012 and the average prevalence was 0.087%. The prevalence decreased over this period in some countries, but did not change significantly in others. In the U.S., the prevalence of scrapie has dropped from approximately 0.5%, in 2003, to 0.015% as of 2013. S

Scrapie is much less common in goats than sheep; however, active surveillance programs have revealed that there may be significant numbers of infected goats in some areas. Between 2002 and 2009, surveillance programs in the E.U. identified approximately 3300 scrapie-infected goats (compared to about 15,000 infected sheep). The overall prevalence of infection was 0.098%, in the eight E.U. countries that reported goat scrapie in 2002-2012. However, most of these cases occurred in one country and the average prevalence in the other seven countries was 0.02%. Surveillance of goats in the U.S., targeted at certain animal populations, suggested that the prevalence was < 0.1% in 2007-2008.

Atypical Scrapie

Sheep and goats with atypical scrapie tend to be older than those with classical scrapie. While infections have been reported in all ages over 18 months (the lower age limit for testing in the E.U.), several studies found that more than half of all infected animals were more than 5 years old and one study reported increasing prevalence with age. Typically, only a single animal is infected in each herd or flock, although additional cases are occasionally reported in large groups of animals.

References

- Appearance-of-the-healthy-animal, agriculture-livestock-general-management-practices-of-livestock: vikas-pedia.in, Retrieved 18 January, 2019

- Animal-health, animal-health-animal-welfare: animalsmart.org, Retrieved 26 June, 2019

- How-you-can-help-keep-wildlife-safe, urban-wildlife: citywildlife.org, Retrieved 12 July, 2019

- Animal-disease, science: britannica.com, Retrieved 19 May, 2019

- Animal-health-management: schoolmattazz.com, Retrieved 06 April, 2019

- Detection-and-diagnosis, science-animal-disease: britannica.com, Retrieved 17 March, 2019

- Common-animal-diseases-and-their-prevention-and-treatments, agriculture-livestock-general-management-practices-of-livestock: vikaspedia.in, Retrieved 15 February, 2019

Permissions

All chapters in this book are published with permission under the Creative Commons Attribution Share Alike License or equivalent. Every chapter published in this book has been scrutinized by our experts. Their significance has been extensively debated. The topics covered herein carry significant information for a comprehensive understanding. They may even be implemented as practical applications or may be referred to as a beginning point for further studies.

We would like to thank the editorial team for lending their expertise to make the book truly unique. They have played a crucial role in the development of this book. Without their invaluable contributions this book wouldn't have been possible. They have made vital efforts to compile up to date information on the varied aspects of this subject to make this book a valuable addition to the collection of many professionals and students.

This book was conceptualized with the vision of imparting up-to-date and integrated information in this field. To ensure the same, a matchless editorial board was set up. Every individual on the board went through rigorous rounds of assessment to prove their worth. After which they invested a large part of their time researching and compiling the most relevant data for our readers.

The editorial board has been involved in producing this book since its inception. They have spent rigorous hours researching and exploring the diverse topics which have resulted in the successful publishing of this book. They have passed on their knowledge of decades through this book. To expedite this challenging task, the publisher supported the team at every step. A small team of assistant editors was also appointed to further simplify the editing procedure and attain best results for the readers.

Apart from the editorial board, the designing team has also invested a significant amount of their time in understanding the subject and creating the most relevant covers. They scrutinized every image to scout for the most suitable representation of the subject and create an appropriate cover for the book.

The publishing team has been an ardent support to the editorial, designing and production team. Their endless efforts to recruit the best for this project, has resulted in the accomplishment of this book. They are a veteran in the field of academics and their pool of knowledge is as vast as their experience in printing. Their expertise and guidance has proved useful at every step. Their uncompromising quality standards have made this book an exceptional effort. Their encouragement from time to time has been an inspiration for everyone.

The publisher and the editorial board hope that this book will prove to be a valuable piece of knowledge for students, practitioners and scholars across the globe.

Index

www.ingramcontent.com/pod-product-compliance
Lightning Source LLC
Chambersburg PA
CBHW082049190326
41458CB00010B/3491